GABBE'S
OBSTETRICS
STUDY GUIDE

A Companion to the 8th Edition

GABBE'S
OBSTETRICS
STUDY GUIDE

A Companion to the 8th Edition

Anthony Sciscione

Vanita D. Jain

Audrey A. Merriam

Eva K. Pressman

Rini Banerjee Ratan

Alyssa Stephenson-Famy

Thaddeus P. Waters

ELSEVIER

Elsevier
1600 John F. Kennedy Blvd.
Ste 1800
Philadelphia, PA 19103-2899

GABBE'S OBSTETRICS STUDY GUIDE A COMPANION TO THE 8TH EDITION   ISBN: 978-0-323-68330-2

Notice

ISBN: 978-0-323-68330-2

Content Strategist: Sarah Barth
Content Development Specialist: Meredith Madeira
Publishing Services Manager: Shereen Jameel
Project Manager: Nadhiya Sekar
Design Direction: Renee Duenow

Printed in China

Last digit is the print number: 9 8 7 6 5 4 3 2 1

CONTRIBUTORS

Vanita D. Jain
Medical Director, Antepartum & High Risk Unit
Managing Partner, Delaware Center for Maternal Fetal
    Medicine
Christiana Care
Newark, DE
Clinical Assistant Professor
Maternal Fetal Medicine
Sidney Kimmel School of Medicine, Thomas Jefferson
    University
Philadelphia, PA

Audrey Merriam
Assistant Professor
Obstetrics, Gynecology and Reproductive Sciences
Yale University
New Haven, CT

Eva K. Pressman
Professor
Obstetrics and Gynecology
University of Rochester
Rochester, NY

Rini Banerjee Ratan
Vice Chair of Education
Obstetrics and Gynecology
Columbia University Vagelos College of Physicians & Surgeons
New York, NY

Anthony Sciscione, DO
Director of Maternal-Fetal Medicine and the OB/GYN
    Residency Program
Christiana Health System
Newark, DE
Professor
Department of Obstetrics and Gynecology
Jefferson Medical College
Philadelphia, PA

Alyssa Stephenson-Famy
Associate Professor
Obstetrics & Gynecology
University of Washington
Seattle, WA

Thaddeus P. Waters, MD
Director of Maternal Fetal Medicine and Inpatient Obstetrics
Department of Obstetrics and Gynecology
Rush University Medical Center
Chicago, IL

This book is dedicated to my wife,
who time after time has had to donate her time so that I could give my time
to my wonderful students.

To all of the learners the authors have had the privilege to educate.
We hope you will exceed every one of our accomplishments.

Lastly, to our mentors who gave tirelessly and unwaveringly to our education.

Anthony Sciscione

Welcome to the first edition of the Study Guide for the Gabbe's Obstetrics textbook. The Gabbe's textbook has become one of the most used and trusted obstetric resources and educational tools in the world. As with any exceptional reference, the scope and volume of educational information is tremendous; however, within each chapter there are areas that are considered clinically more applicable. The other authors and I have focused on these areas when creating the questions contained in this book. Furthermore, in order to reinforce the subject matter, a concise explanation of the answer to each question, using content from the Gabbe's textbook, has been provided along with a link to the specific area within the textbook. Each of the authors of this study guide are passionate career-long educators; as such the questions have been carefully and thoughtfully prepared for all learners. We hope that you will find this resource as useful as the time and effort that went into its creation by our devoted team.

Anthony Sciscione
Residency Director
OB/GYN
Christiana Care
Newark, DE

CONTENTS

SECTION VI Pregnancy and Coexisting Disease

SECTION I

Physiology

Placental Anatomy and Physiology

Anthony Sciscione

(see *Gabbe's Obstetrics: Normal and Problem Pregnancies*, 8e: ch1)

QUESTIONS

1. The original wall of the blastocyst becomes:

  a. Chorionic plate

  b. Decidual plate

  c. Basal plate

  d. Amnionic plate

  e. Chorionic plate

2. As the placenta models and establishes access to the maternal blood flow, the resistance to flow through the spiral arteries and placenta drops significantly, creating a low-resistance/high-capacitance system. As a result, the amount of maternal cardiac output increases by what percentage by term?

  a. 5%–9%

  b. 10%–15%

  c. 16%–20%

  d. 21%–25%

  e. 25%–30%

3. A 20-year-old nulliparous woman presents at 26 weeks gestation with severe range hypertension and laboratory evidence of Hemolysis, Elevated Liver Enzymes and Low Platelets (HELLP) syndrome. A sonogram reveals a severely growth-restricted fetus with a category III fetal heart tracing. She is started on magnesium sulfate, and after maternal stabilization, the patient is prepared for cesarean delivery. It appears that defects in early trophoblast invasion predicated on spiral artery development predispose pregnancies for the above scenario. What percentage of spiral arteries are fully converted to normal function in women with preeclampsia and fetal growth restriction?

  a. 10%

  b. 15%

  c. 20%

  d. 25%

  e. 30%

4. The endometrium has a key role in regulating receptivity at the time of implantation through signaling that occurs from the uterine epithelium and secretions. Uterine glands secrete into the intervillous space "uterine milk," which supplies key substances. Which of the following is one of the components of "uterine milk?"

  a. Fetal proteins

  b. Glucose

  c. Lipid droplets

  d. Fatty acids

5. Which of the following chemicals stimulate cytotrophoblastic fusion?

  a. TGF-β

  b. Human chorionic gonadotropin (hCG)

  c. Endothelin

  d. Leukemia inhibiting factor

  e. Estrogen

6. A 26-year-old nulliparous patient at 34 weeks gestation presents for a routine prenatal visit. Her fundal height is 30 cm and a fetal sonogram is ordered. The fetus is under the fifth percentile for estimated fetal weight. Doppler flow studies reveal reverse flow in the umbilical artery. The patient is sent to labor and delivery for admission and fetal monitoring. The patient meets criteria for preeclampsia with severe features and there is a category III fetal heart rate tracing. Immediate delivery is performed and the placenta is sent for pathological examination. The placenta is small and the placental pathologist diagnosis chronic hypoxia. Which chemical interacts with ASCT2 to result in an increased number of cytotrophoblastic cells observed in the placentas of hypoxic pregnancies?

  a. Syncytin

  b. Prostacyclin

  c. Thromboxane A2 (TXA2)

  d. VEGF

  e. Placental Growth factor (PGF)

7. The development of fetal vasculature begins how many weeks after conception?

   a. 2

   b. 3

   c. 4

   d. 5

   e. 6

8. The yolk sac is the initial site of which of the following?

   a. Hormone production

   b. Hematopoiesis

   c. Immunoglobulins

   d. Amniotic fluid

   e. hCG

ANSWERS

1. Answer: **a**

(see *Gabbe's Obstetrics* 8e: ch1)

The original wall of the blastocyst becomes the chorionic plate, the cytotrophoblastic shell is the precursor of the basal plate, and the lacunae form the IVS. The trabeculae are the forerunners of the villous trees, and repeated lateral branching gradually increases their complexity.

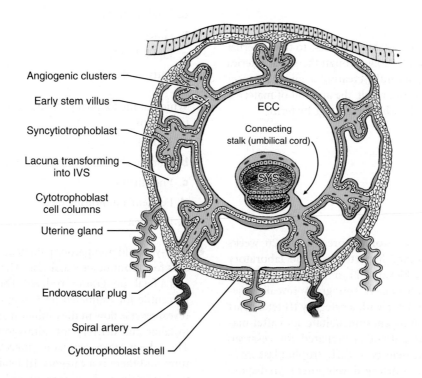

2. Answer: **b**

(see *Gabbe's Obstetrics* 8e: ch1)

The most proximal part of the spiral arteries, where they arise from the uterine arcuate arteries, always remain unconverted, unlike the terminal ends, and will act as the rate-limiting segment. These segments gradually dilate in conjunction with the rest of the uterine vasculature during early pregnancy, most probably under the effects of estrogen; as a result, the resistance of the uterine circulation falls, and uterine blood flow increases from approximately 45 mL/min during the menstrual cycle to around 750 mL/min at term or 10% to 15% of maternal cardiac output. Studies in the mouse have demonstrated that the radial arteries account for ~90% of the total uteroplacental vascular resistance.[1]

3. Answer: **a**

(see *Gabbe's Obstetrics* 8e: ch1)

Many complications of pregnancy are associated with defects in extravillous trophoblast invasion and failure to establish the maternal placental circulation correctly. In the most severe cases, the cytotrophoblastic shell is thin and fragmented; this is observed in approximately two-thirds of spontaneous miscarriages. In milder cases, the pregnancy may continue but be complicated later by preeclampsia, intrauterine growth restriction, or a combination of the two. The physiologic changes are either restricted to the superficial endometrial parts of the spiral arteries or are absent all together. In the most severe cases of preeclampsia associated with major fetal growth restriction, only 10% of the arteries may be fully converted, compared with 96% in normal pregnancies.[2]

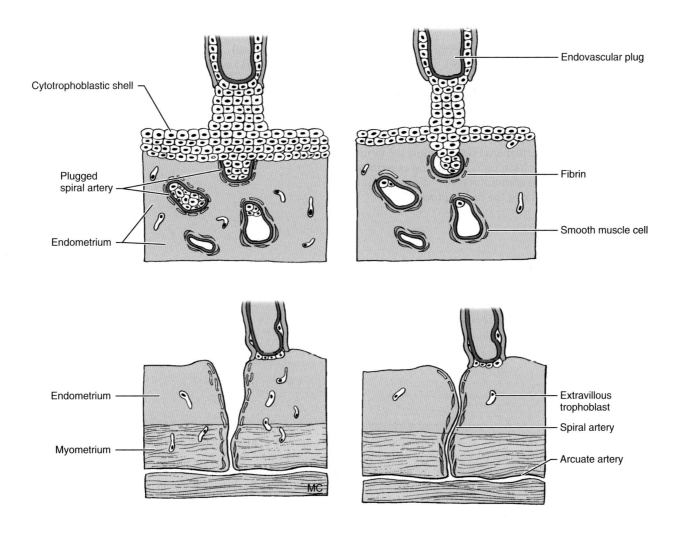

4. Answer: d

(see *Gabbe's Obstetrics* 8e: ch1)

Glycodelin-A, formerly referred to as *PP14* or α_2-*PEG*, is derived from the glands and yet accumulates within the amniotic fluid, with concentrations that peak at around 10 weeks gestation, indicating that the placenta must be exposed to glandular secretions extensively throughout the first trimester. This exposure was confirmed by a review of archival placenta in situ hysterectomy specimens that demonstrated glands discharging their secretions into the IVS through openings in the basal plate throughout the first trimester (see the figure in Answer 1).[3] Their secretions, referred to as "uterine milk," are a heterogeneous mix of maternal proteins; carbohydrates, including glycogen; and lipid droplets phagocytosed by the syncytiotrophoblast.

5. Answer: b

(see *Gabbe's Obstetrics* 8e: ch1)

The factors that regulate and mediate cytotrophoblastic fusion are uncertain. Growth factors such as EGF, GM-CSF, and VEGF are able to stimulate fusion in vitro, as are the hormones estradiol and hCG. By contrast, TGF-β, leukemia inhibitory factor, and endothelin inhibit the process, which suggests that the outcome in vivo depends on a balance between these opposing influences. One of the actions of hCG at the molecular level is to promote the formation of gap junctions between cells, and strong experimental evidence suggests that communication via gap junctions is an essential prerequisite in the fusion process.[4]

6. Answer: a

(see *Gabbe's Obstetrics* 8e: ch1)

Syncytin interacts with the amino acid transporter protein ASCT2, and the expression of both is influenced by hypoxia in trophoblast cell lines in vitro. This could provide an explanation for the increased number of cytotrophoblast cells observed in placentae from hypoxic pregnancies.

7. Answer: b

(see *Gabbe's Obstetrics* 8e: ch1)

The development of the fetal vasculature begins during the third week after conception (the fifth week of pregnancy) with the de novo formation of capillaries within the villous stromal core. Hemangioblastic cell cords differentiate under the influence of growth factors such as basic fibroblast growth factor and VEGF.[5] By the beginning of the fourth week, the cords have developed lumens, and the endothelial cells become flattened. Surrounding mesenchymal cells become closely apposed to the tubes and differentiate to form pericytes. During the next few days, connections form between neighboring tubes to form a plexus, and this ultimately unites with the allantoic vessels developing in the connecting stalk to establish the fetal circulation to the placenta.

8. Answer: b

(see *Gabbe's Obstetrics* 8e: ch1)

Phylogenetically, the oldest membrane is the yolk sac, and the SYS plays a major role in the embryonic development of all mammals. The function of the yolk sac has been most extensively studied in laboratory rodents. It has demonstrated that it is one of the initial sites of hematopoiesis, that it synthesizes a variety of proteins, and that it is involved in maternal-fetal transport.

REFERENCES

1. Rennie MY, Whiteley KJ, Adamson SL, et al. Quantification of gestational changes in the uteroplacental vascular tree reveals vessel specific hemodynamic roles during pregnancy in mice. *Biol Reprod.* 2016;95:43.
2. Brosens IA. The utero-placental vessels at term - the distribution and extent of physiological changes. *Trophoblast Res.* 1988;3:61-67.
3. Burton GJ, Watson AL, Hempstock J, et al. Uterine glands provide histiotrophic nutrition for the human fetus during the first trimester of pregnancy. *J Clin Endocrinol Metab.* 2002;87:2954-2959.
4. Frendo JL, Cronier L, Bertin G, et al. Involvement of connexin 43 in human trophoblast cell fusion and differentiation. *J Cell Sci.* 2003;116:3413-3421.
5. Aplin JD, Whittaker H, Jana Lim YT, et al. Hemangioblastic foci in human first trimester placenta: Distribution and gestational profile. *Placenta.* 2015;36:1069-1077.

Fetal Development and Physiology/ Cellular Programming Epi-Clinical

Vanita D. Jain

(see *Gabbe's Obstetrics: Normal and Problem Pregnancies*, 8e: ch2)

QUESTIONS

1. Umbilical blood flow to the fetus is maintained despite changes in maternal blood flow or hypoxia?
   a. True
   b. False

2. At what gestational age does mean amniotic fluid volume (AFV) peak?
   a. 26 weeks
   b. 28 weeks
   c. 30 weeks
   d. 32 weeks
   e. 34 weeks

3. What is the primary source of amniotic fluid in the second trimester?
   a. Transudate of maternal plasma through chorion-amnion interface
   b. Transudate of fetal plasma through fetal skin
   c. Fetal lung fluid
   d. Fetal urine

4. All of the following factors found in maternal serum are directly correlated with fetal growth except:
   a. Insulin-like growth factor 1 (IGF-1)
   b. Insulin
   c. Corticosteroids
   d. Epidermal growth factor (EGF)
   e. Insulin-like growth factor 2 (IGF-2)

5. Well-oxygenated blood is preferentially directed into the foramen ovale in fetal circulation from the ductus venosus by which pathway?
   a. Tricuspid valve
   b. Aortic semilunar valve
   c. Superior vena cava
   d. Inferior vena cava and crista dividens
   e. Pulmonary vein

6. The fetal right ventricle (RV) and left ventricle (LV) function as two pumps in series.
   a. True
   b. False

7. Which of the following fetal organs receives the largest amount of biventricular cardiac venous output?
   a. Hepatic artery of the liver
   b. Fetal body (abdomen/thorax)
   c. Placenta
   d. Fetal brain
   e. Fetal gastrointestinal tract

8. One of the key factors that maintain adequate fetal tissue oxygenation besides higher fetal cardiac output and organ blood flows is the increased oxygen carrying capacity of fetal hemoglobin. What key chemical is responsible for the leftward shift in the fetal oxygen dissociation curve?
   a. 2,3-Diphosphoglycerate (DPG)
   b. Alpha melanocyte stimulating hormone (Alpha-MSH)
   c. Angiotensin converting enzyme (ACE)
   d. Vascular endothelial growth factor (VEGF)

ANSWERS

1. Answer: a

(see *Gabbe's Obstetrics* 8e: ch2)

Short-term changes in umbilical blood flow are regulated by perfusion pressure and there is a linear relationship between flow and perfusion pressure. Small (2 to 3 mmHg) increases in umbilical vein pressure evoke proportional decreases in umbilical blood flow, but increases in uterine tone affect both vessels without changing umbilical blood flow. The fetoplacental circulation is resistant to the vasoconstrictive effects of infused pressor agents, although endogenous vasoactive autacoids including nitric oxide and endothelin-1 may be important.[1] Thus, despite changes in fetal blood flow distribution and increases in blood pressure during acute hypoxia, umbilical blood flow is maintained over a wide range of oxygen tensions unless cardiac output decreases.

2. Answer: d

(see *Gabbe's Obstetrics* 8e: ch2)

AFV increases from 250 to 800 mL from 16 to its peak at 32 weeks gestation, remains stable up to 39 weeks, and declines to 500 mL at 42 weeks.

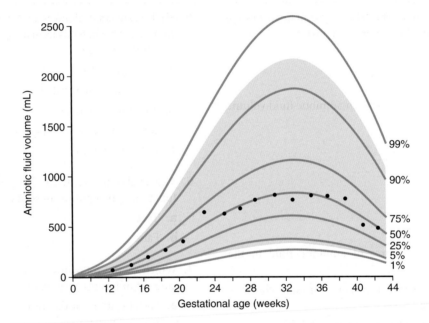

3. Answer: d

(see *Gabbe's Obstetrics* 8e: ch2)

Fetal urine is the primary source of amniotic fluid between 20 and 40 weeks gestation, with values of 400 to 1200 mL/day at term compared with the first trimester, which is not dependent on fetal urine production. A clinically useful example of this is that fetuses with bilateral agenesis have normal amounts of amniotic fluid in the first trimester but anhydramnios in the second trimester.

4. Answer: e

(see *Gabbe's Obstetrics* 8e: ch2)

IGF, together with IGF-binding proteins and IGF receptors, has the largest impact on fetal growth. IGF-1 and IGF-2 are present in human fetal-tissue extracts after 12 weeks gestation and levels begin to increase by 32 to 34 weeks gestation. IGF-1 levels correlate with fetal size and reduced IGF-1 levels are associated with growth restriction.[2] In contrast, serum IGF-2 levels and fetal growth do not correlate. However, IGF-2 may regulate placental growth and nutrient permeability.

5. Answer: **d**

(see *Gabbe's Obstetrics* 8e: ch2)

Placental gas exchange provides well-oxygenated blood to the umbilical vein, which delivers blood to the ductus venosus, small branches to the left lobe of the liver, and a major branch to the right lobe.

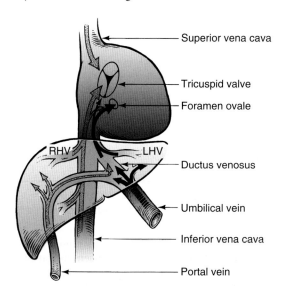

Although both the ductus venosus blood and the hepatic portal/fetal trunk bloods enter the inferior vena cava entering the right atrium, little mixing occurs. This stream of well-oxygenated ductus venosus blood is preferentially directed across the interatrial septum via the foramen ovale into the left atrium (see figures).

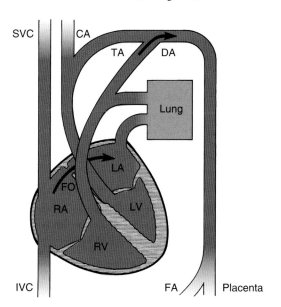

Thus, left atrial filling results from umbilical vein–ductus venosus blood, with a small contribution from pulmonary venous flow. As a result, blood with the highest oxygen content is delivered to the left atrium, LV, and ultimately the carotid and vertebral circulations and the brain.

6. Answer: **b**

(see *Gabbe's Obstetrics* 8e: ch2)

In the fetus, unique vascular shunts provide an unequal distribution of venous return to the respective atria, and ventricular output represents a mixture of oxygenated and deoxygenated blood. Thus, the fetal RV and LV function as two pumps in parallel, rather than in series, and cardiac output is described as the combined ventricular output (CVO). RV output exceeds 60% of biventricular output[3] and is directed through the ductus arteriosus to the descending aorta (see the second figure in Answer 5).

7. Answer: **c**

(see *Gabbe's Obstetrics* 8e: ch2)

The placenta receives approximately 40% of the CVO.[4] Third trimester umbilical blood flow increases proportionate to fetal growth. The placenta is a large recipient of blood flow and necessary to support fetal growth. The right ventricle output is about 66% of the CVO, but only 7% of this enters the pulmonary circulation. The 59% enters the aorta (via the ductus arteriosus). An additional 10% enters the aorta as well from the LV. Of this 69% of the CVO that reaches the descending aorta, 40% goes to the placenta, with the remainder distributed to the abdominal organs and lower body.

8. Answer: a

(see *Gabbe's Obstetrics* 8e: ch2)

The fetus exists in a state of aerobic metabolism, despite arterial blood PO_2 values in the 20 to 35 mm Hg range. Adequate fetal tissue oxygenation occurs by several mechanisms. Higher fetal cardiac output and organ blood flows are primary, but higher hemoglobin concentration and increased oxygen-carrying capacity of fetal hemoglobin also contribute. The leftward shift in the fetal oxygen dissociation curve shows increased fetal blood oxygen saturation relative to oxygen tension.

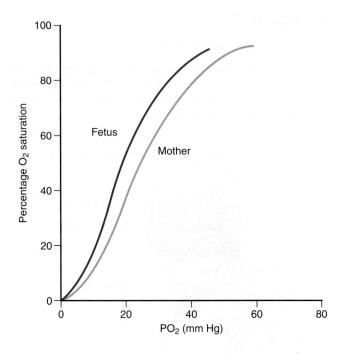

At a partial pressure of 26.5 mm Hg, adult blood oxygen saturation is 50%, whereas fetal oxygen saturation is 70%. The basis for fetal hemoglobin increased oxygen affinity is the effect of organic phosphate 2,3-DPG.

REFERENCES

1. Thaete LG, Dewey ER, Neerhof MG. Endothelin and the regulation of uterine and placental perfusion in hypoxia-induced fetal growth restriction. *J Soc Gynecol Investig.* 2004;11:16-21.
2. Forbes K, Westwood M. The IGF axis and placental function. a mini review. *Horm Res.* 2008;69:129-137.
3. Anderson DF, Bissonnette JM, Faber JJ, Thornburg KL. Central shunt flows and pressures in the mature fetal lamb. *Am J Physiol.* 1981;241:H60.
4. Rudolph AM, Heymann MA. Circulatory changes during growth in the fetal lamb. *Circ Res.* 1970;26:289-299.

Maternal Physiology

Anthony Sciscione

(see *Gabbe's Obstetrics: Normal and Problem Pregnancies*, 8e: ch 3)

QUESTIONS

1. Maternal cardiac output (CO) increases between 30% and 50% during pregnancy. At which gestational age does it peak?

   a. 13–19 weeks

   b. 20–24 weeks

   c. 25–30 weeks

   d. 31–36 weeks

   e. 37 weeks until delivery

2. A 31-year-old G1P0 patient presents to the labor and delivery unit with a complaint of a headache at 28 weeks gestation. A blood pressure (BP) is taken, and it is 120/82 in the lateral recumbent position. Which of the following is NOT true about taking BP in pregnancy?

   a. BP should be taken in the sitting position.

   b. Use Korotkoff sound 4.

   c. Taking BP in the lateral recumbent position can falsely lower results.

   d. Korotkoff 4 sound cannot be identified in the majority of pregnant patients.

3. CO in pregnancy reaches its peak at which point in pregnancy?

   a. First trimester

   b. Second trimester

   c. Third trimester

   d. Postpartum

4. A 41-year-old G3P2002 presents for her first prenatal visit at 12 weeks gestation. She states that she is on iron supplementation from prior to her pregnancy due to iron deficiency anemia. Her laboratory workup by hematology confirmed the diagnosis. You counsel her about iron needs in pregnancy. Which of the following is correct?

   a. Iron requirement of pregnancy is 500 mg.

   b. The normal pregnant woman absorbs 2.5 mg/day.

   c. Iron requirements in the first trimester are 0.5 mg/day.

   d. Iron requirements in the third trimester are 6 mg/day.

   e. Iron requirements stay constant across gestation.

5. The risk for thromboembolism increases by how many fold in the pregnant woman?

   a. 1–2

   b. 3–4

   c. 5–6

   d. 7–8

   e. 9–10

6. A 26-year-old nulliparous patient presents at 28 weeks with the complaint of shortness of breath. Her prenatal course had been uncomplicated. A workup is positive for pulmonary embolus. Before starting therapy, laboratories for thrombophilia are ordered. Which of the following is true for the laboratory changes in pregnancy?

   a. Protein S decreases

   b. Protein C decreases

   c. Antithrombin III decreases

   d. Bleeding time decreases

   e. Fibrinogen decreases

7. Which of the following pulmonary functions increases the most in pregnancy?

   a. Vital capacity

   b. Tidal volume

   c. Total lung capacity

   d. Inspiratory reserve volume

   e. Inspiratory capacity

8. There is an increase in renal blood flow and glomerular filtration rate during pregnancy. As a result many plasma levels decrease, which of the following levels go down in pregnancy?

   a. Blood urea nitrogen (BUN)

   b. Creatinine

   c. Uric acid

   d. All the above

9. A 21-year-old woman presents for her second prenatal visit at 18 weeks gestation. She has no medical issues. However, on her routine laboratory work, her urine culture was found to be positive for *Escherichia coli*. She has no symptoms. You counsel her that of women with asymptomatic bacteriuria, what percentage go on to develop pyelonephritis?

   a. 10%

   b. 20%

   c. 30%

   d. 40%

   e. 50%

10. A 31-year-old woman at 18 weeks gestation is having her routine anatomy ultrasound. She feels well. Her prenatal care has been uneventful. She has no significant medical or surgical history. You receive the report and it states that gallstones are noted in the gallbladder. The patient is concerned due to the technician advising the patient of the finding. You counsel the patient that this is an incidental finding and what percentage of pregnant women have gallstones noted on sonogram?

    a. 1%

    b. 5%

    c. 10%

    d. 15%

    e. 20%

11. A 34-year-old woman is diagnosed with Graves disease and opts for ablative therapy with radioactive iodine. Two weeks after the procedure, she presents to your office with complaints of nausea. A pregnancy test is positive. A sonogram reveals a gestational age of 8 weeks. The patient is concerned about the effects of the radioactive iodine on the fetus. You reassure her that the fetal thyroid cannot concentrate iodine until what gestational age?

    a. 6 weeks

    b. 8 weeks

    c. 10 weeks

    d. 12 weeks

    e. 14 weeks

ANSWERS

1. **Answer: c**

   (see *Gabbe's Obstetrics* 8e: ch3)

   Although the literature is not clear regarding the exact point in gestation at which CO peaks, most studies point to a range between 25 and 30 weeks.[1,2] The data on whether the CO continues to increase in the third trimester are very divergent, with equal numbers of good longitudinal studies showing a mild decrease, a slight increase, or no change.[1] Thus, little to no change is likely during this period.

2. **Answer: b**

   (see *Gabbe's Obstetrics* 8e: ch3)

   The position when the BP is taken and what Korotkoff sound is used to determine the diastolic BP are important. BP is lowest in the lateral recumbent position, and the BP of the superior arm in this position is 10 to 12 mm Hg lower than that in the inferior arm. In the ambulatory setting, BP should be measured in the sitting position, and the Korotkoff 5 sound should be used. This is the diastolic BP when the sound disappears, as opposed to the Korotkoff 4, when a muffling of the sound is apparent. In a study of 250 gravidas, the Korotkoff 4 sound could only be identified in 48% of patients, whereas the Korotkoff 5 sound could always be determined.

3. Answer: d

(see *Gabbe's Obstetrics* 8e: ch3)

In the immediate postpartum period (10 to 30 minutes after delivery), with a further rise in CO of 10% to 20%, CO reaches its maximum. This increase is accompanied by a fall in the maternal heart rate (HR) that is likely secondary to increased Stroke volume (SV). Traditionally, this rise was thought to be the result of uterine auto-transfusion, as described earlier with contractions, but the validity of this concept is uncertain. In both vaginal and elective cesarean deliveries, the maximal increase in CO occurs 10 to 30 minutes after delivery and returns to the prelabor baseline 1 hour after delivery. The increase was 37% with epidural anesthesia and 28% with general anesthesia. Over the next 2 to 4 postpartum weeks, the cardiac hemodynamic parameters return to near-preconceptional levels.

4. Answer: d

(see *Gabbe's Obstetrics* 8e: ch3)

The iron requirements of gestation are about 1000 mg. This includes 500 mg used to increase the maternal red blood cell (RBC) mass (1 mL of erythrocytes contains 1.1 mg iron), 300 mg transported to the fetus, and 200 mg to compensate for the normal daily iron losses by the mother. Thus, the normal expectant woman needs to absorb an average of 3.5 mg/day of iron. In actuality, the iron requirements are not constant but increase remarkably during the pregnancy from 0.8 mg/day in the first trimester to 6 to 7 mg/day in the third trimester. The fetus receives its iron through active transport via transferrin receptors located on the apical surface of the placental syncytiotrophoblast.[3]

5. Answer: c

(see *Gabbe's Obstetrics* 8e: ch3)

Pregnancy places women at a five- to six-fold increased risk for thromboembolic disease. This greater risk is caused by increased venous stasis, vessel wall injury, and changes in the coagulation cascade that lead to hypercoagulability. The increase in venous stasis in the lower extremities is due to compression of the inferior vena cava (IVC) and the pelvic veins by the enlarging uterus. The hypercoagulability is caused by an increase in several procoagulants, a decrease in the natural inhibitors of coagulation, and a reduction in fibrinolytic activity. These physiologic changes provide defense against peripartum hemorrhage.

6. Answer: a

(see *Gabbe's Obstetrics* 8e: ch3)

Pregnancy has been shown to cause a progressive and significant decrease in the levels of total and free protein S from early in pregnancy, but it has no effect on the levels of protein C and antithrombin III.[4] If a workup for thrombophilias is performed during gestation, the clinician should use caution when attempting to interpret these levels, if they are abnormal. Ideally, the clinician should order DNA testing for the Leiden mutation instead of testing for activated Protein C (APC). For protein-S screening during pregnancy, the free protein-S antigen level should be tested, with normal levels in the second and third trimesters being identified as greater than 30% and 24%, respectively. The Prothrombin time (PT), activated Partial Thromboplastin time (PTT), and thrombin time all fall slightly but remain within the limits of normal nonpregnant values, whereas the bleeding time and whole blood clotting times are unchanged.

7. Answer: b

(see *Gabbe's Obstetrics* 8e: ch3)

TABLE 3.1	Pulmonary Changes of Pregnancy		
Measurement	**Definition**		**Change in Pregnancy**
Respiratory rate	Number of breaths per minute		Unchanged
Vital capacity (VC)	Maximal amount of air that can be forcibly expired after maximal inspiration (IC + ERV)		Unchanged
Inspiratory capacity (IC)	Maximal amount of air that can be inspired from resting expiratory level (TV + IRV)		Increased 5%–10%
Tidal volume (TV)	Amount of air inspired and expired with a normal breath		Increased 30%–40%
Inspiratory reserve volume (IRV)	Maximal amount of air that can be inspired at the end of normal inspiration		Unchanged
Functional residual capacity	Amount of air in lungs at resting expiratory level (ERV + RV)		Decreased 20%
Expiratory reserve volume (ERV)	Maximal amount of air that can be expired from resting expiratory level		Decreased 15%–20%
Residual volume (RV)	Amount of air in lungs after maximal expiration		Decreased 20%–25%
Total lung capacity	Total amount of air in lungs at maximal inspiration (VC + RV)		Decreased 5%

From Cruickshank DP, Wigton TR, Hays PM. Maternal physiology in pregnancy. In Gabbe SG, Niebyl JR, Simpson JL, eds. *Obstetrics: Normal and Problem Pregnancies*. 3rd ed. New York: Churchill Livingstone; 1996.

8. Answer: d

(see *Gabbe's Obstetrics* 8e: ch3)

The clinical consequence of glomerular hyperfiltration is a reduction in maternal plasma levels of creatinine, BUN, and uric acid. Serum creatinine decreases from a nonpregnant level of 0.8 to 0.5 mg/dL by term. Likewise, BUN falls from nonpregnant levels of 13 to 9 mg/dL by term. Serum uric acid declines in early pregnancy because of the rise in Glomerular Filtration rate (GFR) and reaches a nadir by 24 weeks with levels of 2 to 3 mg/dL. After 24 weeks, the uric acid level begins to rise, and by the end of pregnancy, the levels in most women are essentially the same as before conception. The rise in uric acid levels is caused by increased renal tubular absorption of urate and increased fetal uric acid production.

9. Answer: c

(see *Gabbe's Obstetrics* 8e: ch3)

The normal pregnancy-related changes in the kidneys and urinary tract can have profound clinical implications. From 2% to 8% of pregnancies are complicated by asymptomatic bacteriuria, and risk is increased among multiparous women; those of a low socioeconomic class; and women with diabetes, sickle cell disease, and history of previous urinary tract infections. Although this prevalence is approximately equivalent to that in the nonpregnant population, in pregnancy, 30% of these progress to pyelonephritis. This rate is three to four times higher in pregnancy compared with that of nonpregnant controls; overall, 1% to 2% of all pregnancies are complicated by urinary tract infections.[5]

10. Answer: c

(see *Gabbe's Obstetrics* 8e: ch3)

Because of progesterone, the rate at which the gallbladder empties is much slower. After the first trimester, the fasting and residual volumes of the gallbladder are twice as great. In addition, the biliary cholesterol saturation is increased, and the chenodeoxycholic acid level is decreased. This change in the composition of the bile fluid favors the formation of cholesterol crystals, and with incomplete emptying of the gallbladder, the crystals are retained and gallstone formation is enhanced. Furthermore, the progesterone acts to inhibit smooth muscle contraction of the gallbladder, thereby predisposing to formation of sludge or gallstones. By the time they deliver, up to 10% of women have gallstones on ultrasonographic examination; however, only 1 in 6000 to 1 in 10,000 pregnancies ultimately require cholecystectomy.

11. Answer: d

(see *Gabbe's Obstetrics* 8e: ch3)

Because iodine is actively transported across the placenta and the concentration of iodide in the fetal blood is 75% that of the maternal blood, the fetus is susceptible to iodine-induced goiters when the mother is given pharmacologic amounts of iodine. Similarly, radioactive iodine crosses the placenta, and if given after 12 weeks gestation when the fetal thyroid is able to concentrate iodine, profound adverse effects can occur. These include fetal hypothyroidism, mental retardation, attention-deficit disorder, and a 1% to 2% increase in the lifetime cancer risk.

REFERENCES

1. Meah VL, Cockcroft JR, Backx K, Shave R, Stöhr EJ. Cardiac output and related haemodynamics during pregnancy: a series of meta-analyses. *Heart*. 2016;102(7):518-526. doi:10.1136/heartjnl-2015-308476
2. Robson S, Hunter S, Boys R. Serial study of factors influencing changes in cardiac output during human pregnancy. *Am J Physiol*. 1989;256:H1060-H1065.
3. Koenig MD, Tussing-Humphreys L, Day J, Cadwell B, Nemeth E. Hepcidin and iron homeostasis during pregnancy. *Nutrients*. 2014;6(8):3062-3083. doi:10.3390/nu6083062.
4. Clark P, Brennand J, Conkie JA, Mccall F, Greer IA, Walker ID. Activated protein C sensitivity, protein C, protein S and coagulation in normal pregnancy. *Thromb Haemost*. 1998;79:1166-1170.
5. Gilstrap LC, Cunningham FG, Whalley PJ. Acute pyelonephritis in pregnancy: an anterospective study. *Obstet Gynecol*. 1981;57(4):409-413.

Maternal-Fetal Immunology

Alyssa Stephenson-Famy

(see *Gabbe's Obstetrics: Normal and Problem Pregnancies*, 8e: ch4)

QUESTIONS

1. Which elements are important for the maternal adaptive immune system to target specific antigens?
   a. Macrophages
   b. Dendritic cells
   c. Natural killer cells
   d. Eosinophils
   e. T-cells

2. Susceptibility to *Neisseria gonorrhea* and *Neisseria meningitidis* has been associated with genetic deficiencies in which component of the innate immune system?
   a. Complement proteins C5–C9
   b. Complement protein C1q
   c. Lectin binding protein
   d. Decidual natural killer cells

3. The fetal inflammatory response syndrome is associated with high levels of which of the following in fetal blood?
   a. Chemokine inhibitors
   b. Antiinflammatory cytokines (including interleukin [IL]-10)
   c. Proinflammatory cytokines (including IL-1β, tumor necrosis factor-α [TNF-α], and IL-6)
   d. Major histocompatibility complex molecules
   e. Autoantibodies

4. What is the first antibody to be produced during an immune response?
   a. IgA
   b. IgD
   c. IgE
   d. IgG
   e. IgM

5. What is the principle substance transmitted through breast milk that provides the neonatal humoral immunity from the mother?
   a. Neutrophils
   b. Regulatory T-cells (T_{REG})
   c. IgA
   d. Cytokines
   e. Chemokines

6. T_{REG} are involved in establishing fetal tolerance by suppressing CD8+ T cells but disrupt the maternal immune response to which of the following infections?
   a. *Mycobacterium tuberculosis*
   b. *Listeria monocytogenes*
   c. *Yersinia pestis*
   d. *Brucella abortus*
   e. HIV

7. A-24-year old healthy G1P0 is considering private umbilical cord blood banking based on advertisements in her maternity magazines. She has no family history of hematologic disorders or malignancy. What counseling for this patient most accurately reflects the American College of Obstetrics and Gynecology (ACOG) recommendation regarding umbilical cord blood banking?
   a. Routine umbilical cord blood banking is recommended for all patients
   b. Public umbilical cord blood banking has wide applications for use in adult autoimmune conditions
   c. Private umbilical cord blood banking is cost-effective only for children with high likelihood of a stem cell transplant
   d. Public umbilical cord blood banking has the lowest utility for patients in underrepresented racial or ethnic groups

8. Expression of major histocompatibility class (MHC) molecules on extravillous fetal trophoblast cells is limited to:

   a. Class I antigens (e.g., Human Leukocyte Antigen [HLA-C])

   b. Class II antigens (e.g. HLA-DR, -DQ, and -DP)

   c. Polymorphic genes that are often matched for transplantation

   d. Antigens expressed from maternal genes

9. What percentage of women with rheumatoid arthritis (RA) experience improvement of their symptoms during the second and third trimesters of pregnancy?

   a. 10%

   b. 30%

   c. 50%

   d. 70%

   e. 90%

10. A 34-year-old woman with RA demonstrates remission of her symptoms during the third trimester and has recurrent symptoms postpartum. What immunologic process likely explains temporary amelioration of her symptoms during pregnancy?

   a. Increase in sex hormones

   b. Placental production of gamma globulin

   c. Maternal-fetal HLA disparity

   d. Immunologic weakness of the mother

ANSWERS

1. **Answer: e**

   (see *Gabbe's Obstetrics* 8e: ch4)

   Adaptive immunity results in the clonal expansion of lymphocytes (T cells and B cells) and antibodies against a specific antigen and is capable of eradicating an infection that has overwhelmed the innate immune system (macrophages, dendritic cells, NK cells, basophils, and eosinophils).

2. **Answer: a**

   (see *Gabbe's Obstetrics* 8e: ch4)

   Genetic deficiencies in C5–C9 complement proteins have been associated with susceptibility to *N. gonorrhea* and *N. meningitidis*.

3. **Answer: b**

   (see *Gabbe's Obstetrics* 8e: ch4)

   Proinflammatory cytokines such as IL-1β, TNF-α, and IL-6 have also been identified in the amniotic fluid, maternal and fetal blood, and vaginal fluid of women with intraamniotic infection and are associated with the **fetal inflammatory response syndrome.**

4. **Answer: e**

   (see *Gabbe's Obstetrics* 8e: ch4)

   The first antibody to be produced during an immune response is IgM, because it is expressed before isotype switching.

5. **Answer: c**

   (see *Gabbe's Obstetrics* 8e: ch4)

   IgA is the predominant antibody class in epithelial secretions and is the principal antibody in breast milk, providing the neonate with humoral immunity from the mother.

6. **Answer: b**

   (see *Gabbe's Obstetrics* 8e: ch4)

   T_{REG} cells act to suppress the function of $CD8^+$ T cells, which is necessary for fetal tolerance, but secondarily disrupts the maternal immune response towards *L. monocytogenes*. The placenta becomes highly infected with *L. monocytogenes* perhaps due to the initial immunosuppressive actions of T_{REG} cells, which is necessary for bacterial eradication.

7. **Answer: c**

   (see *Gabbe's Obstetrics* 8e: ch4)

   Private umbilical cord blood banking is controversial as it is expensive and has a limited number of clinical uses. ACOG recommends private cord blood banking for families with children with high likelihood of needing a stem cell transplant. Public umbilical cord blood banking especially for under-represented racial or ethnic groups is important.

8. Answer: a

(see *Gabbe's Obstetrics* 8e: ch4)

HLA-C, a class Ia molecule that is highly polymorphic, expressed primarily by extravillous trophoblast, and is thought to interact with dNK cells to facilitate uterine spiral artery remodeling.

9. Answer: d

(see *Gabbe's Obstetrics* 8e: ch4)

Nearly three-quarters of pregnant women with RA experience improvement in symptoms during the second and third trimesters, with a return of symptoms postpartum.

10. Answer: c

(see *Gabbe's Obstetrics* 8e: ch4)

Maternal-fetal HLA disparity is the strongest predictor of RA amelioration/remission in human pregnancy.

Preconception and Prenatal Care

Audrey Merriam

(see *Gabbe's Obstetrics: Normal and Problem Pregnancies*, 8e: ch5)

QUESTIONS

1. All of the following screening tests are recommended during a preconception visit or at the first prenatal visit, EXCEPT:
   a. HIV
   b. Hepatitis B
   c. Blood type and Rh status
   d. Cytomegalovirus (CMV)
   e. Genetic carrier screening

2. Which of the following recommendations about exercise in pregnancy is correct?
   a. Women should be counseled that 30 minutes or more of moderate exercise daily is recommended in pregnancy in the absence of medical or obstetric contraindications.
   b. Women should be counseled that only 10 minutes of light exercise daily is safe in pregnancy regardless of medical or obstetric comorbidities.
   c. Women should not be encouraged to begin an exercise program during pregnancy.
   d. Women should be counseled that no amount of exercise in pregnancy is safe.
   e. There are no recommendations regarding exercise in pregnancy.

3. During interconception care, patients should be counseled that pregnancy spacing of _____ can decrease the risk of preterm birth and low birth weight.
   a. 12 months
   b. 6 months
   c. 24 months
   d. 18 months
   e. 36 months

4. A "Reproductive Life Plan" references the following:
   a. The number and anticipated space of children a woman plans to have
   b. Family history
   c. Maternal and paternal ages
   d. Maternal medical comorbidities
   e. All of the above

5. Risk assessment for maternal morbidity and mortality should occur when?
   a. Only prior to pregnancy
   b. Once a woman is in labor
   c. In the first trimester
   d. Continuously throughout the preconception, antepartum, intrapartum, and postpartum periods
   e. In the second trimester, between 24 and 28 weeks gestation

6. Discussion of environmental exposures during pregnancy is discouraged during the preconception or pregnancy time period because:
   a. There is no way to mitigate these so women should not be needlessly frightened.
   b. There are only a handful of exposures/chemicals that cause harm during pregnancy.
   c. No environmental exposures have been proven to cause complications during pregnancy or for the developing fetus.
   d. Only a few women are exposed to potentially harmful exposures/chemicals so not all women need to have this discussion.
   e. All women should have a discussion about toxic environmental exposures because there may be ways to prevent or reduce exposure.

7. Interconception care or preconception care is crucial for all of the following reasons, except:

   a. Potentially modifiable behaviors may be addressed that affect the risk for genetic anomalies in the fetus.

   b. Potentially modifiable behaviors may be addressed that affect maternal health.

   c. Potentially modifiable behaviors may be addressed that affect the health of the fetus later in life.

   d. Potentially modifiable behaviors may be addressed that affect the risk of congenital anomalies in the fetus.

   e. Potentially modifiable behaviors may be addressed that affect the risk of low birth weight infants.

8. Which of the following statements is true regarding prenatal care?

   a. Group prenatal care or centering is associated with worse outcomes for mothers and infants.

   b. Prenatal care is important because pregnancy is considered to be a teachable moment.

   c. The frequency of prenatal visits should be every 4 weeks until 28 weeks gestation, every 2–3 weeks between 28 and 36 weeks gestation, and then weekly from 36 weeks gestation until delivery for all women.

   d. Prenatal care should just involve care between a woman and her obstetric provider

   e. Evaluating barriers to care and socioeconomic status is not part of prenatal care

9. The term prenatal care refers to the following time period:

   a. The period from the first prenatal visit until delivery

   b. The period from the first prenatal visit until the 6-week postpartum visit

   c. The period from preconception through postpartum care, extending up to 1 year after the infant's birth

   d. The period from conception through the 6-week postpartum visit

   e. The period from conception through postpartum care, extending up to 1 year after the infant's birth

10. Preconception counseling should be considered for the following patient:

    a. A 28-year-old woman with a history of Crohn disease

    b. A 21-year-old woman with a history of a 23-week delivery 11 months ago

    c. A 32-year-old woman with an uncomplicated medical history

    d. A 43-year-old woman with a body mass index (BMI) of 48 kg/m^2 with a history of type 2 diabetes and chronic hypertension, not requiring medication after gastric bypass surgery

    e. All of the above

11. A 36-year-old G2P0101 African American woman comes in for a "well-woman" examination. She has one child aged 10 years old who was born at 34 weeks after preterm premature rupture of membranes. She is recently remarried and would like to have another child. She has been using combined oral contraceptives for contraception. Her BMI is 34 kg/m^2 and her blood pressure at this visit is 142/89. She states she does not have high blood pressure, and review of her previous vital signs in your office show normal blood pressures. She mentions to you that she has been stressed because of her daughter's frequent doctor visits due to sickle cell disease and thinks that may be why her blood pressure is elevated. She admits to social alcohol use. She does not exercise but she does cook most of her meals at home. She does not remember if she has received Tetanus, diphtheria, pertussis vaccine (Tdap) in the past. Given this information, what should your next steps be?

    a. Refer her to an internal medicine physician for chronic hypertension management.

    b. Tell the patient this is her well-woman examination and she will need to return for a preconception counseling visit.

    c. Tell her that she is healthy enough for pregnancy and she can stop her oral contraceptive pills and attempt conception.

    d. Use this visit as an opportunity to discuss many issues related to optimizing her health prior to conception, including, but not limited to, her BMI, alcohol use, exercise, blood pressure, age, genetic disease screening, and immunization status.

    e. Refer her to a maternal-fetal medicine specialist for preconception counseling.

12. A 27-year-old G0 comes to see you for an annual examination. She states she is only here for her Pap smear. Her BMI is 17 kg/m² and her medical history is significant for cystic fibrosis with pancreatic insufficiency and she is currently on multiple medications. She has been in a relationship with her boyfriend for the past 2 years and feels safe in the relationship. She is not currently on contraception because her pulmonologist told her that it is unlikely that she would ever become pregnant. She is not upset about this as she does not think that she would ever want children given her medical history, but she is not certain. What is the appropriate next step?

a. Tell her you agree with her pulmonologist and perform her Pap smear.

b. Counsel the patient that although her chance of fertility is likely lower than a woman without cystic fibrosis, she could still become pregnant and discuss contraceptive options with her in addition to performing her Pap smear and discussing the importance of optimization of her health if she did desire a future pregnancy.

c. Tell the patient she should be using condoms "just in case."

d. Refer her to a family planning specialist to discuss contraception and perform her Pap smear.

e. Refer her to a maternal-fetal medicine specialist to discuss pregnancy and cystic fibrosis because the patient is uncertain about desiring children in the future.

ANSWERS

1. Answer: d

(see *Gabbe's Obstetrics* 8e: ch5)

Routine screening for prior infection with CMV is only recommended for at-risk populations and should not be a part of routine screening for women contemplating pregnancy or who are pregnant.

2. Answer: a

(see *Gabbe's Obstetrics* 8e: ch5)

Recreational exercises should be encouraged in pregnancy. Unfortunately, many women are routinely told to decrease their physical activity, even though research on moderate aerobic activity shows no negative impact on pregnancy outcomes. The American College of Obstetricians and Gynecologists recommends 30 minutes or more of moderate exercise daily during pregnancy. Women may start an exercise program in the absence of contraindications under supervision of a medical provider.

3. Answer: c

(see *Gabbe's Obstetrics* 8e: ch5)

The World Health Organization recommends waiting 24 months between delivery and conception as this has been shown to decrease the risk of preterm birth and low-birth-weight (PTB/LBW) infants, especially in women with a history of these complications during a prior pregnancy. This interconception interval has been associated with decreased risk of PTB/LBW and decreased risk for uterine rupture among women attempting a vaginal birth after a cesarean delivery.

4. Answer: e

(see *Gabbe's Obstetrics* 8e: ch5)

The key elements of a reproductive life plan include (1) the desire or lack of desire to have children, (2) parental ages, (3) maternal health and coexisting medical conditions, (4) the desired number of children and anticipated spacing of children, (5) risk tolerance for genetic or medical/obstetric complications, (6) family history, and (7) life context.

5. Answer: d

(see *Gabbe's Obstetrics* 8e: ch5)

Risk of maternal morbidity and mortality changes throughout the pregnancy, in addition to the preconception and postpartum period. Providers should reassess risk factors before pregnancy, during pregnancy, in labor, and postpartum to identify those at highest risk. However, it should be emphasized that the majority of morbidity and mortality occurs in women without identifiable risk factors.

6. Answer: e

(see *Gabbe's Obstetrics* 8e: ch5)

All pregnant women are exposed to and have detectable levels of chemicals that can be harmful to reproduction or human development. These exposures may be mitigated or prevented, and all women should be made aware of known toxic substances because all women are at risk.

7. Answer: a

(see *Gabbe's Obstetrics* 8e: ch5)

Human health status in adulthood is dictated by microenvironmental and macroenvironmental conditions around the time of conception; therefore, the first prenatal visit may be too late to address modifiable behaviors that could optimize not only pregnancy outcome for the mother but the health of the child and future adult. A second significant contribution to adverse pregnancy outcome is related to congenital anomalies, PTB, and LBW. The risk for genetic anomalies is not considered a modifiable risk factor.

8. Answer: b

(see *Gabbe's Obstetrics* 8e: ch5)

Pregnancy qualifies as a teachable moment because it meets the following criteria: perception of personal risk and outcome expectancies is increased, the perceptions are associated with strong affective or emotional responses, and the event is associated with a redefinition of self-concept or social role. Studies looking at changing the prenatal visit schedule frequency and the use of group prenatal care have shown no difference in outcomes when compared to traditional models of care. Due to the impact of socioeconomic status on access to care and health literacy, this should be addressed at prenatal visits and additional specialists should be utilized as needed due to the depth and breadth or information that need to be covered.

9. Answer: c

(see *Gabbe's Obstetrics* 8e: ch5)

The breadth of prenatal care does not end with delivery but rather includes preconception care and postpartum care that extends up to 1 year after the infant's birth.

10. Answer: e

(see *Gabbe's Obstetrics* 8e: ch5)

All women should be offered preconception care to promote the health of women before conception in order to reduce preventable adverse pregnancy outcomes by facilitating risk screening, health promotion, and effective interventions as part of routine health care, and by emphasizing those factors requiring action before conception or early in pregnancy to have maximal impact.

11. Answer: d

(see *Gabbe's Obstetrics* 8e: ch5)

All health care practitioners should approach every health care encounter with a reproductive-age woman as an opportunity to maximize her health and that of her future offspring. A visit where potential future child bearing is discussed should be seen as a teachable opportunity and topics to be discussed should include the woman's reproductive life plan, age, BMI, substance use/abuse, weight gain, exercise, chronic medical conditions, genetic and family history, and intimate partner violence. Other topics may be discussed as they apply to the patient.

12. Answer: b

(see *Gabbe's Obstetrics* 8e: ch5)

When a woman does not desire conception within the near future, reliable contraception should be prescribed, and the importance of compliance reinforced. Data suggest that many women with complex medical problems who are advised against pregnancy conceive unintentionally and/or do not use contraception because of low perceived risk of conceiving. All health care practitioners should approach every health care encounter with a reproductive-age woman as an opportunity to maximize her health and that of her future offspring.

Prenatal Care

6

Nutrition During Pregnancy

Thaddeus P. Waters

(see *Gabbe's Obstetrics: Normal and Problem Pregnancies*, 8e: ch6)

QUESTIONS

1. A vegan diet may be insufficient for pregnancy for all of the following except:

   a. Iron

   b. Essential amino acids

   c. Trace minerals

   d. Fat

2. To avoid listeriosis, pregnant women should be advised to do all of the following except:

   a. Wash all fruits and vegetables.

   b. Avoid all cold cuts.

   c. Avoid all cheeses.

   d. Cook meat to minimum safe temperatures.

3. All of the following are contributors to constipation in pregnancy except:

   a. Increased smooth muscle tone

   b. Increase in water reabsorption from the large intestine

   c. Slower gastrointestinal (GI) motility

   d. Iron supplementation

4. Which of the following is most accurate regarding nausea and vomiting of pregnancy?

   a. Vitamin B_6 is a first-line treatment for nausea and vomiting.

   b. A potential cause is human placenta lactogen.

   c. More than half of women have symptoms of nausea and vomiting in the third trimester.

   d. It is more common for women with heartburn.

5. All of the following are accurate regarding maternal anemia in pregnancy except:

   a. Ferritin levels <10 µg/L have the highest sensitivity and specificity for diagnosing iron deficiency.

   b. It is defined as hemoglobin less than 11 g/dL in all trimesters.

   c. Iron supplementation for women multiple gestations is higher than for women with a singleton gestation.

   d. Intravenous iron can significantly increase maternal hemoglobin levels within 7 days of administration.

6. A 23-year-old G2P0010 presents at 6 weeks with a missed period. She reports a history of a prior pregnancy complicated by anencephaly. Which of the following is the most appropriate recommendation for this patient?

   a. An early dating ultrasound to evaluate for a neural tube defect

   b. Prescribing 4000 µg/day of supplemental folate

   c. Referral for genetic counseling

   d. A daily prenatal vitamin with folate

7. A-24-year old G1P0 presents for prenatal care at 8 weeks. She reports no significant past medical history. Her weight is 128 lb and she is 65 inches tall. All of the following are appropriate recommendations for this patient except

   a. The patient should have a total gestational weight gain of 28 to 40 lb.

   b. The patient should anticipate up to an additional 300 kcal/day of intake during pregnancy.

   c. Dietary protein intake should be increased from 0.8 g/kg/day to 1.1 g/kg/day during pregnancy.

   d. The daily recommended intake for folate in pregnant women is 600 µg/day.

8. All of the following are accurate regarding vitamin D during pregnancy except
   a. To evaluate vitamin D concentrations, a serum 25-hydroxy-D level is needed.
   b. The daily requirement for vitamin D in pregnancy is 600 IU/day.
   c. Vitamin D supplementation is often not required during pregnancy.
   d. Low vitamin D levels are associated with several adverse pregnancy outcomes, including depression.

ANSWERS

1. Answer: **d**

   (see *Gabbe's Obstetrics* 8e: ch6)

   Vegan diets—those that exclude all animal products, including eggs and dairy—may provide insufficient iron, essential amino acids, trace minerals (zinc), vitamin B_{12}, vitamin D, calcium, and Polyunsaturated fatty acids (PUFA) to support normal embryonic and fetal development. Thus, it is recommended that patients who follow a vegan diet meet with a dietitian early during the pregnancy to analyze their nutritional intake and assess any necessary supplementation that should be added. For example, fortified vegetarian food products are now widely available and include some nondairy milks with added calcium and vitamin D, meat substitutes that contain protein, and fortified juice and breakfast cereals.[1]

2. Answer: **c**

   (see *Gabbe's Obstetrics* 8e: ch6)

   To avoid listeriosis, pregnant women should be advised to wash vegetables and fruits well; cook all meats to minimum safe internal temperatures; avoid processed, precooked meats (cold cuts, smoked seafood, pâté) and soft cheeses (brie, blue cheese, Camembert, and Mexican queso blanco [white cheese]); and only consume dairy products that have been pasteurized.

3. Answer: **a**

   (see *Gabbe's Obstetrics* 8e: ch6)

   Fifty percent of pregnant women experience constipation at some point during their pregnancy, which is often associated with straining, hard stools, and incomplete evacuation rather than infrequent defecation. Constipation during pregnancy is associated with smooth muscle relaxation, an increase in water reabsorption from the large intestine, and slower GI motility. Pregnant women often note overall GI discomfort, a bloated sensation, an increase in hemorrhoids and heartburn, and decreased appetite. Constipation can also be aggravated by iron supplements. Strategies for managing constipation during pregnancy are shown in Box 6.1.

   BOX 6.1   Strategies for Managing Constipation in Pregnancy

   - Increase fluid intake by drinking water, herbal teas, and noncaffeinated beverages.
   - Increase daily fiber intake by eating high-fiber cereals, whole grains, legumes, and bran.
   - Use a psyllium fiber supplement (e.g., Metamucil).
   - Increase consumption of fresh, frozen, or dried fruits and vegetables.
   - Participate in moderate physical activity such as walking, swimming, or yoga.
   - Take stool softeners in conjunction with iron supplementation.

   Courtesy Lisa Hark, PhD, RD

4. Answer: **a**

   (see *Gabbe's Obstetrics* 8e: ch6)

   Women with hyperemesis may vomit multiple times throughout the day, lose more than 5% of their prepregnancy body weight, and usually require hospitalization for dehydration and electrolyte replacement. After following these recommendations, vitamin B_6 (10 to 25 mg three times daily) can be considered as first-line treatment for nausea and vomiting during pregnancy. Ginger and acupuncture may also be helpful to treat nausea during pregnancy.[2,3]

5. Answer: b

(see *Gabbe's Obstetrics* 8e: ch6)

Hemoglobin less than 11 g/dL or hematocrit below 33% in the first or third trimester indicates anemia. Hemoglobin less than 10.5 g/dL or hematocrit below 32% in the second trimester also indicates anemia (Table 6.1).

TABLE 6.1	Diagnosis of Anemia in Pregnancy.		
Lab Test	First Trimester	Second Trimester	Third Trimester
Hemoglobin (g/dL)	<11	10.5	<11
Hematocrit (%)	<33	32	<33

Data from U.S. Centers for Disease Control and Prevention (www.cdc.gov)

6. Answer: b

(see *Gabbe's Obstetrics* 8e: ch6)

In women with a previous pregnancy affected by an neural tube defect (NTD), research has shown that supplementation with 4000 µg/day (4 mg/day of folate initiated at least 1 month prior to attempting to conceive and continued throughout the first trimester of pregnancy reduced the risk of a repeat NTD by 72%.[4] Whereas no definitive evidence proves that other high-risk groups such as close family members of affected individuals, diabetics, or women on antiseizure medications will benefit from higher levels of supplementation, many experts recommend a higher dose of folate—at least 1000 µg/day—before conception and in early pregnancy. For these women, a separate folate supplement should be prescribed; additional doses of multivitamins should not be used as this could lead to toxicity of other vitamins, particularly vitamin A, which is teratogenic to the developing fetus.[5]

7. Answer: a

(see *Gabbe's Obstetrics* 8e: ch6)

The 2009 Institute of Medicine guidelines recommend that overweight women with a singleton pregnancy gain a total of 15 to 25 lb during pregnancy (compared with 25 to 35 lb for normal-weight women). Obese women are advised to gain only 11 to 20 lb during the course of their pregnancy.

8. Answer: c

(see *Gabbe's Obstetrics* 8e: ch6)

Recent studies have shown that low maternal vitamin D levels are common during pregnancy, even in patients who take daily prenatal vitamins that contain 400 IU of vitamin D (50% of mothers and 65% of newborn infants were significantly vitamin D deficient at the time of birth, despite daily supplementation with 400 IU of vitamin D and drinking two glasses of vitamin D fortified milk).

REFERENCES

1. Craig WJ, Mangels AR, American Dietetic Association. Position of the American Dietetic Association: vegetarian diets. *J Am Diet Assoc.* 2009;109:1266.
2. Chittumma P, Kaewkiattikun K, Wiriyasiriwach B. Comparison of the effectiveness of ginger and vitamin B6 for treatment of nausea and vomiting in early pregnancy: a randomized double-blind controlled trial. *J Med Assoc Thai.* 2007;90:15.
3. Jewell D, Young G. Interventions for nausea and vomiting in early pregnancy. *Cochrane Database Syst Rev.* 2003;CD000145.
4. Molloy AM, Kirke PN, Brody LC, et al. Effects of folate and vitamin B12 deficiencies during pregnancy on fetal, infant, and child development. *Food Nutr Bull.* 2008;29:101.
5. US Preventive Services Task Force, Agency for Healthcare Research and Quality. Folic acid for the prevention of neural tube defects: US Preventive Services Task Force recommendation statement. *Ann Intern Med.* 2009;150:626.

7

Medications and Environmental Agents in Pregnancy and Lactation

Alyssa Stephenson-Famy

(see *Gabbe's Obstetrics: Normal and Problem Pregnancies*, 8e: ch7)

QUESTIONS

1. What is the incidence of major congenital malformations in the general population?
   a. 0.5%
   b. 2%
   c. 5%
   d. 12%
   e. 20%

2. What is the classic teratogenic period following the last menstrual period (for a 28-day cycle) in which major organs are forming?
   a. 0–15 days
   b. 16–30 days
   c. 31–71 days
   d. 72–100 days
   e. 101–130 days

3. In research studies, mice develop specific teratogenic malformations after a drug exposure throughout the first trimester. This drug is known to rapidly diffuse across the placenta. Similar studies in other mammalian species (similar dose/timing) did not demonstrate the same teratogenic effect. Which of Wilson's six principles of teratogenesis best describes this observation?
   a. Genotype of the embryo
   b. Timing of the exposure
   c. Dose effect
   d. Efficiency of placental transfer
   e. Mechanism of drug

4. A postpartum woman undergoes a dental procedure and receives a prescription for acetaminophen with codeine for pain. She is breastfeeding her 3-week-old newborn. The pharmacist warns against using the medication while breastfeeding. What is the pharmacist's primary concern regarding use of this medication during lactation?
   a. Ultra-rapid metabolism
   b. Neonatal allergy to codeine
   c. Excessive neonatal gastric absorption
   d. Drug concentration in colostrum

5. A 26-year-old woman with endometriosis is taking danazol. Due to a long history of irregular periods, she does not determine that she is pregnant until 12 weeks gestation. The timing of danazol exposure is 7–10 weeks gestation. What is the most likely teratogenic effect?
   a. No effect, given known medication safety in pregnancy
   b. No effect, given timing of exposure in first trimester
   c. Ambiguous genitalia, if the fetus is female
   d. Ambiguous genitalia, if the fetus is male

6. A 30-year-old female with long-standing epilepsy is planning a pregnancy. Which antiepileptic drug (AED) is least likely to cause congenital malformations and would be the safest drug during pregnancy?
   a. Carbamazepine
   b. Valproic acid
   c. Phenytoin
   d. Topiramate
   e. Lamotrigine

7. A 36-year-old woman with a mechanical mitral heart valve due to rheumatic heart disease is anticoagulated with warfarin prior to learning that she is pregnant. What disorder is associated with first trimester warfarin exposure?

    a. Neural tube defect

    b. Cleft lip/palate

    c. Hydrocephalus

    d. Ebstein anomaly

    e. Chondrodysplasia punctata

8. A 28-year-old woman with hyperthyroidism presents for preconception care. She was told she should take propyl-thiouracil (PTU) in the first trimester and then should take methimazole in the second and third trimesters. What is the reason for this recommendation?

    a. Fetal teratogenic effect of PTU

    b. Maternal liver toxicity of PTU

    c. Safety of methimazole with breastfeeding

    d. Radioactive iodine (^{131}I or ^{125}I) concentration in fetal thyroid

9. A woman with a urinary tract infection has a positive pregnancy test. The urine culture shows pan-sensitive *Escherichia coli*. Which antibiotic should be avoided given the diagnosis of pregnancy?

    a. Cephalosporins

    b. Sulfonamides

    c. Nitrofurantoin

    d. Tetracycline

    e. Metronidazole

10. A 25-year-old woman with chronic back pain takes non-steroidal antiinflammatory drugs (NSAIDs) throughout her pregnancy. Which outcome is the fetus/neonate most likely to develop?

    a. Ventral septal defect

    b. Patent ductus arteriosus

    c. Oligohydramnios

    d. Polyhydramnios

    e. Neonatal withdrawal

11. A newborn is evaluated after delivery due to being small for gestational age and having facial anomalies, including small palpebral fissures, short philtrum, epicanthic folds, flattened nasal bridge, and short low-set ears. His mother was known to have polysubstance use during her pregnancy. Heavy use of which substance most likely caused the findings in this newborn?

    a. Alcohol

    b. Marijuana

    c. Cocaine

    d. Opioids

    e. Methamphetamine

12. An 18-year-old woman is in a car accident and requires multiple imaging studies for evaluation of pelvic fractures. During her hospitalization, she has a positive pregnancy test. Which threshold amount of radiation should be avoided during early pregnancy due to risk of congenital anomalies?

    a. 0.1 rad

    b. 0.5 rad

    c. 1 rad

    d. 5 rad

    e. 10 rad

ANSWERS

1. **Answer: b**

   (see *Gabbe's Obstetrics* 8e: ch7)

   The incidence of major malformations in the general population is 2% to 3%.[1] These are malformations incompatible with survival (anencephaly), those requiring major surgery (cleft palate or congenital heart disease), or causing permanent disability (developmental delays). The malformation rate may be as high as 7% to 10 % if minor defects are counted (ear tags, extra digits).

2. Answer: c

(see *Gabbe's Obstetrics* 8e: ch7)

The classic teratogenic period is from day 31 after the last menstrual period in a 28-day cycle to 71 days from the last period. During this critical period, organs are forming and teratogens may cause malformations that are usually overt at birth. Administration of drugs early in this period may affect heart or neural tube; later exposure affects ear and palate formation.

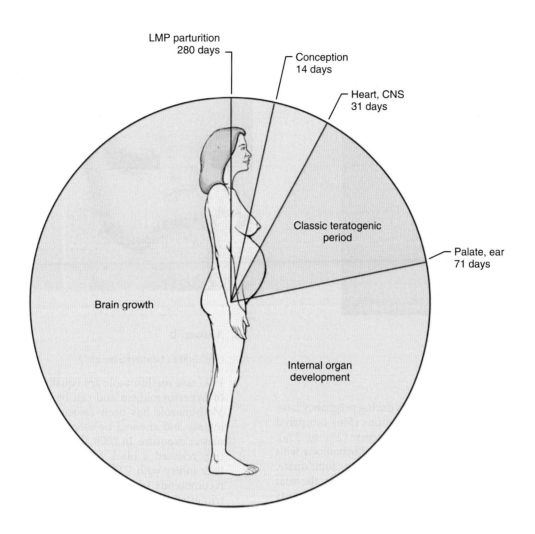

3. Answer: a

(see *Gabbe's Obstetrics* 8e: ch7)

Wilson's six general principles of teratogenesis[2] provide a framework for understanding how structural or functional teratogens may act: Genotype and Interaction With Environmental Factors, Timing of Exposure, Mechanisms of Teratogenesis, Manifestation, Age, and Dose Effect. Susceptibility of a species to a teratogen depends on the *genotype of the conceptus* and the manner in which the genetic makeup of the conceptus interacts with environmental factors. This most likely explains many species-specific effects of drugs during pregnancy (timing of exposure, dose effect, placental drug transfer, and drug metabolism may also alter the effect on any teratogen the developing embryo).

4. Answer: a

(see *Gabbe's Obstetrics* 8e: ch7)

Drugs such as codeine and tramadol have variations in maternal metabolism that can lead to adverse neonatal effect. Mothers who receive codeine and are "ultra-rapid" metabolizers will convert codeine to high concentrations of morphine, which easily passes into the breast milk and can cause neonatal respiratory depression.

5. Answer: c

(see *Gabbe's Obstetrics* 8e: ch7)

Danazol is an androgenic steroid which may masculinize a developing female fetus. Danazol (Danocrine) has been reported to produce clitoral enlargement and labial fusion when given inadvertently for the first 9 to 12 weeks after conception.

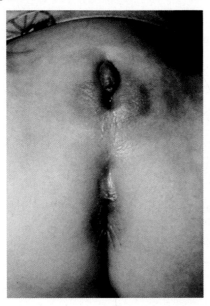

6. Answer: e

(see *Gabbe's Obstetrics* 8e: ch7)

Women with epilepsy taking AEDs during pregnancy have nearly double the risk of malformations (5%) compared with pregnant women without epilepsy (2% to 3%). There is an increased risk of major malformations with valproate, phenytoin, carbamazepine, and topiramate. Published studies on lamotrigine exposures in the first trimester have shown no increased risk of birth defects overall.

7. Answer: e

(see *Gabbe's Obstetrics* 8e: ch7)

Warfarin has been associated with *chondrodysplasia punctata* and includes nasal hypoplasia, bone stippling seen on radiologic examination, ophthalmologic abnormalities including bilateral optic atrophy, and developmental delay.

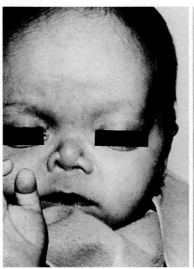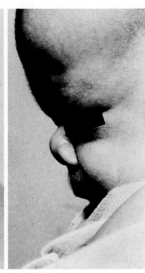

8. Answer: b

(see *Gabbe's Obstetrics* 8e: ch7)

PTU and methimazole are equally effective for treatment of hyperthyroidism and can be used with breastfeeding. Methimazole has been associated with scalp defects in infants and choanal or esophageal atresia with first trimester exposure. In 2009, the Food and Drug Administration released a black box warning highlighting serious liver injury with PTU treatment. The Endocrine Society recommends treatment with PTU only during the first trimester and switching to methimazole for the remainder of the pregnancy.

9. Answer: d

(see *Gabbe's Obstetrics* 8e: ch7)

Tetracyclines readily cross the placenta and are firmly bound by chelation to calcium in developing bone and tooth structures, which can cause teeth discoloration, hypoplasia of the enamel, and inhibition of bone growth. Alternate antibiotics are currently recommended during pregnancy because of these concerns.

10. Answer: c

(see *Gabbe's Obstetrics* 8e: ch7)

No evidence of teratogenicity has been reported for other NSAIDs; however, chronic use may lead to oligohydramnios and constriction of the fetal ductus arteriosus or neonatal pulmonary hypertension.

11. Answer: a

(see *Gabbe's Obstetrics* 8e: ch7)

Fetal alcohol syndrome includes growth restriction before and/or after birth; characteristic facial anomalies, including small palpebral fissures, indistinct or absent philtrum, epicanthic folds, flattened nasal bridge, short length of nose, thin upper lip, low-set, uneven ears, and mid-face hypoplasia; and central nervous system dysfunction including microcephaly, varying degrees of developmental disabilities, or other evidence of abnormal neurobehavioral development.

12. Answer: d

(see *Gabbe's Obstetrics* 8e: ch7)

Prenatal exposure to ionizing radiation less than 5 rad has not been shown to increase the risk of congenital malformations. Exposures are expressed as Gray (Gy): 10 mGy equals 1 rad. Fortunately, virtually no single diagnostic test produces a substantive risk (Table 7.1). Only multiple CT scans and fluoroscopies would lead to cumulate exposures of 100 mGy or 10 rad.

TABLE 7.1 Approximate Fetal Doses From Common Diagnostic Procedures.

Examination	Mean (mGY)	Maximum (mGY)
Conventional X-ray examinations		
Abdomen	1.4	4.2
Chest	<0.01	<0.01
Intravenous urogram	1.7	10
Lumbar spine	1.7	10
Pelvis	1.1	4
Skull	<0.01	<0.01
Thoracic Spine	<0.01	<0.01
Fluoroscopic examinations		
Barium meal Upper gastrointestinal series (UGI)	1.1	5.8
Barium enema	6.8	24
Computed tomography		
Abdomen	8.0	49
Chest	0.06	0.96
Head	<0.005	<0.005
Lumbarspine	2.4	8.6
Pelvis	25	79

0 mGY = 1 rad.
From Lowe SA. Diagnostic radiography in pregnancy: risks and reality. *Aust N Z J Obstet Gynaecol* 2004;44:191.

REFERENCES

1. Wilson JG, Fraser FC: *Handbook of Teratology*. New York: Plenum; 1979.

2. Wilson JG: Current status of teratology—general principles and mechanisms derived from animal studies. In: Wilson JG, Fraser FC (eds). *Handbook of Teratology*. New York: Plenum; 1977:47.

3. Answer: a

(see *Gabbe's Obstetrics* 8e: ch8)

Exposure to drugs or alcohol during adolescence may result in different neuroadaptations than when exposures occur in adulthood, and the process of addiction is more likely to be triggered in the adolescent brain. Perhaps rendering adolescents vulnerable is the lack of development of the frontal cortex, with executive control, motivation, and decision making more able to be influenced by drug exposure.

4. Answer: b

(see *Gabbe's Obstetrics* 8e: ch8)

Adverse childhood experiences include neglect; physical, emotional, and sexual abuse; a parent with a mental illness; being a victim of (or a witness to) violence in the home; divorce; substance abuse within the home; or an incarcerated family member. For every adverse childhood experience identified, there is a two- to four-fold lifetime increase in SUD.

5. Answer: a

(see *Gabbe's Obstetrics* 8e: ch8)

While universal screening for SUD is currently recommended, universal testing is not necessarily recommended. One has to adhere to state laws for drug testing and seek consent to do so in those states where consent is required. Pregnant women should be informed of the potential ramifications of a positive test result, including any mandatory reporting requirements. Current recommendations are that universal screenings rely on validated tools, such as the 4Ps, National Institute on Drug Abuse quick screen, and Car, Relax, Alone, Forget, Friends, Trouble (CRAFFT) CRAFFT for women 26 years of age or younger.

6. Answer: c

(see *Gabbe's Obstetrics* 8e: ch8)

It is common to use the skills of motivational interviewing when pursuing a brief intervention. The clinician practices motivational interviewing with five general principles in mind: (1) express empathy through reflective listening; (2) develop discrepancy between clients' goals or values and their current behavior; (3) avoid argument and direct confrontation; (4) adjust to client resistance rather than opposing it directly; and (5) support self-efficacy and optimism.

7. Answer: b

(see *Gabbe's Obstetrics* 8e: ch8)

Neonatal abstinence syndrome will occur in 40%–80% of neonates exposed to chronic opiate use. Neonatal abstinence syndrome is difficult to observe at the patient level; therefore, many efforts in the maternal care of opiate use disorder revolve around mitigating neonatal abstinence syndrome, including smoking cessation and breastfeeding. Breastfeeding should also be recommended to women with OUD. Babies benefit from the nurturing behavior required for breastfeeding, receive the benefits of human milk, receive a trace amount of opiate in human milk, and are less likely to suffer severe neonatal abstinence syndrome. In addition, the oxytocin release encountered with lactation is of benefit to the mother in combatting postpartum depression and relapse.

8. Answer: b

(see *Gabbe's Obstetrics* 8e: ch8)

There is a reported association between first-trimester exposure to benzodiazepines and cleft lip and palate. Marijuana use has not been consistently associated with any congenital birth defect. Cocaine readily crosses the placenta and fetal blood brain barrier, and numerous reports of congenital malformations have been reported to be associated with this exposure. However, such studies have methodologic flaws, and current literature suggests that such information was overreported during the years of the cocaine and crack epidemic, due to publication bias of positive findings. Therefore, teratogenicity has not been definitively associated with cocaine exposure. Similarly, amphetamines and methamphetamines cross the placenta, without clear demonstration of associated fetal structural defects. Opiates are not historically thought to be teratogenic, but recent reports have raised the possibility of an association. Some reports have found that the odds of having a child with atrial or ventricular septal defects, hypoplastic left heart syndrome, spina bifida, and gastroschisis are higher in fetuses with opioid exposures in utero than those without exposure. However, studies to date are significantly limited by size, design, and recall bias, making interpretation challenging. Thus, the possible teratogenicity associated with opiate exposure in the first trimester remains under investigation.

Obstetrical Ultrasound: Imaging, Dating, Growth, and Anomaly

Vanita D. Jain

(see *Gabbe's Obstetrics: Normal and Problem Pregnancies*, 8e: ch9)

QUESTIONS

1. A 21-year-old G1P0 presents for her "anatomy ultrasound" at 20 weeks gestational age. Her prenatal course has been uncomplicated; however, her body mass index is noted to be 50 kg/m². In order to optimize your scanned image, you attempt to use "windows" in the abdominal wall near the umbilicus. In addition to this technique, starting with which frequency probe may improve your penetration?
   a. 2 Mhz
   b. 3 Mhz
   c. 5 Mhz
   d. 8 Mhz

2. While imaging a patient for fetal anatomy, you have difficulty visualizing the fetal heart adequately. The image appears too "dark." Which of the following maneuvers would improve your image quality?
   a. Turning off tissue harmonics
   b. Choosing a higher frequency probe
   c. Adjusting your power
   d. Increasing or adjusting your gain

3. A 32-year-old G1P1001 is at 22 weeks gestation when her Anti-D titer returns as 1:64. She is referred to the Maternal Fetal Medicine department for fetal anemia screening. The Doppler flow study that is most useful in diagnosing fetal anemia is:
   a. Umbilical vein peak systolic velocity
   b. Systolic to diastolic ratio of the ductus venosus
   c. Resistance index of the fetal middle cerebral artery
   d. Peak systolic velocity of the fetal middle cerebral artery
   e. Pulsatility index of the fetal middle cerebral artery

4. One of the first steps in fetal imaging is to establish the position of the fetus and orientation or "situs." To do so, probe orientation is imperative. Which of the following statements is correct?
   a. Utilize the side of the stomach to define the position of the fetus.
   b. Utilize the axis of the fetal heart to define the position of the fetus.
   c. Confirm in the sagittal view that the right of the screen corresponds superior aspect of the patient.
   d. Confirm that the notch on the ultrasound probe corresponds to the left side of the monitor.
   e. Confirm that the notch on the ultrasound probe corresponds to the right side of the monitor.

5. A 21-year-old presents with a positive urine hCG. Based on her last menstrual period (LMP) she should be about 10 weeks pregnant. Ultrasound is performed in your office to confirm the pregnancy and for dating. The best measure for gestational-age determination in the first trimester is the:
   a. Measurement of the gestational sac
   b. Measurement of the yolk sac
   c. Measurement of the cerebral falx
   d. Measurement of the crown-rump length (CRL)
   e. Measurement of the biparietal diameter

6. A 32-year-old G2P1001 presents to your office with vaginal bleeding. An ultrasound is performed and reveals a viable 11-week fetus with a fetal heart rate of 166 beats per minute. The patient reports no significant medical or surgical history. Her prior pregnancy was uncomplicated and delivered full term. This was a spontaneous conception. She is tearful and wishes to know the risk of losing the pregnancy due to her vaginal bleeding. You counsel her:

   a. About 80% of women with bleeding will miscarry in the setting of a normal ultrasound with a live embryo.

   b. About 50% of women with bleeding will miscarry in the setting of a normal ultrasound with a live embryo.

   c. Only 10% of women with bleeding will miscarry in the setting of a normal ultrasound with live embryo.

   d. Only 1% of women with bleeding will miscarry in the setting of a normal ultrasound with live embryo.

7. A 29-year-old G4P3003 presents for an obstetrician appointment after her home urine pregnancy test. An ultrasound is performed in the office, and a fetus is seen with a CRL, measuring 46 mm. No fetal heart motion is noted. The mean sac diameter is 22 mm. The patient has not had an ultrasound previously. Based on these findings, you would recommend:

   a. Repeat ultrasound in 7–10 days

   b. Counseling regarding a failed intrauterine pregnancy and recommend a dilation and currettage (D&C)

   c. Counseling regarding a failed intrauterine pregnancy and recommend methotrexate

   d. A beta-HCG quantitative value via blood draw and repeat ultrasound and office evaluation in 4 weeks

8. A 26-year-old G2P1001 with an uncomplicated, otherwise normal pregnancy presents at 36 weeks to your office. Last week in the office, the midwife performing her visit noted that the fetus appeared to be in the breech position, based on Leopold maneuvers. She is here to confirm this finding and consider her options. She has had a previous anatomy ultrasound that was normal and her dating was confirmed by first trimester ultrasound. Which is the correct type of ultrasound to perform to confirm fetal position?

   a. CPT code 76805 A standard 2nd/3rd trimester

   b. CPT code 76811 A specialized anatomy ultrasound

   c. CPT code 76815 A limited examination

   d. CPT code 76816 A follow-up examination

9. In determining the amniotic fluid volume during an ultrasound examination, which of the following statements is correct:

   a. The line between calipers should not cross through loops of cord or fetal parts.

   b. Each pocket of fluid should measure at least 4 cm in width.

   c. Polyhydramnios is defined as an amniotic fluid index (AFI) >20 cm.

   d. Oligohydramnios is defined as an AFI <10 cm.

10. An 18-year-old presents for her anatomy ultrasound at 18 weeks gestational age. The fetus appears normal on anatomy evaluation. However, the placental edge is noted to be 18 mm from the internal os on transvaginal evaluation. The correct next step in management is:

   a. Diagnosing a low lying placenta previa and counseling the patient for a repeat examination in 4 weeks

   b. Diagnosing a low-lying placenta previa and counseling that there is an 80% likelihood this will not resolve

   c. Diagnosing a low-lying placenta previa and counseling that a follow-up evaluation in the third trimester at 32 weeks is recommended

   d. Counseling that this a low-lying placenta and the risk of bleeding is so great immediate hospitalization is warranted

11. A 24-year-old G1P0 at 20 weeks gestation has a basic ultrasound performed in her general obstetrician's office. During the examination, the technician and the supervising physician suspect a single umbilical artery (SUA). A specialized sonogram is performed and confirms the finding. Which of the following is a true statement about SUA?

   a. SUA affects 1.4% of fetuses

   b. There is a higher rate of trisomy 16

   c. The rate of associated anomalies is 50%

   d. There is a 20% risk of fetal growth restriction

12. A 16-year-old presents for an ultrasound after a positive home pregnancy test. She does not recall the date of her last menstrual period (LMP). She also reports very irregular cycles since she started menstruating. She also notes she did get a Depo Provera injection approximately 6 months ago. She thinks she had spotting 5–6 weeks ago. You refer her for a formal ultrasound to confirm dating. Which of the following statements is correct?

   a. Dating should be derived from the fetal biometry (biparietal diameter = BPD, head circumference = HC, femur length = FL, abdominal circumference = AC) if the pregnancy on ultrasound appears >14 weeks.

   b. Dating should be obtained by utilizing the LMP date as the date of spotting 5–6 weeks prior.

   c. Dating should be obtained by utilizing the Depo Provera date 4 months prior.

   d. Dating should be based on CRL if the pregnancy on ultrasound appears >14 weeks.

13. When calculating an estimated fetal weight (EFW) on ultrasound, a large number of formulas exist. However, all formulas incorporate which measurement:

   a. BPD

   b. HC

   c. AC

   d. FL

14. A 32-year-old G4P3003 presents at 32 weeks for an ultrasound to measure growth as her fundal height in the office was only 26 cm. An EFW notes the fetus to be small for gestational age measuring at the ninth centile, and the diagnosis of fetal growth restriction is made. Doppler studies and the AFI are normal. The BPP is 8 out of 8. A repeat growth ultrasound is recommended in:

   a. 48 hours

   b. 7–10 days

   c. 3–4 weeks

   d. 6–8 weeks

15. A 25-year-old G1P0 asks about the safety of ultrasound at her first prenatal visit when you make the recommendation for a sonographic fetal anatomy evaluation. You counsel her:

   a. As long as the TI remains under 10, no adverse effect is noted.

   b. No independently confirmed adverse effect is caused from exposure to ultrasound in human subjects.

   c. All ultrasound is considered to be of moderate risk to the fetus.

   d. The sonographer will follow the ALARA principle and increase the acoustic output from the transducer as much as possible to keep the fetus safe.

16. A 39-year-old G1P0 who had conception achieved through in vitro fertilization and is at 12 weeks gestation presents for her first prenatal. When discussing her options for aneuploidy testing via first trimester screen, you review with her various options. You explain that on first trimester ultrasound, which of the following is the most important sonographic component in aneuploidy detection:

   a. Reverse ductus venosus flow

   b. Nasal bone measurement

   c. Measurement of the nuchal translucency

   d. Presence of tricuspid regurgitation

17. Which of the following is the least common neural tube defect?

   a. Anencephaly

   b. Meningomyleocele

   c. Holoprosencephaly

   d. Encephalocele

18. A 29-year-old G2P1001 is carrying a fetus diagnosed with cerebral ventriculomegaly. The fetal lateral ventricle measurement is noted to be 11 mm. After counseling, a full anatomy evaluation, and appropriate work-up, the patient is most interested in the likelihood of a normal outcome. You explain you will refer the patient to pediatric neurology for further counseling; however, in general, when the lateral ventricle measurement at the atrium measures in the mild range, the chances of a normal outcome are:

   a. <10%

   b. 20%

   c. 50%

   d. >90%

19. An anatomy ultrasound is performed at 20 weeks gestation and notes the following findings: thickened nuchal fold of 10 mm, absent nasal bone, an EIF, and an AV canal defect. You counsel the patient and recommend amniocentesis. The patient asks what condition you suspect. Based on the constellation of findings, the most likely concern is for:

   a. Trisomy 13

   b. Monosomy X

   c. Trisomy 18

   d. Trisomy 21

ANSWERS

1. **Answer: a**

   (see *Gabbe's Obstetrics* 8e: ch9)

   Available ultrasound probes operate over a range of frequencies (e.g., 1–5 Mhz and 4–8 Mhz for abdominal probes).

   Lower-frequency sound waves improve tissue penetration but at the expense of better resolution versus higher-frequency probes, which have less tissue penetration with better resolution. In general, start with the lowest-frequency probe available and increase frequency until a balance between penetration and resolution can be found.

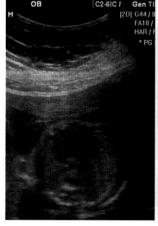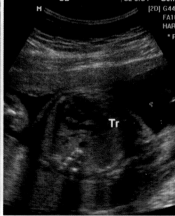

2. Answer: d

(see *Gabbe's Obstetrics* 8e: ch9)

"Gain" refers to the lightness or darkness of ultrasound images. Acceptable images demonstrate the full range of grays that the machine is capable of producing. The proper amount of gain varies by patient and situation. Gain is controlled by simply adjusting the setting on the machine console, usually a knob or a toggle switch. Increasing the gain will brighten or "lighten up" your image and improve resolution.

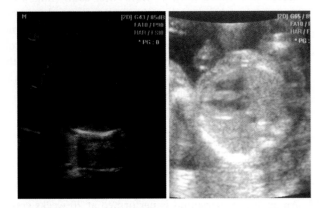

3. Answer: d

(see *Gabbe's Obstetrics* 8e: ch9)

Doppler ultrasound is used to demonstrate the presence, direction, and velocity of blood flow. The machine displays moving blood as color superimposed on the two-dimensional gray-scale image. Pulse-wave Doppler continuously measures the relative velocity of flow within a designated gate inside a vessel. Flow velocity waveforms are used to calculate the systolic/diastolic (S/D) ratio, the pulsatility index, and the resistance index. These indexes are primarily used to assess downstream resistance in the vessel being examined. For some applications, the absolute flow velocity is needed. For example, when screening for fetal anemia, the peak systolic velocity in the fetal middle cerebral artery is measured, which correlates with the degree of fetal anemia. Importantly, the angle of insonation (θ) should be in line with the direction of blood flow.

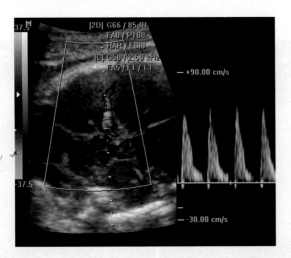

4. Answer: d

(see *Gabbe's Obstetrics* 8e: ch9)

The notch or ridge demarcates the side of the probe that will correspond to the left side of the monitor. The probe is always started with the notch up and then rotated counterclockwise to turn from sagittal to the transverse view. With the notch up, turning counter clockwise, the notch will point to the operators left side, also corresponding to the left side of the monitor on the ultrasound machine. Answer c is incorrect, because for sagittal views the right of the screen represents, by definition, the inferior aspect of the patient. Answers a and b are wrong, as one cannot depend on the side of the stomach or the axis of the heart to define the position of the fetus, as these structures are not always in a normal position (for example, situs inversus).

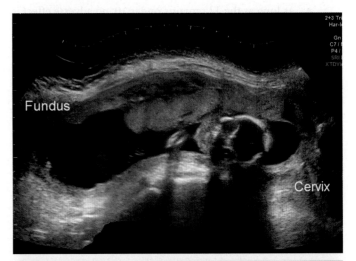

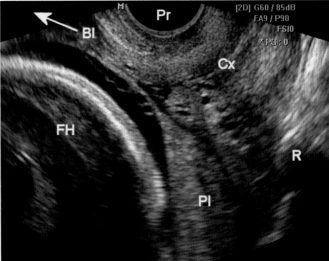

5. Answer: d

(see *Gabbe's Obstetrics* 8e: ch9)

Until 12 weeks, the CRL should be measured for gestational age determination. Care should be taken to measure the full length of the fetus. The gestational age can be significantly underestimated if an oblique plane is used.

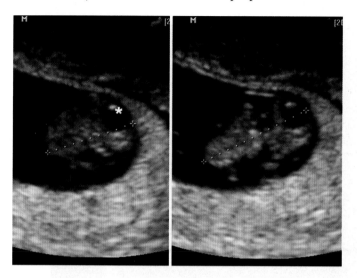

6. Answer: c

(see *Gabbe's Obstetrics* 8e: ch9)

When cardiac activity has been demonstrated, the miscarriage rate is reduced to 2% to 4% in asymptomatic low-risk women. However, in women >35 years old with a history of fertility treatment, the miscarriage rate in asymptomatic women was still 16% after a heartbeat was documented. Of women <35 years old who present with bleeding, 5%–15% miscarry if the ultrasound is normal and shows a live embryo. If an intrauterine clot is present coexistent with an otherwise normal-appearing pregnancy, the miscarriage rate is 15%.

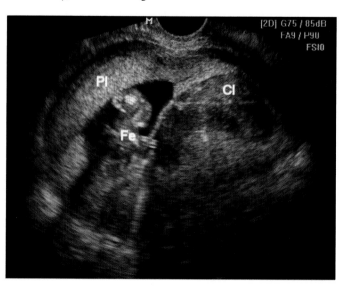

7. Answer: b

(see *Gabbe's Obstetrics* 8e: ch9)

Because no significant medical risk attends waiting for certainty when a failed pregnancy is suspected, a cautious approach is always advisable. However, criteria for deciding that an intrauterine pregnancy of uncertain viability is in fact a failed pregnancy were recommended by a multi-specialty panel convened by the Society of Radiologists in Ultrasound. These include:

1. The presence of a fetus with a CRL of more than 7 mm and no heartbeat;

2. The absence of an embryo when the mean sac diameter is greater than 25 mm;

3. The absence of an embryo with a heartbeat more than 2 weeks after a scan showed a gestational sac without a yolk sac; and

4. The absence of an embryo with a heartbeat more than 11 days after a gestational sac with a yolk sac was seen.

These criteria have been endorsed by American and Canadian practice guidelines.

8. Answer: c

(see *Gabbe's Obstetrics* 8e: ch9)

Limited ultrasound examinations, also performed by an individual with appropriate training, are used to obtain a specific piece of information about the pregnancy. Examples include the determination of fetal cardiac activity and fetal lie, assessment of amniotic fluid volume, and measurement of cervical length.

9. Answer: a

(see *Gabbe's Obstetrics* 8e: ch9)

The AFI is the sum of the measurements of the deepest vertical pocket (DVP) of fluid in each of the uterine quadrants. Each pocket should measure at least 1 cm in width. The line between the calipers should not cross through loops of cord or fetal parts. Polyhydramnios and oligohydramnios can be defined by either the AFI or measurement of the single DVP. Polyhydramnios is typically defined as an AFI greater than 24 cm or DVP of greater than 8 cm, and oligohydramnios, as an AFI less than 5 cm or DVP less than 2 cm.

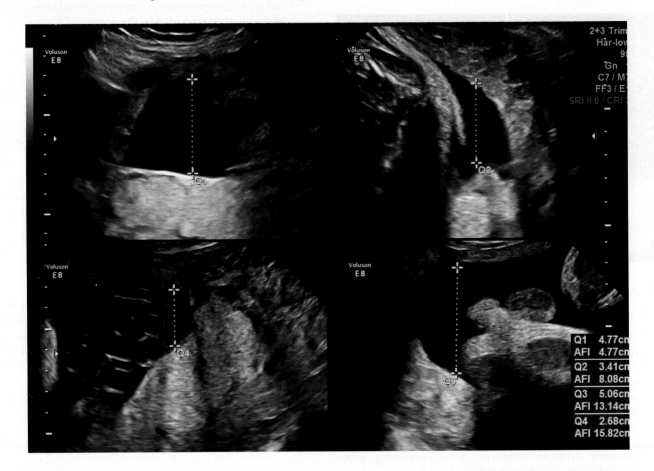

10. Answer: c

(see *Gabbe's Obstetrics* 8e: ch9)

Between 18 and 23 weeks gestation, the edge of the placenta extends to or covers the internal os of the cervix in about 2% of patients. A joint statement by the major ultrasound and obstetric societies in the United States and Canada recommended a classification that retains only the terms *placenta previa* and *low-lying placenta*. The distance that the edge of the placenta covers or ends short of the internal cervical os should be measured and reported. This quantitative description is more helpful than a report of "complete" or "partial" previa for predicting the future placental position and in planning management. For pregnancies greater than 16 weeks, if the placental edge ends 2 cm or more from the cervix, the placental location should be reported as normal. If the placental edge is less than 2 cm from the internal os but not covering the internal os, the placenta should be labeled as low lying, and follow-up ultrasonography is recommended at 32 weeks gestation. (answer c) When the degree of overlap is 15 mm or greater, 19% persist as placenta previa, whereas if the overlap is 25 mm or greater, 40% remain. Another study found that when placenta previa is present at 15 to 19 weeks, only 12% persist. The rate of persistence gradually increases as the gestational age advances, up to 73% if placenta previa is present at 32 to 35 weeks. The risk of bleeding with a low lying placenta is low, as such immediate hospitalization is NOT warranted

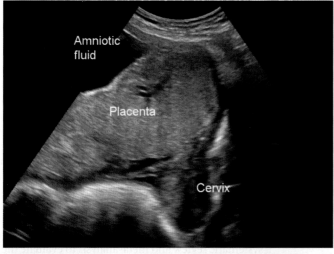

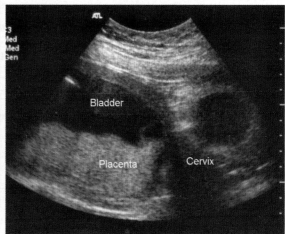

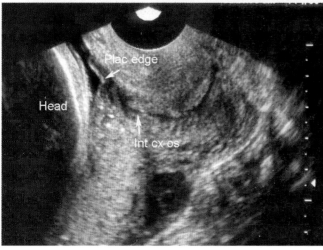

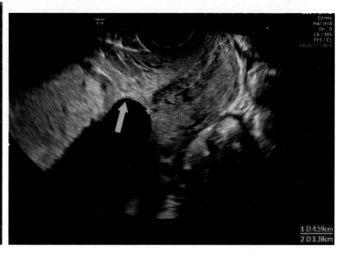

11. Answer: d

(see *Gabbe's Obstetrics* 8e: ch9)

An SUA is present in about 0.5% of all newborns. Since there is a 20% incidence of associated malformations, including aneuploidy, this finding should prompt a detailed fetal survey. Fetuses with an SUA have a 20% chance of growth restriction. Additionally, the rate of polyhydramnios, abruption, placenta previa, structural placental abnormalities, cesarean delivery, low Apgar scores, and fetal death are all increased.[1] For this reason, follow-up growth ultrasounds and testing for fetal well-being should be considered.

12. Answer: a

(see *Gabbe's Obstetrics* 8e: ch9)

Agreement is near universal that in pregnancies in which the menstrual dates are uncertain or thought to be unreliable because of uncertain recall, irregular cycles, recent hormonal contraception use, or an abnormally light LMP, dates derived from ultrasound biometry are preferred. A joint committee opinion issued in 2014 from American College of Obstetricians and Gynecologists, AIUM, and SMFM entitled "Method for Estimating Due Date" made very specific recommendations that extend through the entire pregnancy (Table 9.1).

TABLE 9.1   Guidelines for Redating Based on Ultrasonography.

Gestational Age Range*	Method of Measure-ment	Discrepancy Between Ultrasound Dating and LMP Dating That Supports Redating
≤13 6/7 wk	CRL	
• ≤8 6/7 wk		More than 5 d
• 9 0/7 wk to 13 6/7 wk		More than 7 d
14 0/7 wk to 15 6/7 wk	BPD, HC, AC, FL	More than 7 d
16 0/7 wk to 21 6/7 wk	BPD, HC, AC, FL	More than 10 d
22 0/7 wk to 27 6/7 wk	BPD, HC, AC, FL	More than 14 d
28 0/7 wk and beyond†	BPD, HC, AC, FL	More than 21 d

AC, abdominal circumference; *BPD*, biparietal diameter, *CRL*, crown-rump length; *FL*, femur length; *HC*, head circumference; *LMP*, last menstrual period.
*Based on LMP.
†Because of the risk of redating a small fetus that may be growth restricted, management decisions based on third-trimester ultrasonography alone are especially problematic and need to be guided by careful consideration of the entire clinical picture and close surveillance.
Reprinted with permission from Methods for estimating the due date. Committee Opinion No. 700. American College of Obstetricians and Gynecologists. Obstet Gynecol 2017;129:e150–4.

13. Answer: c

(see *Gabbe's Obstetrics* 8e: ch9)

Several formulas for calculating the EFW are in use. The most popular of these have been compiled in a review by Nyberg and colleagues.[2] All incorporate the abdominal circumference because this is the standard measurement most susceptible to the variations in fetal soft tissue mass. Although the AC alone is a fairly good marker of abnormal fetal growth, the addition of other standard measurements to estimated weight formulas increases their accuracy.

14. Answer: c

(see *Gabbe's Obstetrics* 8e: ch9)

If the EFW is less than the 10th or greater than the 90th percentile, the fetus is said to be small or large for the gestational age. **Repeated ultrasound examinations for growth should be usually be performed at least 3 to 4 weeks apart.** Performing growth assessment at less than 2-week intervals should be avoided because the inherent errors associated with ultrasonographic measurements make it difficult to tell if apparent trends are due to the real growth or variations in the measurement technique.

15. Answer: b

(see *Gabbe's Obstetrics* 8e: ch9)

Since diagnostic ultrasound was introduced for clinical use, attention has appropriately been given to ensuring its safety. It has been recognized that the energy from sound waves is converted into heat as the sound waves are attenuated. The numbers pertinent to users of obstetric ultrasound are the thermal indexes (TIs) for soft tissue (TIs) and bone (TIb). The TI denotes the potential for increasing the temperature of tissue being insonated with that power output. It is determined by the settings and ultrasound modalities being used. A TI of 1.0 indicates that given certain conditions, the temperature of the tissue may be increased by 1°C. A 2015 official statement from the AIUM on ultrasound bioeffects states that no effects have been observed from unfocused beam spatial-peak temporal-average intensities below 100 mW/cm^2 or TI values less than 2. In 2009, the World Health Organization sponsored a systematic review and meta-analysis to evaluate the safety of human exposure to ultrasonography in pregnancy. This study showed no adverse maternal or perinatal effects, impaired physical or neurologic development, increased risk for malignancy in childhood, subnormal intellectual performance, or mental diseases. This analysis concluded that according to the available evidence, exposure to diagnostic ultrasonography during pregnancy appears to be safe. In another official statement, the AIUM propounds the as low as reasonably achievable (ALARA) principle.[3] This means that the potential benefits and risks of each examination should be considered, and equipment controls should be adjusted to reduce as much as possible the acoustic output from the transducer.

16. Answer: **c**

(see *Gabbe's Obstetrics* 8e: ch9)

Ultrasound assessment of the fetal nuchal translucency is an important part of first-trimester aneuploidy screening and has a detection rate of 70% when used solely for screening[4].

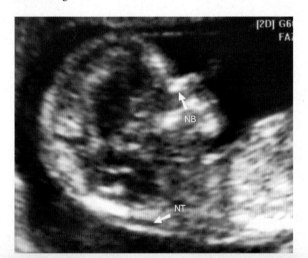

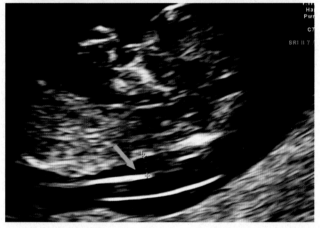

There are rigorous criteria for appropriate nuchal translucency and nasal bone images, and individuals who wish to perform the ultrasound component of the first-trimester screen must be certified to do so. Using cardiac flow indices in the first trimester remains experimental.

17. Answer: **d**

(see *Gabbe's Obstetrics* 8e: ch9)

Encephalocele is the least common type of neural tube defect and is manifested by a protrusion of the meninges, and sometimes brain tissue, through a defect in the cranium.

18. Answer: d

(see *Gabbe's Obstetrics* 8e: ch9)

The accepted upper limit of the transverse diameter of the lateral ventricles at the atrium in an axial view is 10 mm.

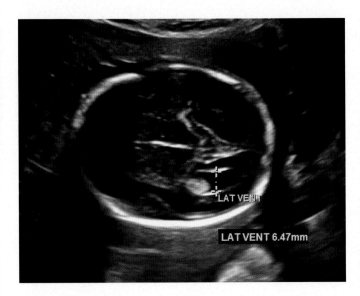

Ventriculomegaly is described as "mild" (10 to 12 mm) (top figure) "moderate" (12 to 14 mm) (middle figure), and "severe" (greater than 15 mm) (bottom figure).

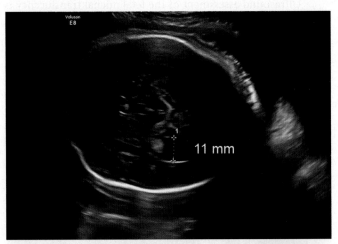

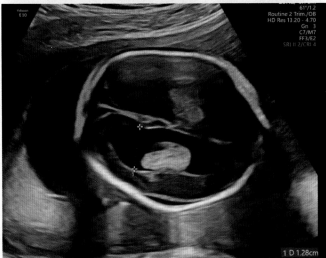

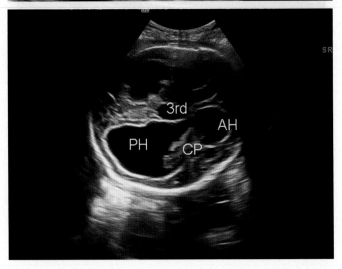

When the ventricles measure between 10 and 12 mm, the chance of a normal neurologic outcome is 96%, and it is 86% with a measurement between 12 and 15 mm.

19. Answer: d

(see *Gabbe's Obstetrics* 8e: ch9)

The presence of an AV canal defect has a strong association with Down syndrome, present in about 50% of cases of fetuses with this condition. The presence of a thick nuchal fold (top figure), hypoplastic or absent nasal bone (middle figure), and echogenic intracardiac focus (bottom figure) is associated with trisomy 21.

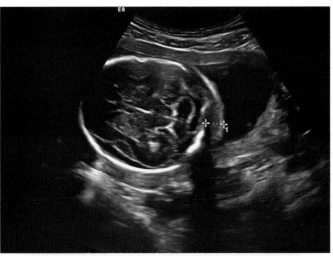

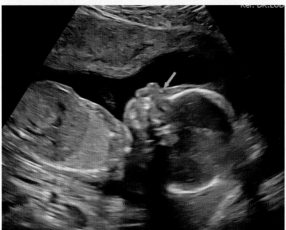

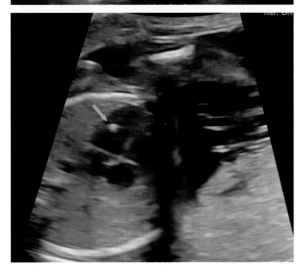

REFERENCES

1. Hua M, Odibo AO, Macones GA, et al. Single umbilical artery and its associated findings. *Obstet Gynecol.* 2010;115:930-934.

2. Nyberg DA, Abuhamad A, Ville Y. Ultrasound assessment of abnormal fetal growth. *Semin Perinatol.* 2004;28:3-22.

3. American Institute of Ultrasound in Medicine. Official Statement, As Low As Reasonably Achievable (ALARA) Principle. Approved 4/2/2014.

4. ACOG Practice Bulletin 163. Screening for fetal aneuploidy. May 2016. *Obstet Gynecol.* 2016 May;127(5):e123-37

10

Genetic Screening and Prenatal Genetic Diagnosis

Alyssa Stephenson-Famy

(see *Gabbe's Obstetrics: Normal and Problem Pregnancies*, 8e: ch10)

QUESTIONS

1. What is the rate of major congenital anomaly in the general population?
   a. 0.5%
   b. 1%
   c. 3%
   d. 5%
   e. 10%

2. A 24-year-old G1P0 woman at 10 weeks at her first prenatal visit reports that two first-degree maternal family members required cardiac surgery in infancy. What is the most appropriate evaluation?
   a. Cell-free fetal DNA
   b. Expanded carrier testing for both parents
   c. Routine anatomy ultrasound
   d. Referral to clinical geneticist or genetic counselor

3. A 28-year-old woman presents for preconception counseling with her husband who is 59 years old. What genetic disorder would the fetus be at increased risk for?
   a. Autosomal dominant disorders
   b. Autosomal recessive disorders
   c. Balanced translocations
   d. Uniparental disomy
   e. Sex chromosome aneuploidy

4. A 34-year-old woman presents for counseling following a 7-week missed abortion for which she underwent dilation and curettage. Cytogenetic analysis of the products of conception showed 47,XX,+18. Parental karyotypes are normal. What is the recurrence risk for her in a future pregnancy?
   a. 0.1%
   b. 0.5%
   c. 1%
   d. 5%
   e. 10%

5. A couple presents for evaluation of recurrent pregnancy loss. Maternal testing included negative antiphospholipid antibody syndrome testing, and pelvic sonography revealed no abnormalities. Maternal karyotype showed 45t(14q;21q) and paternal karyotype was normal. What is the empiric risk for having an offspring with Down syndrome?
   a. 0.1%
   b. 0.5%
   c. 1%
   d. 5%
   e. 10%

6. A 3-year-old child undergoes an evaluation for developmental delay which included a chromosomal microarray analysis and is found to have a small deletion (<1 Mb) which was reported as potentially a pathogenic copy number variant. What is the next recommended evaluation?
   a. Karyotype of the child
   b. Karyotype of both parents
   c. Chromosomal microarray of unaffected siblings
   d. Chromosomal microarray of both parents

7. A 17-year-old girl undergoes evaluation for primary amenorrhea. She is short in stature (148 cm) and is found to have streak gonads by MRI. She has a normal IQ and has no other identifiable congenital abnormalities. What is the most likely karyotype?
   a. 46,XX
   b. 45,X/46,XX
   c. 47,XX,+21
   d. 47,XXY
   e. 48,XXXX

8. A 21-year-old male is evaluated for hypospadias and small testes. His karyotype is 47,XXY. Evaluation of his sex signaling hormones would most likely show which result?

    a. Elevated luteinizing hormone (LH), elevated follicle-stimulating hormone (FSH), normal testosterone

    b. Elevated LH, elevated FSH, elevated testosterone

    c. Elevated LH, elevated FSH, decreased testosterone

    d. Decreased LH, decreased FSH, normal testosterone

    e. Decreased LH, decreased FSH, elevated testosterone

    f. Decreased LH, decreased FSH, decreased testosterone

9. Which aneuploidy screening test has the highest detection rate and lowest false-positive rate for detection of trisomy 21?

    a. First-trimester nuchal translucency, pregnancy-associated plasma protein A (PAPP-A), free β-human chorionic gonadotropin (hCG)

    b. Second-trimester quad (maternal serum α-fetoprotein [MSAFP], hCG, unconjugated estriol [uE_3], inhibin)

    c. Sequential (first- and second-trimester quad)

    d. Serum integrated (PAPP-A, quad screen)

    e. Cell-free DNA (cfDNA)

10. A 30-year-old nondiabetic, nonsmoking woman undergoes second trimester serum screening at 16 weeks. Her dates were confirmed by 6-week ultrasound and she is known to have a singleton gestation. Fetal anatomic ultrasound has not yet been performed. The results of her serum analytes show MSAFP, 3.6 multiples of the median (MoM); hCG, 0.95 MoM; uE_3, 1.05 MoM; inhibin, 1.1 MoM. What is the most likely cause of this result?

    a. Trisomy 13

    b. Trisomy 18

    c. Trisomy 21

    d. Monosomy X

    e. Open neural tube defect

11. During routine prenatal care, a 24-year-old woman who is of non-Hispanic European ancestry is found to be a carrier of the cystic fibrosis delta-F-508 mutation. Her 26-year-old husband is also found to be a carrier of this mutation. What is the risk that the couple will have a fetus affected with cystic fibrosis?

    a. 1/4

    b. 1/100

    c. 1/400

    d. 1/800

    e. 1/2000

12. G-banded karyotype can detect numeric abnormalities, balanced translocations, and structural abnormalities greater than what size?

    a. 0.25 million base pairs (Mb)

    b. 0.5 Mb

    c. 1 Mb

    d. 2.5 Mb

    e. 5 Mb

13. A 37-year-old woman at 20 weeks gestation undergoes routine anatomic ultrasound, which shows a complex congenital cardiac defect and bilateral fetal pyelectasis. She would like to proceed with amniocentesis. Based on current American College of Obstetricians and Gynecologists (ACOG) and Society for Maternal Fetal Medicine (SMFM) guidelines, what is the most appropriate test?

    a. Karyotype

    b. Chromosomal microarray

    c. Quantitative polymerase chain reaction

    d. Placental mosaicism studies

    e. Single gene testing

14. A 20-year-old G1P0 of Greek descent presents to establish prenatal care. Her complete blood count shows a mean corpuscular volume (MCV) of 73%. She has normal iron studies. What additional testing should be performed?

    a. Hemoglobin electrophoresis

    b. Expanded carrier screening

    c. DNA-based globin gene testing

    d. Folate level

    e. Lead level

ANSWERS

1. Answer: c

(see *Gabbe's Obstetrics* 8e: ch10)

Approximately 3% of liveborn infants will have a major congenital anomaly.

2. Answer: d

(see *Gabbe's Obstetrics* 8e: ch10)

The clinician should inquire into the health status of first-degree relatives (siblings, parents, offspring), second-degree relatives (nephews, nieces, aunts, uncles, grandparents), and third-degree relatives (first cousins, especially maternal). A positive family history of a genetic disorder may warrant referral to a clinical geneticist or genetic counselor who can accurately assess the risk of having an affected offspring and review genetic screening and testing options.

3. Answer: a

(see *Gabbe's Obstetrics* 8e: ch10)

A paternal-age effect is associated with a small aggregate increased risk (0.3% to 0.5% or less in men over 40 years of age) for sporadic gene mutations for certain autosomal-dominant conditions such as achondroplasia and craniosynostosis. No specific screening tests exist for anomalies associated with advanced paternal age, although some of these conditions may be detected by ultrasonography.

4. Answer: c

(see *Gabbe's Obstetrics* 8e: ch10)

Autosomal trisomies have a recurrence risk of approximately 1% following either trisomy 18 or 21.

5. Answer: e

(see *Gabbe's Obstetrics* 8e: ch10)

Translocations most commonly associated with Down syndrome involve chromosomes 14 and 21. One parent may have the same translocation, [45t(14q;21q)], referred to as a *Robertsonian translocation*. Empiric risks for having an offspring with Down syndrome are approximately 10% for female Robertsonian translocation carriers.

6. Answer: d

(see *Gabbe's Obstetrics* 8e: ch10)

Chromosomal microarray analysis has been recommended as a first-tier test for the postnatal evaluation of individuals with undiagnosed developmental delay, intellectual disabilities, autism spectrum disorder, and/or multiple congenital anomalies. As copy number variants (CNVs) can be familial, parental studies are recommended when a CNV is identified in a child or fetus.

7. Answer: b

(see *Gabbe's Obstetrics* 8e: ch10)

Common features of Monosomy X, or Turner syndrome include primary ovarian failure, absent pubertal development due to gonadal dysgenesis (streak gonads), and short stature (<150 cm). Mosaicism (i.e., 45,X/46,XX) is frequent. Various somatic anomalies can occur, but overall IQ is considered normal.

8. Answer: c

(see *Gabbe's Obstetrics* 8e: ch10)

Klinefelter syndrome, most commonly 47,XXY chromosome complement, are undervirilized and have small testes, azoospermia, elevated FSH and luteinizing hormone levels, and decreased testosterone.

9. Answer: e

(see *Gabbe's Obstetrics* 8e: ch10)

cfDNA has a 99% detection rate for trisomy 21 and a less than 1% false-positive rate. The other tests listed, which use serum hormone testing and/or first trimester ultrasound findings, have an 81%–95% detection rate for trisomy 21 and a 5% false-positive rate. It is important to remember with cfDNA testing that it is necessary to perform a confirmatory diagnostic testing to confirm positive screening results (Table 10.1).

TABLE 10.1 Aneuploidy Screening Tests.

Screening Test	Trisomy 21 Detection Rate (%)	False-Positive Rate (%)
First-trimester NT, PAPP-A, free β-hCG	82 to 87	5
Second-trimester quad (MSAFP, hCG, uE₃, INHA)	81	5
Sequential (first- and second-trimester quad)	95	5
Serum integrated (PAPP-A, quad screen)	85 to 88	5
cfDNA	99	<1

cfDNA, Cell-free DNA; *hCG*, human chorionic gonadotropin; *INHA*, inhibin A; *MSAFP*, maternal serum α-fetoprotein; *NT*, nuchal translucency; *PAPP-A*, pregnancy-associated plasma protein A; *uE₃*, unconjugated estriol.

10. Answer: e

(see *Gabbe's Obstetrics* 8e: ch10)

Serum hCG and inhibin A levels are increased in women carrying fetuses with Down syndrome. Levels of α-fetoprotein (AFP) and uE₃ in maternal serum are lower in pregnancies affected with Down syndrome compared with unaffected pregnancies. Typically, levels of AFP, uE₃, and hCG are reduced in trisomy 18. Open neural tube defects cause an elevated MSAFP but does not affect the other serum analytes.

11. Answer: a

(see *Gabbe's Obstetrics* 8e: ch10)

When both parents are carriers for an autosomal recessive disorder, the risk of having an affected offspring is 25%. Genetic counseling is recommended, and the couple is informed of the availability of prenatal diagnostic testing, preimplantation genetic testing (PGT), donor gametes (eggs or sperm), and adoption to avoid the risk of having an affected child. In addition, the parents should be informed that their relatives are at risk and should also be informed of the availability of carrier screening (Table 10.2).

TABLE 10.2 Likelihood of Affected Fetus After Cystic Fibrosis Carrier Screening.

	Non-Hispanic European White	Ashkenazi Jew
No screening	1/2500	1/2304
Both partners negative	1/173,056	1/640,000
One partner negative, one untested	1/20,800	1/38,400
One partner positive, one negative	1/832	1/1600
One partner positive, other untested	1/100	1/96
Both partners positive	1/4	1/4

12. Answer: e

(see *Gabbe's Obstetrics* 8e: ch10)

Karyotyping can detect numeric abnormalities, balanced translocations, and structural abnormalities greater than 5 to 10 Mb (5 to 10 million base pairs). Higher-resolution tests are required for detecting chromosome rearrangements less than 5 Mb, such as chromosomal microarray analysis (CMA).

13. Answer: b

(see *Gabbe's Obstetrics* 8e: ch10)

ACOG and SMFM recommend that chromosomal microarray analysis replace conventional cytogenetic analysis in patients undergoing invasive diagnostic testing for the evaluation of a fetus with one or more structural abnormalities.

14. Answer: a

(see *Gabbe's Obstetrics* 8e: ch10)

MCV values of less than 80% are indicative of either iron deficiency anemia or thalassemia heterozygosity; therefore, it is necessary to test for iron deficiency. If a deficiency is not found, an elevated hemoglobin A₂ and hemoglobin F will confirm β-thalassemia. DNA-based testing may be necessary to detect α-globin deletions.

11

Normal and Abnormal Labor and Delivery

Rini Banerjee Ratan

(See *Gabbe's Obstetrics: Normal and Problem Pregnancies*, 8e: ch11)

QUESTIONS

1. A 19-year-old G1P0 woman at 41 weeks gestation presents to the labor and delivery unit with painful, regular contractions. Her pregnancy has been uncomplicated. Her cervix is 7 cm dilated and 90% effaced. The leading edge of the fetal head is palpable 1 cm below the maternal ischial spines. Fetal heart rate (FHR) tracing is category I. What is the station of the fetus at this time?

   a. −1/5

   b. −1/3

   c. 0/5

   d. +1/3

   e. +1/5

2. Which cardinal movement refers to passage of the widest diameter of the presenting part to a level below the plane of the pelvic inlet?

   a. Descent

   b. Flexion

   c. Extension

   d. Engagement

   e. Expulsion

3. Which shape of the female bony pelvis is more often associated with delivery in the occiput posterior (OP) position?

   a. Gynecoid

   b. Anthropoid

   c. Android

   d. Platypelloid

   e. None of the above

4. A 42-year-old G5P4 at 41 weeks gestation presents to the labor and delivery unit with painful, regular contractions. Her pregnancy has been uncomplicated. On admission she was examined and her cervix found to be 4 cm dilated, 80% effaced, with the vertex at −2/5 station. Her past obstetric history is notable for four prior uncomplicated spontaneous vaginal deliveries at term. FHR tracing is category I. Four hours later she is examined and her cervix is found to be 8 cm dilated, 90% effaced, with the vertex at 0/5 station and fetal occiput directly posterior. Which of the following best describes this fetal position?

   a. Malpresentation

   b. Asynclitism

   c. Malposition

   d. Funic presentation

   e. Oblique fetal lie

5. A 28-year-old G1P0 at 39 weeks gestation presents to the labor and delivery unit with painful, regular contractions. Her pregnancy has been uncomplicated. Her cervix is 3 cm dilated, 70% effaced, with the vertex at −2/5 station. FHR tracing is category I. She is uncomfortable, requesting pain relief. She has a labor doula who is on her way to the hospital. Which of the following statements regarding common interventions in normal labor is true?

   a. Epidural use significantly increases the mean duration of the second stage

   b. Ambulation in early labor significantly decreases the need for oxytocin

   c. Upright rather than recumbent positioning is associated with a significantly longer first stage of labor

   d. Administration of IV fluid is not beneficial

   e. The presence of a labor doula is associated with a significant increase in operative vaginal delivery

6. How is fetal macrosomia defined by the American College of Obstetricians and Gynecologists (ACOG)?

   a. Birthweight greater than or equal to the 95th percentile for a given gestational age

   b. Birthweight greater than 5000 g for any gestational age

   c. Birthweight greater than 4000 g to 4500 g for any gestational age

   d. Birthweight greater than one standard deviation above the mean for gestational age

   e. Birthweight greater than 4000 g for any gestational age with maternal diabetes

7. A 37-year-old G2P1 at 39 weeks gestation presents to the labor and delivery unit for scheduled induction of labor in the setting of gestational diabetes. Her body mass index is 48. Her past obstetric history is notable for one prior vaginal delivery at term. Her cervix is 1 cm dilated, 50% effaced, with the vertex at −2/5 station. FHR tracing is category I. She reports occasional, intermittent contractions. She appears comfortable at present. Which of the following is the most appropriate initial method to assess uterine activity?

   a. Observation

   b. Manual palpation

   c. External tocodynamometry

   d. Intrauterine pressure catheter (IUPC)

   e. Intermittent auscultation

8. What is the biologic half-life of oxytocin?

   a. 3–4 minutes

   b. 30–40 minutes

   c. 3–4 hours

   d. 30–40 hours

   e. 3–4 days

9. A 20-year-old G1P0 at 38 weeks gestation presents to the labor and delivery unit with mild, irregular contractions. Her pregnancy has been uncomplicated. Her cervix is long and closed and the fetal vertex is at −3/5 station. FHR tracing is category I. She appears comfortable at present. She is eager to have a vaginal delivery as she would like to have many children in the future. Which of the following is the most appropriate next step in management to minimize her risk of cesarean delivery?

   a. Perform early artificial rupture of membranes

   b. Administer high-dose oxytocin augmentation

   c. Encourage early epidural analgesia

   d. Discourage the use of epidural analgesia

   e. Delay admission until active labor has been established

10. A 33-year-old G2P2 undergoes an uncomplicated normal spontaneous vaginal delivery of a vigorous live born infant at term. Her pregnancy has been uncomplicated. The patient is a Jehovah's Witness and is not willing to accept blood products. Which of the following is the most appropriate next step in management to minimize her risk of postpartum hemorrhage?

    a. Apply downward umbilical cord traction while massaging the uterine fundus.

    b. Administer oxytocin after delivery of the fetus and prior to delivery of the placenta.

    c. Allow delivery of the placenta by gravity without applying traction on the cord.

    d. Delay umbilical cord clamping until at least 2 minutes after delivery.

    e. Defer administration of uterotonic agents until after delivery of the placenta.

11. A 30-year-old G2P1 at 40 weeks gestation presents to the labor and delivery unit in spontaneous active labor. She reports rupture of membranes with lightly stained greenish fluid approximately 1 hour earlier. Her pregnancy has been uncomplicated. FHR tracing shows a baseline 140 with moderate variability, spontaneous accelerations, and intermittent variable decelerations with a nadir to 110 lasting approximately 30 seconds with spontaneous return to baseline. She is found to be fully dilated and progresses quickly to spontaneous vaginal delivery of a vigorous live born female infant. The infant is noted to cry spontaneously at birth, and meconium-stained fluid is noted at the time of delivery. Which of the following is the most appropriate course of action after cord clamping?

    a. Immediate bulb suction of the infant's oropharynx.

    b. Transient intubation and tracheal suctioning of meconium from the oropharynx.

    c. Place the naked infant directly on mother's bare chest and cover with towels.

    d. Wipe the infant dry and transfer to the warmer immediately.

    e. Swaddle the infant in a warm blanket and encourage immediate breastfeeding.

12. A 37-year-old G2P1 at 40 weeks gestation is admitted to the labor and delivery unit in spontaneous active labor, now in the second stage. FHR tracing has been category II, with moderate variability and intermittent variable decelerations. She has a history of inflammatory bowel disease with multiple abdominal surgeries in the past, but her symptoms have been largely quiescent during this pregnancy. She has been pushing for the last 20 minutes with good descent of the fetal head. The fetal vertex is crowning in left occiput anterior position. Which of the following is the most appropriate next step in management?

    a. Passive perineal support

    b. Immediate cesarean delivery

    c. Midline episiotomy

    d. Fundal pressure

    e. Mediolateral episiotomy

13. A 20-year-old G1P0 at 40 weeks gestation presents to the labor and delivery unit with regular, painful contractions. Her pregnancy has been uncomplicated. Her cervix is 3 cm dilated, 50% effaced, and −2/5 station. FHR tracing is category I. Her cervix is reexamined 2 hours later and found to be 6 cm dilated, 90% effaced, and 0/5 station. This patient is currently in which stage of labor?

    a. First stage, latent phase

    b. First stage, active phase

    c. Second stage

    d. Third stage

    e. Fourth stage

14. A 39-year-old G1 P0 undergoes a vacuum-assisted vaginal delivery of a vigorous live born infant at term. The newborn's weight is 4250 g. Examination of the patient's perineum after delivery of the placenta reveals a midline laceration extending into the perineal body with superficial disruption of the external anal sphincter.
    Which of the following terms best classifies this patient's perineal injury?

    a. Intact perineum

    b. First-degree tear

    c. Second-degree tear

    d. Third-degree tear

    e. Fourth-degree tear

ANSWERS

1. Answer: e

(see *Gabbe's Obstetrics* 8e: ch11)

Station is a measure of descent of the bony presenting part of the fetus through the birth canal. The current standard classification (−5 to +5) is based on a quantitative measure in centimeters of the distance of the leading bony edge from the ischial spines. The midpoint (0 station) is defined as the plane of the maternal ischial spines.

2. Answer: d

(see *Gabbe's Obstetrics* 8e: ch11)

In the cephalic presentation with a well-flexed head, the largest transverse diameter of the fetal head is the biparietal diameter (9.5 cm). In the breech, the widest diameter is the bitrochanteric diameter. Clinically, engagement can be confirmed by palpation of the presenting part, both abdominally and vaginally. With a cephalic presentation, engagement is achieved when the leading bony presenting part is at zero station on vaginal examination.

3. Answer : b

(see *Gabbe's Obstetrics* 8e: ch11)

The anthropoid pelvis—with its exaggerated oval shape of the inlet, largest antero-posterior (AP) diameter, and limited anterior capacity—is more often associated with delivery in the OP position.

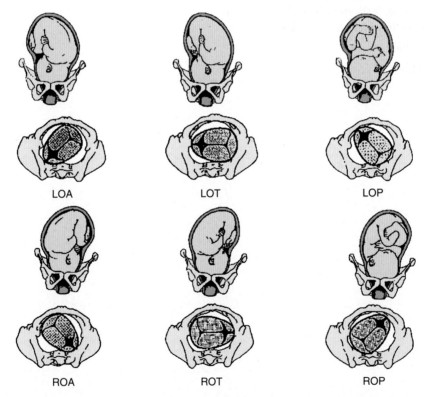

• **Fig. 11.1** Fetal presentations and positions in labor. *LOA,* Left occiput anterior; *LOP,* left occiput posterior; *LOT,* left occiput transverse; *ROA,* right occiput anterior; *ROT,* right occiput transverse; *ROP,* right occiput posterior. (From Challis JRG: Characteristics of parturition. In Creasy RK, Resnik R [eds]: Maternal-Fetal Medicine, 4th ed, p 484. Philadelphia, WB Saunders, 1999.)

4. **Answer: c**

(see *Gabbe's Obstetrics* 8e: ch11)

Malposition refers to any position in labor that is not occipput anterior (OA), left occiput anterior (LOA), or right occiput anterior (ROA). Malpresentation is a term used for any presentation other than vertex. Asynclitism occurs when the sagittal suture is not directly central relative to the maternal pelvis. Funic presentation refers to presentation of the umbilical cord and is rare at term. Fetal lie refers to the longitudinal axis of the fetus relative to the longitudinal axis of the uterus. In a singleton pregnancy, only a fetus in a longitudinal lie can be safely delivered vaginally.

5. **Answer: a**

(see *Gabbe's Obstetrics* 8e: ch11

Epidural use significantly increases the mean duration of the second stage. A well-designed randomized trial of women in early labor compared ambulation with usual care and found no differences in the duration of the first stage, need for oxytocin, use of analgesia, neonatal outcomes, or route of delivery. Upright rather than recumbent positioning during labor is associated with a significantly shorter first stage of labor. The presence of a labor doula is associated with a significant reduction in the use of analgesia, oxytocin, and operative vaginal delivery. The available data suggest that IV fluid is beneficial in labor.

6. **Answer: c**

(see *Gabbe's Obstetrics* 8e: ch11)

Fetal macrosomia is defined by ACOG as birthweight greater than 4000 g to 4500 g for any gestational age. However, ACOG does not recommend considering prophylactic cesarean delivery until an estimated fetal weight of >5000 g in women without diabetes and >4500 g in women with diabetes.

7. **Answer: c**

(see *Gabbe's Obstetrics* 8e: ch11)

External tocodynamometry measures the change in shape of the abdominal wall as a function of uterine contractions. It is a qualitative measure rather than quantitative. Although it permits graphic display of uterine activity and allows for accurate correlation of FHR patterns with uterine activity, external tocodynamometry does not allow measurement of contraction intensity or basal uterine tone. The most precise method for determination of uterine activity is the direct measurement of intrauterine pressure with an IUPC. However, this procedure should not be performed unless indicated, given the small, but finite associated risks of uterine perforation, placental disruption, and intrauterine infection.

8. **Answer: a**

(see *Gabbe's Obstetrics* 8e: ch11)

Oxytocin is a peptide hormone synthesized in the hypothalamus and released from the posterior pituitary in a pulsatile fashion. At term, oxytocin serves as a potent uterotonic agent.

9. **Answer: e**

(see *Gabbe's Obstetrics* 8e: ch11)

In a recent Cochrane review, a metaanalysis of 11 trials concluded that early oxytocin augmentation in women with spontaneous labor was associated with a significant decrease in cesarean delivery. A metaanalysis of eight trials determined that early amniotomy and oxytocin augmentation was associated with a significantly shortened duration of labor. Amniotomy alone did not affect labor length or the rate of cesarean delivery. Perhaps the most important factor in active management is delaying admission until active labor has been established.

10. **Answer: b**

(see *Gabbe's Obstetrics* 8e: ch11)

A Cochrane review and several additional studies support the role of oxytocin as a key component in the active management strategy to reduce blood loss with delivery.[1,2] ACOG, the World Health Organization, the American Academy for Family physicians, and the Association of Women's Health, Obstetric and Neonatal Nurses (AWHONN) recommend prophylactic use of a uterotonic (preferably oxytocin) after all births for the prevention of postpartum hemorrhage. Given the available evidence, at least oxytocin, probably with the addition of misoprostol or Methergine as appropriate per patient, or carbetocin where available, should be given to all women upon delivery of the baby, either at the anterior shoulder or full body delivery, but certainly before placental delivery.

11. **Answer: c**

(see *Gabbe's Obstetrics* 8e: ch11)

For infants born with meconium-stained amniotic fluid, the ACOG Committee on Obstetric Practice and the American Academy of Pediatrics (AAP) no longer recommend routine intubation and tracheal suctioning. Rather, the presence of meconium should prompt notification and availability of an appropriately credentialed team. The vigorous infant may remain on the mother's chest for skin-to-skin and initial newborn care, while routine resuscitation measures should be performed for the nonvigorous infant.

12. Answer: a

(see *Gabbe's Obstetrics* 8e: ch11)

Based on the lack of consistent evidence that episiotomy is of benefit, and may in fact cause more harm, routine episiotomy has no role in modern obstetrics. Midline episiotomy does not protect the perineum from further tearing, and data do not show that it improves neonatal outcome. Furthermore, midline episiotomy has been associated with a significant increase in third- and fourth-degree lacerations in nulliparous women with both spontaneous and operative vaginal delivery. Neither episiotomy type has been shown to reduce severe perineal tears compared with no episiotomy.

13. Answer: b

(see *Gabbe's Obstetrics* 8e: ch11)

The first stage of labor is from labor onset until full dilation of the cervix; the second stage is from full cervical dilation until delivery of the baby; and the third stage begins with delivery of the baby and ends with delivery of the placenta. The first stage of labor is divided into two phases: the first is the latent phase and the second is the active phase. The latent phase begins with the onset of labor and is characterized by regular, painful uterine contractions and a slow rate of cervical change. The active phase of labor is defined as the period in which the greatest rate of cervical dilation occurs.

14. Answer: d

(see *Gabbe's Obstetrics* 8e: ch11)

A first-degree tear is defined as a superficial tear confined to the epithelial layer; it may or may not need to be repaired depending on size, location, and amount of bleeding. A second-degree tear extends into the perineal body, but not into the external anal sphincter. A third-degree tear involves superficial or deep injury to the external anal sphincter, whereas a fourth-degree tear extends completely through the sphincter and the rectal mucosa.

REFERENCES

1. Guidelines for oxytocin administration after birth: AWHONN practice brief number 2. *J Obstet Neonatal Nurs.* 2015;44:161-163

2. Anderson JM, Etches D. Prevention and management of postpartum hemorrhage. *Am Fam Physician.* 2007;75:875-882.

Intrapartum Care

Intrapartum Care

12

Induction of Labor

Anthony Sciscione

(See *Gabbe's Obstetrics: Normal and Problem Pregnancies*, 8e: ch12)

QUESTIONS

1. A 21-year-old G2P1001 presents for a prenatal visit at 38 weeks gestation. Her prenatal care has been uneventful. Her vital signs are normal. A recent ultrasound reveals adequate growth and a biophysical profile of 10/10. The patient asks when induction of labor (IOL) will be recommended because she states "I am tired of being pregnant." The best management strategy is delivery at which gestational age?

   a. Now
   b. 39 weeks
   c. 40 weeks
   d. 41 weeks
   e. >42 weeks

2. A 31-year-old G1P0 patient presents for her prenatal visit at 38 weeks gestation. Her prenatal care has been uncomplicated. You discuss with her induction at 39 weeks gestation and reference the ARRIVE trial. You discuss the potential benefits of IOL over expectant management. Which of the following is significantly decreased in the IOL group?

   a. NICU admission
   b. Neonatal intraventricular hemorrhage
   c. Cesarean delivery
   d. Stillbirth
   e. Operative vaginal delivery

3. A 20-year-old nulliparous woman presents for a prenatal visit at 38 weeks gestation. Her prenatal care has been uneventful. She elects to have her labor induced at 39 weeks gestation after counseling. You decide to use PGE$_z$ to induce her labor. Which of the following is NOT true about PGE$_z$ IOL?

   a. Enhances cervical effacement
   b. Decreases cesarean delivery
   c. Reduces oxytocin use
   d. Shortens the induction to delivery time

4. A 41-year-old nulliparous woman at 37 weeks gestation presents to the labor and delivery unit with elevated blood pressure. Her work-up reveals normal laboratory results, but the diagnosis of gestational hypertension is made and IOL is planned today. Her cervix is long and closed. You elect to induce her labor with 25 micrograms of misoprostol every 4 hours. At what time do vaginal misoprostol serum levels peak?

   a. 10–12 minutes
   b. 30–37 minutes
   c. 40–46 minutes
   d. 65–72 minutes
   e. 90–101 minutes

5. A 21-year-old nulliparous woman presents to the labor and delivery unit at 37 weeks with a complaint of persistent headache. Her prenatal course has been uncomplicated. Her blood pressure is elevated and laboratory tests return with mild elevations in her liver function tests. The diagnosis of preeclampsia with severe features is made, and IOL is planned immediately. Her cervix is unfavorable. You and your partner discuss using the Foley catheter versus a double balloon catheter. Which of the following is an advantage of the Foley catheter?

   a. Decrease in cesarean delivery
   b. Higher cost
   c. Higher patient satisfaction
   d. Quicker expulsion times

6. A 26-year-old nulliparous patient at 39 weeks gestation presents for a routine prenatal visit. Her prenatal course has been uneventful and all her laboratory tests have been normal. Her cervix is 1 centimeter dilated and 50% effaced. She is very worried about IOL, which you have recommended at 41 weeks gestation. She has read about "membrane stripping." You counsel her the benefit of membrane stripping is:

   a. Decrease in cesarean delivery

   b. Decrease in operative delivery

   c. Increase in premature rupture of the membranes

   d. Decrease in IOL at 41 weeks gestation

   e. Increase in significant bleeding

7. A 31-year-old G3P2002 at 38 weeks gestation presents to the labor and delivery unit for IOL for severe cholestasis. Her prenatal course has been otherwise uncomplicated, except for bile acid levels of 20. Her cervix is 2–3 centimeters dilated, 80% effaced, and the fetus is at −2 station. You decide to begin oxytocin induction using a "high-dose" protocol. Which of the following is a typical high-dose oxytocin protocol?

   a. Initial dose of 6 mU/min, increased 10 mU/min every 30 minutes

   b. Initial dose of 4 mU/min, increased 10 mU/min every 10 minutes

   c. Initial dose of 10 mU/min, increased 10 mU/min every 30 minutes

   d. Initial dose of 6 mU/min, increased 6 mU/min every 30 minutes

   e. Initial dose of 6 mU/min, increased 6 mU/min every 10 minutes

8. A 21-year-old nulliparous woman at 37 weeks gestation presents to the labor and delivery unit for IOL for gestational hypertension. Her cervix is 1 centimeter dilated and long. You decide to use a combination of methods. Which one appears to be the best choice?

   a. Foley/misoprostol

   b. Foley/PGE$_2$ gel

   c. Misoprostol/oxytocin

   d. Misoprostol/PGE$_2$ gel

   e. Vaginal and oral misoprostol

9. A 31-year-old nulliparous woman at 41 weeks gestation is having her labor induced for postdates. She had a Foley catheter placed 18 hours ago; it just fell out, and her cervix is now 3 centimeters and 50% effaced with the fetal head at −2 station. You begin a high dose oxytocin protocol and after 2 hours perform an amniotomy. While controversial, what is a reasonable minimum amount of time to make the diagnosis of a failed IOL?

   a. 6 hours

   b. 10 hours

   c. 15 hours

   d. 24 hours

   e. 36 hours

10. A 24-year-old G2P1001 presents at 38 weeks gestation with premature rupture of the membranes for 2 hours. Her cervix is unfavorable, and she is not contracting. Her prenatal course has been uncomplicated. Her vital signs are normal, and there is no evidence of chorioamnionitis. Beta-strep testing has been negative. The fetal heart rate pattern is category I. The patient asks to await labor. You counsel her that proceeding with IOL decreases all of the following EXCEPT:

   a. NICU admission

   b. Cesarean delivery

   c. Chorioamnionitis

   d. Endometritis

ANSWERS

1. Answer: d

(see *Gabbe's Obstetrics* 8e: ch12)

Labor induction between 41 0/7 weeks and 42 0/7 weeks should be considered for women who remain undelivered by this gestational age. A metaanalysis, including 11 randomized controlled trials (RCTs) and 25 observational studies, revealed expectant management of pregnancy was associated with higher odds of cesarean delivery than IOL (OR, 1.22; 95% CI, 1.07 to 1.39).[1] Also, in a 2012 Cochrane metaanalysis of 22 RCTs including 9383 women comparing induction of labor in term/postterm pregnancies vs. expectant management,[2] induction was associated with decreased perinatal death (RR 0.31 95% CI 0.12–0.88), cesarean delivery (RR 0.89 95% CI 0.81–0.97), and meconium aspiration syndrome (RR 0.50 95% CI 0.34–0.73). Lastly, the ARRIVE trial did not include multiparous women, so 39 weeks gestation would not be correct.[3]

2. Answer: c

(see *Gabbe's Obstetrics* 8e: ch12)

The ARRIVE study performed by the Maternal Fetal Medicine Unit Network by Grobman and colleagues randomized 6106 nulliparous women at 41 hospitals with no medical indication for delivery to either planned IOL at 39 0/7 to 39 4/7 or expectant management.[3] The primary outcome was a composite of adverse perinatal events. The proportion of neonates with the primary perinatal outcome was lower in the induction group than in the expectant-management group (4.3% vs. 5.4%, RR 0.80; 95% CI, 0.64 to 1.00; p = 0.049). The rate of cesarean delivery was also decreased in the IOL group (18.6% vs. 22.2%, RR 0.84 95% CI 0.76–0.93) along with the rate of preeclampsia/gestational hypertension (9.1% vs. 14.1%, RR 0.94 95% CI 0.56–0.74). There were no differences in the magnitudes of association of induction with either the primary perinatal outcome or cesarean delivery regardless of cervical status, BMI, maternal age, or race/ethnicity.

3. Answer: b

(see *Gabbe's Obstetrics* 8e: ch12)

Multiple trials have evaluated the effectiveness of intravaginal prostaglandin (PG).[4–7] Rayburn summarized 59 clinical trials with 3313 women in which either intracervical or intravaginal PGE_z was used for cervical ripening before IOL.[7] He concluded that local administration of PGE_z is effective in enhancing cervical effacement and dilation, shortening the induction-to-delivery interval, reducing oxytocin use, and lowering the chance of cesarean delivery for failure to progress when compared to oxytocin alone. These findings were confirmed in a metaanalysis of 44 trials performed worldwide using various PG compounds and dosing regimens. Because no difference in clinical outcomes are apparent when comparing intravaginal or intracervical PGE_z preparations, vaginal administration has been recommended, given its greater ease of administration and patient satisfaction.[5]

4. Answer: d

(see *Gabbe's Obstetrics* 8e: ch12)

It is important to note that different routes of administration of misoprostol have different times to peak concentration, different peak levels, and different changes in their level over time.[8–10] For example, oral misoprostol peaks in 12–28 minutes with levels going to baseline in approximately 2 hours. Vaginal misoprostol peaks in 65–72 minutes and levels continue to remain high for up to 4 hours. For this reason, it is important to be aware that the frequency of dosing is different depending on what route the misoprostol is administered. Most studies demonstrating the efficacy and safety of oral misoprostol use 20–25 mcg oral tablet or oral solution every 2 hours.

5. Answer: c

(see *Gabbe's Obstetrics* 8e: ch12)

Two recent metaanalyses[11,12] determined there was no clinical benefit of the double catheter over the single balloon catheter and showed that the double balloon catheter is associated with lower patient satisfaction. Therefore, without clear clinical benefit and the potential increase in morbidity, patient discomfort, and cost of the double balloon catheter ($200–$300 per catheter), the single balloon catheter should be preferentially used.

6. Answer: d

(see *Gabbe's Obstetrics* 8e: ch12)

A 2005 Cochrane review evaluated routine membrane stripping at 38 or 39 weeks to either prevent prolonged pregnancies or decrease the frequency of more formal inductions after 41 weeks.[13] This review included 22 clinical trials, 20 of which compared membrane sweeping alone versus expectant management. Although the studies were heterogeneous, they found no reduction in cesarean delivery (RR 0.90 95% CI 0.70–1.15) but did find a reduction in the frequency of pregnancy continuing beyond 41 weeks (RR 0.59, 95% CI 0.46–0.74) and 42 weeks (RR 0.28, 95% CI 0.15–0.50). Eight women needed to have membrane sweeping performed to avoid one formal induction (number needed to treat [NNT] = 8). There was an increase in clinically insignificant bleeding and contractions that did not lead to labor and therefore women should be counseled on this prior to having membrane sweeping.

7. Answer: d

(see *Gabbe's Obstetrics* 8e: ch12)

High-dose oxytocin regimens often start with an initial oxytocin dose of 6 mU/min[14] that is increased by 6 mU/min at 15- to 40-minute intervals, or start at 4 mU/min with 4 mU/min incremental increases every 15 minutes. Overall, high-dose protocols have been associated with shorter labor and less chorioamnionitis, whereas low-dose regimens are associated with decreased tachysystole. The overall cesarean delivery rate has been shown to be similar between high- and low-dose protocols.

8. Answer: a

(see *Gabbe's Obstetrics* 8e: ch12)

Choosing a combination method for IOL is reasonable. Data suggest that misoprostol/Foley should be the combination method of choice given the shorter time to delivery, suggestion of a lower risk of morbidity, and more efficient staffing ratios.

9. Answer: c

(see *Gabbe's Obstetrics* 8e: ch12)

Taking all the evidence into account, membrane rupture and oxytocin administration should be a prerequisite before diagnosis of failed IOL. No absolute time cutoff for defining failed induction seems possible, given that there will always be some tradeoff between additional vaginal deliveries achieved and additional morbidities incurred with continued labor induction. Based on the current data, it is reasonable to wait at least 15 hours and up to 24 hours in latent labor after oxytocin and artificial rupture of membranes (AROM) before diagnosing a failed induction. Care must be individualized and take into account other factors to determine the risk benefit balance in continuing labor.

10. Answer: b

(see *Gabbe's Obstetrics* 8e: ch12)

In the setting of PROM at term, defined as rupture of membranes before the onset of labor, labor induction is often recommended because, as found by a metaanalysis of 23 randomized trials, it has been shown to decrease the time from PROM to delivery and the risk of chorioamnionitis, endometritis, and NICU admission without increasing cesarean delivery.[15]

REFERENCES

1. Caughey AB, Sundaram V, Kaimal AJ, et al. Systematic review: elective induction of labor versus expectant management of pregnancy. *Ann Intern Med.* 2009;151(4):252-263.
2. Gulmezoglu AM, Crowther CA, Middleton P, Heatley E. Induction of labour for improving birth outcomes for women at or beyond term. *Cochrane Database Syst Rev.* 2012;13(6).
3. Grobman WA. LB01: A randomized trial of elective induction of labor at 39 weeks compared with expectant management of low-risk nulliparous women. *Am J Obstet Gynecol.* 2018;218(1):S601.
4. Alfirevic Z, Keeney E, Dowswell T, et al. Labour induction with prostaglandins: a systematic review and network meta-analysis. *BMJ.* 2015;5(350).
5. Thomas J, Fairclough A, Kavanagh J, Kelly AJ. Vaginal prostaglandin (PGEz and PGF2a) for induction of labour at term. *Cochrane Database Syst Rev.* 2014;19(6).
6. Fox NS, Saltzman DH, Roman AS, Klauser CK, Moshier E, Rebarber A. Intravaginal misoprostol versus Foley catheter for labour induction: a meta-analysis. *BJOG.* 2011;118(6):647-654.
7. Rayburn WF. Prostaglandin Ez gel for cervical ripening and induction of labor: a critical analysis. *Am J Obstet Gynecol.* 1989;160(3):529-534.
8. Yount SM, Lassiter N. The pharmacology of prostaglandins for induction of labor. *J Midwifery Womens Health.* 2013;58(2):133-144.

9. Tang OS, Schweer H, Seyberth HW, Lee SW, Ho PC. Pharmacokinetics of different routes of administration of misoprostol. *Hum Reprod.* 2002;17(2):332-336.

10. Khan RU, El-Refaey H, Sharma S, Sooranna D, Stafford M. Oral, rectal, and vaginal pharmacokinetics of misoprostol. *Obstet Gynecol.* 2004;103(5 Pt 1):866-870.

11. Salim R, Schwartz N, Zafran N, Zuarez-Easton S, Garmi G, Romano S. Comparison of single- and double-balloon catheters for labor induction: a systematic review and meta-analysis of randomized controlled trials. *J Perinatol.* 2017;4(10):017-0005.

12. Yang F, Huang S, Long Y, Huang L. Double-balloon versus single-balloon catheter for cervical ripening and labor induction: a systematic review and meta-analysis. *J Obstet Gynaecol Res.* 2018;44(1):27-34.

13. Boulvain M, Stan C, Irion O. Membrane sweeping for induction of labour. *Cochrane Database Syst Rev.* 2005;25(1).

14. O'Driscoll K, Foley M, MacDonald D. Active management of labor as an alternative to cesarean section for dystocia. *Obstet Gynecol.* 1984;63(4):485-490.

15. Middleton P, Shepherd E, Flenady V, McBain RD, Crowther CA. Planned early birth versus expectant management (waiting) for prelabour rupture of membranes at term (37 weeks or more). *Cochrane Database Syst Rev.* 2017;4(1).

13

Operative Vaginal Delivery

Thaddeus P. Waters

(See *Gabbe's Obstetrics: Normal and Problem Pregnancies*, 8e: ch13)

QUESTIONS

1. A 33-year-old G2P0 at 37 weeks gestation has a persistent category II tracing in the second stage of labor. The estimated fetal weight (EFW) is 4100g and the patient has an epidural. A vacuum-assisted delivery is recommended to the patient. All of the following are true regarding the fetal risks of a subgaleal hemorrhage except:

    a. The frequency of this complication is 2.5%–4.5%.

    b. The type of cup affects the rate of injury.

    c. The number of "pop-offs" is related to injury, but not the length of time the vacuum is applied.

    d. Fetal morbidity is related to acute hypovolemia.

2. A 27-year-old G3P1 with a prior term vaginal delivery at 38 weeks gestation is diagnosed with arrest of descent in the second stage of labor due to maternal exhaustion. The fetal head is visible on the perineum and in the occiput anterior (OA) position. The fetal tracing is category I and the EFW is 2996g by bedside ultrasound. An operative vaginal delivery is recommended to the patient. As part of the counseling for the procedure, all of the following are accurate except:

    a. Operative vaginal delivery is associated with a lower risk of maternal infection when compared to cesarean delivery.

    b. Long term rates of fecal incontinence are similar for women with an operative vaginal delivery compared to a cesarean delivery.

    c. Fetal risks are related to the type of instrument used (vacuum or forceps).

    d. Use of instruments in combination is not recommended.

3. All of the following are prerequisites for a forceps-assisted vaginal delivery except:

    a. Cervix is fully dilated

    b. Fetal position is precisely known

    c. Adequate maternal analgesia is available

    d. Less than 45-degree rotation required

4. A 24-year-old G1P0 is induced at 40 weeks gestation for suspected fetal growth restriction. Her medical history is significant for a heart murmur with a normal echocardiogram. She has been pushing for 2.5 hours in the second stage with an epidural in place. Which of the following is the most appropriate indication for an operative delivery in this case?

    a. The patient does not have an indication for an operative delivery

    b. A prolonged second stage disorder

    c. Possible fetal compromise due to intrauterine growth restriction

    d. Maternal cardiac disease

5. All of the following are false regarding the frequency of anal sphincter injury with a forceps-assisted vaginal delivery except:

    a. The frequency of injury was estimated at 13%.

    b. The frequency is likely underreported due to recall bias.

    c. Endoanal ultrasound often confirms an injury in women who report altered fecal continence after a forceps delivery.

    d. The overall decrease in forceps use has led to an increase in anal sphincter injury, due to a lack of physician experience and training.

6. A 41-year-old G1P0 in the second stage of labor has a persistent category II tracing. Her station is +4 and the fetus is in the left occipitoanterior (LOA) position. The EFW is 3150g and the pelvis is assessed to be adequate. A vacuum-assisted delivery was attempted with two pop-offs, and the total length of time applied is 5 minutes. Descent was noted with each application. The most appropriate management for this patient is:

    a. A cesarean delivery, as a repeat vacuum placement is contraindicated

    b. A repeat attempt of the vacuum with cesarean if unsuccessful

    c. Operative delivery with forceps

    d. Maternal pushing without operative assistance

7. A 45-year-old G1P0 at 39 weeks and 6 days gestation is in active labor. Her pregnancy has been complicated by maternal obesity with BMI 42 kg/m^2. She has received cervical ripening for 12 hours and oxytocin augmentation for 12 hours. She had artificial rupture of membranes (AROM) 6 hours prior, with meconium-stained amniotic fluid. Her cervix is currently 10 cm dilated, and she has been pushing for 1 hour with poor maternal effort. She has a functioning epidural. Intrauterine pressure catheter demonstrates Montevideo units >200 mm Hg in a 10-minute period. External fetal monitoring has been category I. You examine the patient and note that the biparietal diameter (BPD) is below the level of the ischial spines and the leading point of the fetal head is one finger-breadth from the perineum between contractions. The fetus is occiput anterior and the EFW was normal at 36 weeks. Which of the following is correct?

   a. The patient is currently an appropriate candidate for outlet forceps due to maternal exhaustion.

   b. Vacuum extraction can be correctly performed with vacuum cup placement on the sagittal suture 2 to 3 cm below the posterior fontanel.

   c. The patient is currently an appropriate candidate for outlet forceps due to a prolonged second stage of labor.

   d. Vacuum extraction can be correctly performed with vacuum cup placement on the sagittal suture 2 to 3 cm above the posterior fontanel.

8. A 16-year-old G1P0 at 32 weeks gestation has been transferred to the labor and delivery unit for fetal decelerations. She has been admitted for 1 week due to preterm premature rupture of membranes (PPROM). She is examined. Her cervix is noted to be 10 cm dilated and the fetus is in OA position with the BPD below the level of the ischial spines and the head visible at the perineum. She is contracting painfully every 1–2 minutes. External fetal monitoring demonstrates a fetal bradycardia for 2 minutes. All of the following are appropriate except:

   a. An outlet vacuum extraction can be performed due to NRFHT.

   b. A cesarean delivery should be performed if the fetal bradycardia does not resolve.

   c. Any of the classic forceps are suitable for use on this fetus.

   d. Once adequate anesthesia is obtained, an outlet forceps delivery can be performed, due to NRFHT.

9. A 26-year-old G4P3003 at 37 weeks 3 days is pushing in the labor and delivery unit. Her pregnancy has been complicated by gestational hypertension and A2 gestational diabetes on insulin. The EFW at 36 weeks was appropriate. She has a functioning epidural in place. Her cervix is 10 cm dilated. The fetus is in OP position with fetal scalp visible at the perineum between pushes. She has been pushing for 3 hours. External fetal monitoring is category II, with variables present during contractions. Which of the following statements is correct?

   a. Routine traction with vacuum devices should be maintained in between contractions and can be safely continued, in the absence of a "pop-off" for up to 40 minutes.

   b. Vacuum-assisted delivery has a lower failure rate when compared to forceps.

   c. Detachment of the vacuum cup during traction can be viewed as a safety mechanism of the stainless steel cup.

   d. Operative vaginal delivery should be aborted if descent of the fetal leading point is not noted with a vacuum.

10. A 33-year-old G2P0010 at 39 weeks in the labor and delivery unit has reached the second stage of labor. She was being induced for a known maternal congenital heart defect, with recommendations for an assisted second stage of labor. She has been laboring for the past hour, and her cervix is now 10 cm dilated. The fetus is OA, with BPD below the level of the ischial spines, with the leading point of the fetal head less than a fingerbreadth from the perineum. External fetal monitoring is category I. The tocometer demonstrates contractions every 2–3 minutes. Which of the following is incorrect regarding appropriate placement of forceps for this patient?

   a. When using fenestrated blades, the operator should be able to place two fingertips between the fenestrations and the fetal head.

   b. The posterior fontanel should be one fingerbreadth above the plane of the shanks and midway between the blades.

   c. The sagittal suture should be perpendicular to the plane of the shanks.

   d. The lambdoid sutures should be equidistant from the upper edge of each blade.

ANSWERS

1. Answer: c

(see *Gabbe's Obstetrics* 8e: ch13)

More recent data suggest that subgaleal hemorrhage is highly related to use of the vacuum device,[1-3] with an incidence of subgaleal bleeding of 26 to 45 per 1000.[4] Benaron[5] reported an incidence of 1 per 200 with soft silicone vacuum cups. Subgaleal hemorrhage has an estimated incidence of approximately 4 per 10,000 spontaneous vaginal deliveries.[6] In a 30-month prospective study, Boo[7] evaluated more than 64,000 neonates and found that the incidence per live birth was much higher for vacuum extraction than for other modes of delivery (41/1000 vs. 1/1000). Both the type of cup and the duration of its use are predictors of scalp injury. Soft cups are more likely to be associated with a decreased incidence of scalp injuries but may not be less likely to result in a subgaleal hemorrhage.[8] In one study, vacuum application duration of more than 10 minutes was the best predictor of scalp injury.[9]

2. Answer: b

(see *Gabbe's Obstetrics* 8e: ch13)

In a large longitudinal study that surveyed 3763 women up to 12 years after delivery, 6% self-reported persistent fecal incontinence from either their 3-month or 6-year follow-up survey. Logistic regression analysis demonstrated that any forceps delivery, maternal age between 30 and 34 years, and obesity as defined by BMI were all independently associated with persistent fecal incontinence.

3. Answer: d

(see *Gabbe's Obstetrics* 8e: ch13)

See Box 31.1.

BOX 13.1 Prerequisites For Forceps or Vacuum Extractor Application

- Fetal vertex is engaged.
- Membranes have ruptured.
- Cervix is fully dilated.
- Position is precisely known.
- Assessment of maternal pelvis reveals adequacy for the estimated fetal weight.
- Adequate maternal analgesia is available.
- Bladder is drained.
- Operator is knowledgeable.
- Operator is willing to abandon the procedure if necessary.
- Informed consent has been obtained.
- Necessary support personnel and equipment are present.

---

4. Answer: a

(see *Gabbe's Obstetrics* 8e: ch13)

The following indications are appropriate for consideration of either forceps delivery or vacuum extraction: prolonged second stage (for nulliparous women, lack of continuing progress for 3 hours with regional analgesia or 2 hours without regional analgesia; for multiparous women, lack of continuing progress for 2 hours with regional analgesia or 1 hour without regional analgesia); shortening of the second stage of labor for maternal benefit (i.e., maternal exhaustion, maternal cardiopulmonary or cerebrovascular disease); suspicion of immediate or potential fetal compromise (e.g., nonreassuring fetal heart rate tracing [NRFHT]).

5. Answer: a

(see *Gabbe's Obstetrics* 8e: ch13)

In the largest prospective study to evaluate the prevalence of anal sphincter injury after forceps delivery in nulliparous women using endoanal ultrasound, de Parades and colleagues examined 93 patients 6 weeks after delivery and found a 13% prevalence of anal sphincter injury (Table 13.1).

TABLE 13.1 Prevalence of Anal Sphincter Injury After Forceps Delivery.

Reference	Forceps Deliveries (*N*)	IAS Injury (*N*)	EAS Injury (*N*)	IAS and EAS Injury (*N*)	Total Anal Injury (%)
Sultan[10]	26	7	3	11	81
Sultan[11]	19	MD	MD	MD	79
Abramowitz[12]	35	MD	MD	MD	63
Belmonte-Montes[13]	17	0	11	2	76
Fitzpatrick[14]	61	0	34	0	56
De Parades[15]	93	0	11	1	13

EAS, External anal sphincter; *IAS,* internal anal sphincter; *MD,* missing data.

6. **Answer: b**

(see *Gabbe's Obstetrics* 8e: ch13

Detachment of the vacuum cup during traction should be viewed as an indication for reevaluation of the site of application, direction of axis traction, and fetal maternal pelvic dimensions. Data are limited to provide evidence-based support for the maximum duration of safe vacuum application, the maximum number of pulls required before delivery of the fetal head, and the maximum number of pop-offs or cup detachments before abandonment of the procedure. There is a general consensus, however, that descent of the fetal bony vertex should occur with each pull, and if no descent occurs after three pulls, the operative attempt should be stopped. Most authorities have recommended that the maximum number of cup detachments (pop-offs) be limited to two or three and that the duration of vacuum application before abandonment of the procedure be limited to a maximum of 20 to 30 minutes.

7. **Answer: b**

(see *Gabbe's Obstetrics* 8e: ch13)

Successful use of the vacuum extractor is determined by proper application on the fetal head and traction within the pelvic axis. The leading point of the fetal head is the ideal position for vacuum cup placement. It is labeled the flexion point, or pivot point, and is located on the sagittal suture 2 to 3 cm below the posterior fontanel for the OA position and 2 to 3 cm above the posterior fontanel for the occiput posterior (OP) position.

8. **Answer: a**

(see *Gabbe's Obstetrics* 8e: ch13)

No randomized controlled trials have compared forceps with vacuums or different vacuum types to pass judgment on a gestational age cutoff. American College of Obstetricians and Gynecologists (ACOG) reports that most experts in operative vaginal delivery limit the vacuum procedure to fetuses beyond 34 weeks gestation. This is a reasonable cutoff given that the premature head is likely at greater risk for compression-decompression injuries simply because of the pliability of the preterm skull and the more fragile soft tissues of the scalp.

9. **Answer: d**

(see *Gabbe's Obstetrics* 8e: ch13)

There is a general consensus that descent of the fetal bony vertex should occur with each pull, and if no descent occurs after three pulls, the operative attempt should be stopped. The rapid decompression that results from cup detachment for the soft and rigid vacuum cups has been associated with scalp injury, and it should not be viewed as a safety mechanism that is without potential for fetal risk. Most authorities have recommended that the maximum number of cup detachments (pop-offs) be limited to two or three and that the duration of vacuum application before abandonment of the procedure be limited to a maximum of 20 to 30 minutes.

10. **Answer: a**

(see *Gabbe's Obstetrics* 8e: ch13)

The three criteria needed to confirm proper forceps application are (1) the posterior fontanel should be one fingerbreadth above the plane of the shanks and midway between the blades, or the lambdoid sutures (or anterior fontanel for the OP fetus) should be equidistant from the upper edge of each blade; (2) the sagittal suture should be perpendicular to the plane of the shanks; and (3) if using fenestrated blades, the fenestrations should be barely palpable. The operator should not be able to place more than one fingertip between the fenestration and the fetal head.

REFERENCES

1. Chadwick LM, Pemberton PJ, Kurinczuk JJ. Neonatal subgaleal haematoma: associated risk factors, complications and outcome. *J Paediatr Child Health.* 1996;32:228-232.

2. Benaron DA. Subgaleal hematoma causing hypovolemic shock during delivery after failed vacuum extraction: case report. *J Perinatol.* 1993;12:228-231.

3. Boo N. Subaponeurotic haemorrhage in Malaysian neonates. *Singapore Med J.* 1990;31:207-210.

4. ACOG Practice Bulletin No. 154: Operative Vaginal Delivery. *Obstet Gynecol.* 2015;126(5):e56-65.

5. Teng FY, Sayre JW. Vacuum extraction: does duration predict scalp injury? *Obstet Gynecol.* 1997;89:281-285.

6. Ngan HY, Miu P, Ko L, Ma HK. Long-term neurological sequelae following vacuum extractor delivery. *Aust N Z J Obstetr Gynaecol.* 1990;30:111-114.

7. Whitby EH, Griffiths PD, Rutter S, et al. Frequency and natural history of subdural haemorrhages in babies and relation to obstetric factors. *Lancet.* 2004;363:846-851.

8. DeLee JB. The prophylactic forceps operation. 1920. *Am J Obstet Gynecol.* 2002;187:254.

9. Towner D, Castro MA, Eby-Wilkens E, Gilbert WM. Effect of mode of delivery in nulliparous women on neonatal intracranial injury. *N Engl J Med.* 1999;341:1709-1714.

10. Sultan AH, Kamm MA, Bartram CI, Hudson CN. Anal sphincter trauma during instrumental delivery. *Int J Gynecol Obstet.* 1993;43:263.

11. Sultan AH, Johanson RB, Carter JE. Occult anal sphincter trauma following randomized forceps and vacuum delivery. *Int J Gynecol Obstet.* 1998;61:113.

12. Abramowitz L, Sobhani I, Ganansia R, et al. Are sphincter defects the cause of anal incontinence after vaginal delivery? Results of a prospective study. *Dis Colon Rectum.* 2000;43:590.

13. Belmonte-Montes C, Hagerman G, Vega-Yepez PA, et al. Anal sphincter injury after vaginal delivery in primiparous females. *Dis Colon Rectum.* 2001;44:1244.

14. Fitzpatrick M, Behan M, O'Connell PR, O'Herlihy C. Randomised clinical trial to assess anal sphincter function following forceps or vacuum assisted vaginal delivery. *BJOG.* 2003;110:424.

15. deParades V, Etienney I, Thabut D, et al. Anal sphincter injury after forceps delivery: myth or reality? *Dis Colon Rectum.* 2004;47:24.

14

Shoulder Dystocia

Eva K. Pressman

(See *Gabbe's Obstetrics: Normal and Problem Pregnancies*, 8e: ch14)

QUESTIONS

1. A 29-year-old gravida 2 para 1001 comes to the labor and delivery unit at 39 weeks gestation for induction of labor. Her pregnancy has been complicated by gestational diabetes that was well controlled with diet alone. Her past obstetric history is significant for a vaginal delivery of a 4200g male infant complicated by shoulder dystocia requiring McRoberts maneuver and suprapubic pressure but with a normal neonatal exam. Her prepregnancy BMI was 32 and her weight gain this pregnancy was 10 kg. The estimated fetal weight is 3700g. What is her greatest risk factor for shoulder dystocia in this pregnancy?

   a. Estimated fetal weight

   b. Gestational diabetes

   c. Induction of labor

   d. Obesity

   e. Prior shoulder dystocia

2. A 24-year-old gravida 1 para 0 comes to the labor and delivery unit in active labor at 40 weeks gestation. Her cervix rapidly progresses to 10 cm dilation, 100% effacement, with the vertex at +3 station 30 minutes after arrival. Her pregnancy has been uncomplicated and her fundal height on admission was 37 cm, with an estimated fetal weight of 3500g. At the start of the second stage of labor, the fetal vertex is found to be in a left occiput anterior position. The vertex delivers after pushing over two contractions but then retracts against the maternal perineum and the body does not deliver with the next contraction. What is the most likely anatomic cause for the lack of delivery of the body?

   a. The infant's left shoulder is impacted on the sacral promontory.

   b. The infant's right shoulder is impacted on the sacral promontory.

   c. The infant's left shoulder is obstructed by the pubic symphysis.

   d. The infant's right shoulder is obstructed by the pubic symphysis.

   e. The infant's shoulders are oblique rather than vertical.

3. A 26-year-old gravida 1 para 0 comes to the labor and delivery unit in early active labor at 39 weeks gestation. Her pregnancy has been uncomplicated, with negative screening for gestational diabetes. Her prepregnancy BMI was 22 and she has gained 12 kg this pregnancy. The estimated fetal weight is 3800 g. Her labor progresses slowly and her cervix reaches 10 cm dilation after 22 hours. Epidural analgesia is used. The second stage of labor lasts 3 hours and after the fetal vertex delivers in a left occiput anterior position, the shoulders do not deliver with typical axial traction on the fetal head. What is the most appropriate immediate action?

   a. Instruct the patient to continue pushing.

   b. Discontinue traction on the fetal head.

   c. Initiate oxytocin to increase contractions.

   d. Apply fundal pressure to assist delivery.

   e. Cut an episiotomy to facilitate delivery.

4. A 29-year-old gravida 2 para 1001 comes to the labor and delivery unit in active labor at 40 weeks gestation. Her prior pregnancy was uncomplicated and she had a spontaneous vaginal delivery of a 4200 g male infant 2 years ago. This pregnancy has been uncomplicated. On initial exam her cervix is 6 cm dilated, 50% effaced, and the fetal vertex is at +1 station. She is contracting every 3 minutes and the fetal heart rate (FHR) is in the 140s, with moderate variability and accelerations noted. Her labor progresses well, and 3 hours later, her cervix is fully dilated and the vertex is at +3 station. After 30 minutes of pushing, the fetal vertex delivers in a left occiput anterior position, but the shoulders do not deliver with typical axial traction on the fetal head. McRoberts maneuver is performed and suprapubic pressure is applied. What is likely to be the most effective next step in delivering the fetus without injury to the brachial plexus?

   a. Woods corkscrew maneuver

   b. Extraction of the posterior arm

   c. Maternal knee chest position

   d. Vaginal replacement of the fetal head

   e. Subcutaneous symphysiotomy

5. The use of routine episiotomy in the management of all shoulder dystocia cases has been advocated in the past, but with little scientific evidence in support of this practice. Which of the following patients is most likely to benefit from an episiotomy?

   a. A patient with a narrow vaginal fourchette

   b. A patient with a short perineal body

   c. A patient with four prior vaginal deliveries

   d. A patient with a narrow pubic arch

   e. A patient with a platypoid pelvis

6. Studies have shown that shoulder dystocia simulations improve all of the following outcomes except:

   a. Avoidance of fundal pressure

   b. Communication skills

   c. Documentation

   d. Ineffective suprapubic pressure

   e. Permanent brachial palsy

7. A 27-year-old gravida 1 para 0 undergoes a spontaneous vaginal delivery of a 3400 g male infant in the left occiput anterior position with no noted complications. After delivery, examination of the neonate reveals crepitus over the right clavicle and no spontaneous movement of the right arm. What is the most likely cause of the neonatal findings?

   a. Endogenous forces that pressed the neonatal right shoulder against the maternal symphysis pubis

   b. Endogenous forces that pressed the neonatal right shoulder against the maternal sacral promontory

   c. Excess traction on the fetal head during delivery, leading to stretch of the right shoulder against the perineum

   d. Excess traction on the fetal head during delivery, leading to stretch of the right shoulder against the symphysis pubis

   e. Excess traction on the fetal head during delivery, leading to stretch of the right shoulder against the sacral promontory

8. A 26-year-old gravida 1 para 0 comes to the labor and delivery unit for induction of labor at 41 weeks gestation. Her pregnancy has been complicated by gestational diabetes that was well controlled by diet. Her fundal height is 40 cm and the estimated fetal weight is 3900 g. Her cervix is 3 cm dilated, 80% effaced, with the vertex at −1 station. She is started on an oxytocin infusion that is titrated up to achieve contractions every 3 minutes and progresses to full dilatation after 8 hours. An epidural catheter is in place for pain management. Her second stage lasts 3 hours and after delivery of the fetal head in a left occiput anterior position, the shoulders do not deliver with typical axial traction on the fetal head. McRoberts maneuver and suprapubic pressure allow delivery of the shoulder after 60 seconds. After delivery, examination of the neonate reveals no spontaneous movement of the right arm. What is the most likely clinical course for the neonate?

   a. Recovery of normal right arm function within 1 month

   b. Recovery of normal right arm function after 6 months

   c. Persistence of brachial plexus palsy permanently

   d. Progression of neurologic symptoms to include diaphragm paralysis

   e. Progression of neurologic symptoms to include C8-T1 nerve roots

9. A 30-year-old gravida 3 para 1021 who reports shoulder dystocia of a 4000 g infant in her prior pregnancy presents to labor and delivery at 39 weeks gestation in active labor. The estimated fetal weight for this pregnancy is 3800 g. Her cervix progresses from 5 cm dilation to full dilation over 4 hours, and she pushes for 1 hour before crowning. Due to her history, prophylactic McRoberts positioning is used for delivery. What is the likely benefit of this positioning?

   a. Shorter head to body delivery time

   b. Lower peak force needed to deliver the anterior shoulder

   c. Lower incidence of shoulder dystocia

   d. Lower need for therapeutic maneuvers

   e. No clear benefits for any outcomes

10. A 32-year-old gravida 1 para 0 comes to the labor and delivery unit in active labor at 40 weeks gestation. Her pregnancy has been complicated by gestational diabetes that was well controlled by diet. Her fundal height is 40 cm and the estimated fetal weight is 3800 g. Her cervix is 6 cm dilated, 80% effaced, and −1 station. She progresses to full dilatation after 4 hours. An epidural catheter is in place for pain management. Her second stage lasts 3 hours and the FHR tracing remains category I. After delivery of the fetal head in a left occiput anterior position, the shoulders do not deliver with typical axial traction on the fetal head. Despite multiple maneuvers, including McRoberts, suprapubic pressure, attempted delivery of the posterior arm, Woods corkscrew, and Gaskin positioning, the anterior shoulder cannot be dislodged 5 minutes after delivery of the vertex. What is the greatest risk to the fetus at this time?

    a. Brachial plexus injury

    b. Clavicular fracture

    c. Cervical dislocation

    d. Humeral fracture

    e. Hypoxic brain injury

ANSWERS

1. **Answer: e**
(see *Gabbe's Obstetrics* 8e: ch14)

Women with prior shoulder dystocia are at increased risk for recurrent shoulder dystocia in a subsequent pregnancy. Studies have demonstrated a range of 1%–17% for the occurrence of recurrent shoulder dystocia, with most studies citing an incidence of at least 10%.[1-4] However, since many women with prior shoulder dystocia may not have additional children, or may elect cesarean delivery in a subsequent pregnancy, the actual incidence is difficult to assess but is likely much higher.

2. **Answer: d**
(see *Gabbe's Obstetrics* 8e: ch14)

Shoulder dystocia typically occurs when the descent of the anterior shoulder is obstructed by the symphysis pubis. It can also result from impaction of the posterior shoulder on the maternal sacral promontory. The right arm is typically affected, owing to the fact that the left occiput anterior presentation is more common.

3. **Answer: b**
(see *Gabbe's Obstetrics* 8e: ch14)

When shoulder dystocia is clinically diagnosed, we advise stopping all endogenous (expulsive efforts) and exogenous forces (traction) until an attempt is made to alleviate the obstruction. The woman should be instructed to stop pushing; however, it must be recognized that most likely the gravida will continue to involuntarily exert endogenous expulsive forces, as uterine contractions do not spontaneously abate once the head emerges from the vagina.

4. **Answer: b**
(see *Gabbe's Obstetrics* 8e: ch14)

Delivery of the posterior arm showed a 71% reduction in stretch applied to the anterior nerve plexus, and was the maneuver that required the least force to deliver the anterior shoulder. This decreases the impacted diameter from the bisacromial diameter to the axilloacromial diameter. The endpoint of posterior arm extraction is to substitute the axilloacromial diameter for the bisacromial diameter, with the former being approximately three centimeters shorter than the latter.

5. **Answer: a**
(see *Gabbe's Obstetrics* 8e: ch14)

The need for cutting a generous episiotomy must be based on clinical circumstances, such as a narrow vaginal fourchette in a nulliparous patient. Episiotomy can allow for greater access to the vagina for the performance of the internal manipulations necessary for the rotational maneuvers or for delivery of the posterior shoulder.

6. **Answer: e**
(see *Gabbe's Obstetrics* 8e: ch14)

Studies have shown that shoulder dystocia simulations improve outcomes such as documentation, identification of recurrent mistakes such as ineffective suprapubic pressure or incorrect McRoberts technique, communication skills, and the avoidance of fundal pressure. Marked limitations, however, currently exist with the role of shoulder dystocia simulation: (1) lack of randomized controlled trials, (2) lack of significance with regards to pertinent clinical outcomes such as permanent brachial palsy, (3) involvement of resident physicians, (4) use of simulators that introduce external artificiality, (5) confinement of success to simulated environments only, and (6) lack of transference to a clinical setting.

7. **Answer: a**
(see *Gabbe's Obstetrics* 8e: ch14)

Since 2005, epidemiologic data, case studies, and computer modeling have all provided support to the concept that brachial plexus stretch and injury can result from endogenous forces when the neonate's shoulder presses against the maternal symphysis pubis or sacral promontory. Maternal endogenous forces have been shown to exceed clinician-applied exogenous forces. It has been consistently reported that approximately 50% of brachial plexus palsies occur in the absence of clinically recognized shoulder dystocia.

8. **Answer: a**
    (see *Gabbe's Obstetrics* 8e: ch14)

    Unilateral brachial plexus palsies are the most common neurologic injury sustained by the neonate. Most (75%–85%) of these injuries are transient although permanence is likely if the injury persists beyond 6 months of life. The right arm is typically affected, owing to the fact that the left occiput anterior presentation is more common. Most (80%) of the brachial plexus palsies have been located within the C5-C6 nerve roots (Erb-Duchenne palsy). Other types of brachial plexus palsies that have been described include Klumpke palsy (C8-T1), an intermediate palsy, and complete palsy of the entire brachial plexus. Diaphragmatic paralysis, Horner syndrome, and facial nerve injuries have occasionally been reported to accompany brachial plexus palsy.

9. **Answer: e**
    (see *Gabbe's Obstetrics* 8e: ch14)

    While many women are placed in McRoberts position before delivery, currently available studies do not show clear benefit to these prophylactic measures to prevent shoulder dystocia.

10. **Answer: e**
    (see *Gabbe's Obstetrics* 8e: ch14)

    Shoulder dystocia should be viewed as an obstetric emergency due to the short period of time required to relieve the obstruction prior to the onset of hypoxic brain injury. Not all fetuses have the same baseline reserve during second stage labor, so it is difficult to state an exact length of time in which neonatal encephalopathy will occur if delivery is not completed. Given the considerable overlap in delivery timing for neonates with and without injuries or depression, it is difficult to pinpoint an exact time in which delivery should ideally occur. Based on the current literature, it seems reasonable to consider extraordinary measures to effect delivery once 4–5 minutes have elapsed and the fetus is still undelivered.

REFERENCES

1. Ouzounian JG, Gherman RB, Chauhan S, Battista LR, Lee RH. Recurrent shoulder dystocia: analysis of incidence and risk factors. *Am J Perinatol.* 2012;29:515-518.
2. Smith RB, Lane C, Pearson JF. Shoulder dystocia: what happens at the next delivery? *Br J Obstet Gynaecol.* 1994;101:713-715.
3. Ginsberg NA, Moisidis C. How to predict recurrent shoulder dystocia. *Am J Obstet Gynecol.* 2001;184:1427-1429; discussion: 1429-1430.
4. Lewis DF, Raymond RC, Perkins MB, Brooks GG, Heymann AR. Recurrence rate of shoulder dystocia. *Am J Obstet Gynecol.* 1995;172:1369-1371.

15

Intrapartum Fetal Evaluation

Rini Banerjee Ratan

(See *Gabbe's Obstetrics: Normal and Problem Pregnancies*, 8e: ch15)

QUESTIONS

1. A 27-year-old G2P1 at 39 weeks gestation presents to the labor and delivery unit with painful, regular contractions. Her pregnancy has been uncomplicated. Her cervix is 5 cm dilated, 80% effaced, with the vertex at 0/5 station. Fetal heart rate (FHR) tracing is category I. She is uncomfortable with contractions, but able to tolerate them. She declines pain relief. She requests only intermittent electronic fetal monitoring (EFM) while in labor. Which of the following is the most appropriate course of action?

   a. Ensure that a 1:1 nurse-to-patient ratio can be provided.

   b. Perform fetal monitoring for 20 minutes of every hour in the active phase of labor.

   c. Perform fetal monitoring for 20 minutes of every hour in the second stage of labor.

   d. Advise the patient that American College of Obstetricians and Gynecologists (ACOG) does not support the use of intermittent fetal monitoring for any patients in labor.

2. Which of the following is the most likely physiologic cause of accelerations seen in an FHR tracing?

   a. Fetal head compression

   b. Baroreceptor response

   c. Umbilical cord compression

   d. Fetal movement

   e. Chemoreceptor response

3. Which of the following terms best describes the variability seen in the FHR tracing shown here?

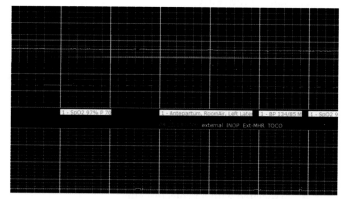

   a. Absent

   b. Minimal

   c. Moderate

   d. Marked

   e. Sinusoidal

4. A 37-year-old G1P0 at 39 weeks gestation presents to the labor and delivery unit with painful, regular contractions. Her pregnancy has been uncomplicated. A bedside ultrasound shows oligohydramnios. She has not had bleeding or leakage of fluid. She reports good fetal movement. Intrapartum fetal monitoring is most likely to demonstrate which of the following types of decelerations in this patient's FHR tracing?

   a. Early

   b. Variable

   c. Late

   d. Prolonged

   e. Bradycardia

5. What percentage of laboring patients in the United States undergo intrapartum EFM?

   a. 100%

   b. 80%

   c. 60%

   d. 40%

   e. 20%

6. Which of the following adjunct technologies has been shown to augment the interpretation of EFM to improve the ability to predict neonatal acidemia?

   a. Fetal blood sampling

   b. Fetal pulse oximetry

   c. ST-segment analysis

   d. Computerized interpretation of EFM

   e. None of the above

7. A 24-year-old G2P1 at 40 weeks gestation has been undergoing induction of labor with oxytocin for 12 hours. Her antenatal course has been uncomplicated. Over the past 30 minutes the FHR tracing has been category II with moderate variability and recurrent late decelerations. Her cervix is 4 cm dilated, 50% effaced, with the vertex at −2/5 station. Artificial rupture of membranes reveals the presence of thin meconium. How does the presence of meconium-stained amniotic fluid influence the interpretation of this category II FHR tracing?

   a. Associated with a protective effect

   b. No increase in adverse outcomes has been reported

   c. Confers an increased risk of neonatal morbidity

   d. Increased risk of morbidity only in the presence of thick meconium

8. A 32-year-old G1P0 woman at 41 weeks gestation is admitted to the labor and delivery unit in active labor, following spontaneous rupture of membranes with clear fluid 2 hours earlier. Her pregnancy has been uncomplicated. On admission her cervix is 5 cm dilated, 80% effaced, with the vertex at 0/5 station. Two hours later, the FHR tracing is category II with moderate variability and recurrent variable decelerations. Her cervix is 8 cm dilated, 90% effaced, with the vertex at +1/5 station. Which of the following is the most appropriate evidence-based next step in management?

   a. Maternal repositioning

   b. Maternal oxygen supplementation

   c. Intravenous fluid bolus administration

   d. Fetal scalp stimulation

   e. Initiation of an amnioinfusion

9. A 27-year-old G1P0 at 39 weeks gestation is undergoing induction of labor for well-controlled gestational diabetes. Her cervix is long and closed on admission, and cervical ripening is initiated with misoprostol. FHR tracing is category I. Eight hours later minimal variability is noted, with no accelerations present. No decelerations are noted either. Her cervix is now 4 cm dilated, 50% effaced, with the vertex at −2/5 station. Which of the following is the most appropriate evidence-based next step in management?

   a. Immediate cesarean delivery

   b. Maternal oxygen supplementation

   c. Fetal scalp stimulation

   d. Maternal repositioning

   e. Initiation of an amnioinfusion

10. Which of the following umbilical cord artery pH values is most strongly associated with neonatal morbidity and mortality?

    a. pH <7.00

    b. pH <7.10

    c. pH <7.20

    d. pH >7.20

    e. pH >7.10

11. A 22-year-old G1P0 at 38 weeks gestation presents to the labor and delivery unit with painful, regular contractions. Her pregnancy has been notable for chronic hypertension, well controlled on labetalol 400 mg twice daily. Her cervix is 2 cm dilated, 50% effaced, with the vertex at −2/5 station. FHR tracing is shown. Which of the following terms best describes this FHR tracing?

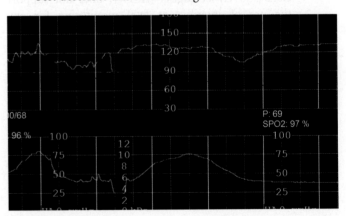

    a. Category I

    b. Category II

    c. Category III

    d. Reactive

12. A 36-year-old G2P1 at 32 weeks gestation is brought to the emergency department by ambulance after being involved in a motor vehicle accident. She sustained direct abdominal trauma and reports significant abdominal pain. Her pregnancy has been otherwise uncomplicated until now. FHR tracing is shown. Which of the following is the most likely underlying etiology of this FHR tracing?

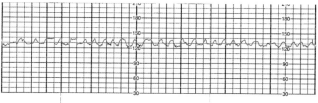
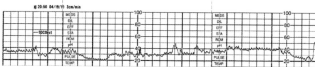

   a. Fetal metabolic acidemia
   b. Uteroplacental insufficiency
   c. Fetal anemia
   d. Umbilical cord compression
   e. Fetal head compression

13. A 25-year-old G3P2 at 39 weeks gestation is undergoing induction of labor for gestational diabetes. Her past obstetric history is notable for two prior normal spontaneous vaginal deliveries at term. Her cervix was 2 cm dilated, 50% effaced, with the vertex at −2/5 station on admission. Oxytocin was initiated 6 hours ago and is now infusing at 12 mU/min. Her fingerstick blood glucose level on admission was 83 mmol/L. FHR tracing is shown. Which of the following is the most appropriate next step in management?

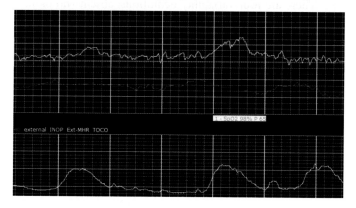

   a. Continue present management
   b. Begin insulin drip
   c. Administer terbutaline
   d. Decrease rate of oxytocin infusion

14. A 39-year-old G2P1 at 36 weeks gestation presents to the labor and delivery unit with the acute onset of severe abdominal pain 30 minutes ago. Her past obstetric history is notable for one prior cesarean delivery for arrest of dilation at term. She appears diaphoretic and extremely uncomfortable. FHR tracing is shown. Which of the following terms best describes this FHR tracing?

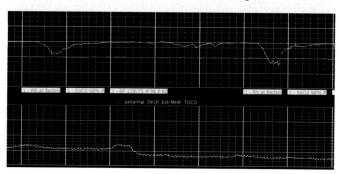

   a. Category I
   b. Category II
   c. Category III
   d. Sinusoidal

15. An 18-year-old G1P0 at 38 weeks gestation is sent to the labor and delivery unit after her blood pressure is found to be 161/107 and 3+ protein on urine dipstick is noted at her routine prenatal visit. She reports intermittent headache for the past day. She reports good fetal movement. She has persistently elevated blood pressure upon admission and a presumptive diagnosis of preeclampsia with severe features is made. FHR baseline is 140 with moderate variability. Spontaneous accelerations are present and no decelerations noted. Magnesium sulfate is initiated for seizure prophylaxis. Which of the following findings may be anticipated in the FHR tracing following the initiation of magnesium sulfate?

   a. Increase in baseline
   b. Decrease in variability
   c. Transient variable decelerations
   d. Increase in spontaneous accelerations
   e. Marked variability

16. A 41-year-old G1P0 at 34 weeks gestation presents to the antenatal testing unit to undergo a routine surveillance ultrasound. Her fetus has been small for gestational age since 28 weeks gestation, now measuring <10th percentile. FHR tracing is shown. Which of the following is the most likely underlying etiology of this FHR tracing?

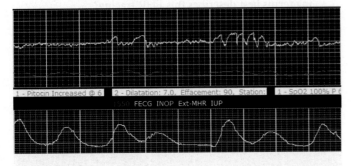

a. Fetal metabolic acidemia

b. Uteroplacental insufficiency

c. Fetal anemia

d. Umbilical cord compression

e. Fetal head compression

ANSWERS

1. Answer: a
(see *Gabbe's Obstetrics* 8e: ch15)

ACOG continues to support intermittent EFM during labor as reasonable for some low-risk patients. If intermittent monitoring is elected, a 1:1 nurse-to-patient ratio is required. ACOG further recommends that fetal monitoring be accomplished for 30 minutes during every hour of the active phase of labor, and every 15 minutes during the second stage of labor based on expert opinion when intermittent monitoring is employed for selected low-risk women.

2. Answer: d
(see *Gabbe's Obstetrics* 8e: ch15)

Accelerations are rises in the FHR above the baseline or at least 15 bpm and last at least 15 seconds before returning to the baseline. At less than 32 0/7 weeks, accelerations are defined less stringently, as an increase of at least 10 bpm that lasts at least 10 seconds before returning to the baseline. Physiologically, accelerations are thought to be due to fetal movement.

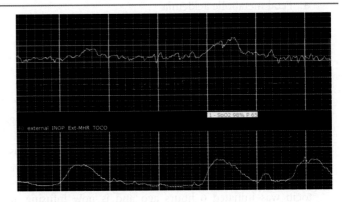

3. Answer: a
(see *Gabbe's Obstetrics* 8e: ch15)

There are four variability definitions: absent (no oscillation) (A), minimal (B), moderate (6–25 bpm) (C), and marked (>25 bpm) (D). A specific pattern of repetitive oscillation is referred to as sinusoidal (E). While rare, it is important to identify as it has been associated with fetal pathology such as anemia.

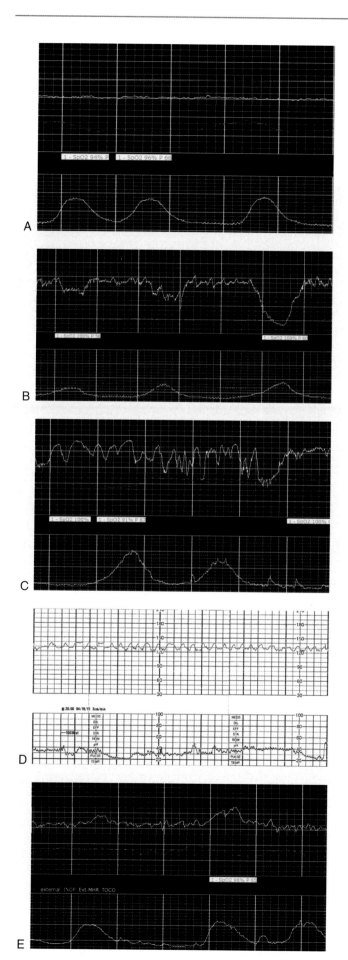

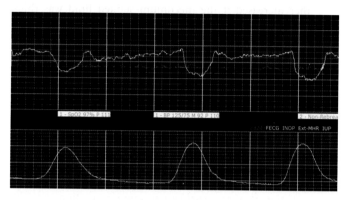

4. Answer: b
(see *Gabbe's Obstetrics* 8e: ch15)

Variable decelerations are characterized by an abrupt descent and an abrupt return to baseline of at least 15 bpm, lasting less than 2 minutes. The nadir of the deceleration is reached in less than 30 seconds, and the shape is often described as a 'V' or 'U' shape. Variable decelerations are caused by umbilical cord compression, which can happen anytime due to the relative movements and positions of mother and fetus, and particularly during labor contractions and the cardinal movements.

5. Answer: b
(see *Gabbe's Obstetrics* 8e: ch15)

Intrapartum fetal monitoring to assess fetal well-being during labor and delivery is a key component of intrapartum management. In fact, over 80% of laboring patients in the United States undergo intrapartum EFM.

6. Answer: e
(see *Gabbe's Obstetrics* 8e: ch15)

Additional high-level evidence may emerge to support the clinical use of fetal scalp sampling to reduce unnecessary cesarean deliveries for concerning EFM, but existing evidence does not support routine clinical use. The lack of significant effect of using fetal pulse oximetry to augment the interpretation of intrapartum EFM in this large multicenter trial prevented fetal pulse oximetry from entering clinical practice. A Cochrane metaanalysis of seven trials comparing S-T segment analysis with EFM to EFM alone, deemed to be moderate to high quality, showed no evidence that S-T segment analysis reduced cesarean delivery, severe metabolic acidosis, or neonatal encephalopathy.[1] To date, there are no studies that demonstrate that computerized interpretation of EFM patterns reduces acidosis or meaningful neonatal morbidity compared with visual interpretation.

7. Answer: c
(see *Gabbe's Obstetrics* 8e: ch15)

Meconium-stained amniotic fluid is common, found to be present in 12% of all laboring patients and in over 20% of patients with category II EFM patterns. In a secondary analysis of a large, prospective cohort study of laboring women at or after 37 weeks with category II patterns, Frey and colleagues found that the presence of meconium was associated with an increased risk of neonatal morbidity compared with those without meconium present. They also found that the increased risk of morbidity was further increased if the meconium-stained fluid was thick compared with thin.[2] The presence or absence of meconium-stained fluid can help risk-stratify patients with a category II FHR tracing for acidemia.

8. Answer: e
(see *Gabbe's Obstetrics* 8e: ch15)

There are no data to support the use of position change to improve category II and III patterns, but the practice is recommended by ACOG, AWHONN, and others due to the physiologic principles and the benign nature of the intervention. Existing data do not provide evidence to support the use of maternal oxygen supplementation and raise the possibility of harm. Intravenous fluid boluses or those given in response to a category II or III pattern without maternal hypotension is not evidence-based. A Cochrane metaanalysis highlighted that in the setting of recurrent variable decelerations, initiation of an amnioinfusion (AI) is a reasonable evidence-based strategy to reduce recurrent decelerations and the chance for cesarean for category II or III EFM patterns.[3]

9. Answer: c
(see *Gabbe's Obstetrics* 8e: ch15)

Large studies have demonstrated that acceleration(s) following scalp stimulation is significantly associated with a normal pH.[4] Scalp stimulation represents a low-risk, inexpensive, and readily available tool to assess for a normal fetal pH in the setting of category II and III patterns.

10. Answer: a
(see *Gabbe's Obstetrics* 8e: ch15)

Umbilical cord pH decreases when persistent hypoxia causes a shift to anaerobic metabolism, and hydrogen ions accumulate and overwhelm the capacity of the fetal buffer system.[5] A metaanalysis of 51 studies demonstrated that an arterial pH <7.00 was strongly associated with neonatal morbidity (odds ratio (OR) 12.5, 95% confidence interval (CI) 6.1–25.6) and mortality (OR 6.1, 95% CI 0.9–41.6).

11. Answer: a
(see *Gabbe's Obstetrics* 8e: ch15)

The combination of features over any 10-minute time interval are considered together and a category is assigned to inform communication, documentation, and management. Category I is considered a normal EFM pattern (see figures and Table 15.1).

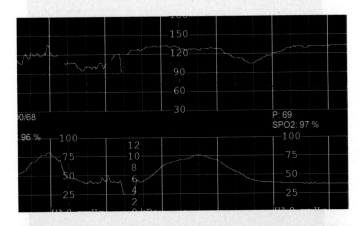

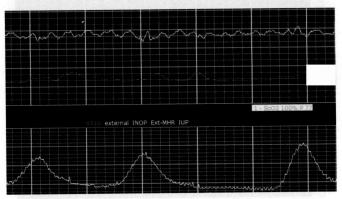

12. Answer: c
(see *Gabbe's Obstetrics* 8e: ch15)

A specific pattern of repetitive oscillation is referred to as sinusoidal. While rare, it is important to identify as it has been associated with fetal pathology such as anemia.

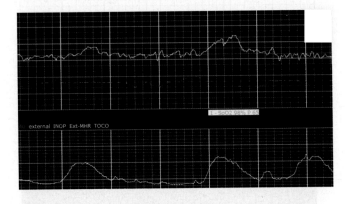

TABLE 15.1   Standard Fetal Heart Rate Definitions.

Pattern	Definition
Baseline	Mean FHR rounded to increments of 5 beats/min in a 10-min window, excluding accelerations, decelerations, and periods of marked FHR variability (>25 beats/min). There must be at least 2 min of identifiable baseline segments (not necessarily contiguous) in any 10-min window or the baseline for that period is indeterminate. • Normal baseline FHR range 110 to 160 beats/min • *Tachycardia* is defined as an FHR baseline >160 beats/min • *Bradycardia* is defined as an FHR baseline <110 beats/min
Variability	Fluctuations in the FHR baseline are irregular in amplitude and frequency and are visually quantitated as the amplitude of the peak to the trough in beats per minute. • Absent: amplitude range undetectable • Minimal: amplitude range detectable but ≤5 beats/min • Moderate (normal): amplitude range 6 to 25 beats/min • Marked: amplitude range >25 beats/min
Accelerations	Abrupt increase (onset to peak <30 s) in the FHR from the most recently calculated baseline. At ≥32 weeks, an acceleration peaks ≥15 beats/min above baseline and lasts ≥15 s but <2 min. At <32 weeks, acceleration peaks ≥10 beats/min above baseline and lasts ≥10 s but <2 min. Prolonged acceleration lasts ≥2 min but <10 min. Acceleration ≥10 min is a baseline change.
Early	Gradual (onset to nadir ≥30 s) decrease in FHR during a uterine contraction. Onset, nadir, and recovery of the deceleration occur at the same time as the beginning, peak, and end of the contraction, respectively.
Late	Decrease in FHR is gradual (onset to nadir ≥30 s) during a uterine contraction. Onset, nadir, and recovery of the deceleration occur after the beginning, peak, and end of the contraction, respectively.
Variable	Decrease in the FHR is abrupt (onset to nadir <30 s) and ≥15 beats/min below the baseline and lasting ≥15 s but <2 min.
Prolonged	Deceleration is ≥15 beats/min below baseline and lasts ≥2 min or more but <10 min. Deceleration ≥10 min is a baseline change.
Sinusoidal pattern	Pattern in FHR baseline is smooth, sine wave–like, and undulating with a cycle frequency of 3–5/min that persists for at least 20 min.

FHR, Fetal heart rate.

13. Answer: d

(see *Gabbe's Obstetrics* 8e: ch15)

It is reasonable to make efforts to resolve tachysystole that occurs in the setting of labor induction or augmentation whenever possible to prevent FHR abnormalities from developing.

14. Answer: c

(see *Gabbe's Obstetrics* 8e: ch15)

Continuous intrapartum EFM is particularly important during TOLAC because of the risk of uterine rupture. While uterine rupture is a rare event, abnormalities in the FHR pattern often precede or accompany uterine rupture. Specifically, there are reports that repetitive variable or prolonged decelerations, or fetal bradycardia, are the most commonly seen patterns preceding or during a uterine rupture.[6,7]

15. Answer: b

(see *Gabbe's Obstetrics* 8e: ch15)

Magnesium exposure is independently associated with a small reduction in average baseline heart rate and a decrease in variability that may or may not persist after the magnesium bolus.

16. Answer: b

(see *Gabbe's Obstetrics* 8e: ch15)

Chronic placental insufficiency can be a cause of growth restriction, and could have a potential impact on FHR pattern. A retrospective cohort study of term infants in the second stage of labor by Epplin et al. found significantly fewer accelerations and more late decelerations among those fetuses with growth restriction compared with those without, but no differences in baseline or variability.[8]

REFERENCES

1. Neilson JP. Fetal electrocardiogram (ECG) for fetal monitoring during labour. *Cochrane Database Syst Rev.* 2015(12):CD000116.

2. Frey HA, Tuuli MG, Shanks AL, Macones GA, Cahill AG. Interpreting category II fetal heart rate tracings: does meconium matter? *American journal of obstetrics and gynecology.* 2014;211(6):644.e641-648.

3. Hofmeyr GJ, Lawrie TA. Amnioinfusion for potential or suspected umbilical cord compression in labour. *Cochrane Database Syst Rev.* 2012;1:CD000013.

4. Elimian A, Figueroa R, Tejani N. Intrapartum assessment of fetal well-being: a comparison of scalp stimulation with scalp blood pH sampling. *Obstet Gynecol.* 1997;89(3):373-376.

5. Uzan S, Berkane N, Verstraete L, Mathieu E, Bréart G. [Acid base balance in the fetus during labor: pathophysiology and exploration methods]. *Journal de Gynécologie, Obstétrique et Biologie de la Reproduction.* 2003;32(1 Suppl):1s68-78.

6. Holmgren C, Scott JR, Porter TF, Esplin MS, Bardsley T. Uterine rupture with attempted vaginal birth after cesarean delivery: decision-to-delivery time and neonatal outcome. *Obstet Gynecol.* 2012;119(4):725-731.

7. Menihan CA. Uterine rupture in women attempting a vaginal birth following prior cesarean birth. *J Perinatol.* 1998;18(6 Pt 1):440-443.

8. Epplin KA, Tuuli MG, Odibo AO, Roehl KA, Macones GA, Cahill AG. Effect of growth restriction on fetal heart rate patterns in the second stage of labor. *Am J Perinatol.* 2015;32(9):873-878.

Obstetrical Anesthesia

Alyssa Stephenson-Famy

(See *Gabbe's Obstetrics: Normal and Problem Pregnancies*, 8e: ch16)

QUESTIONS

1. A 30-year-old G1P1 has a perineal laceration repair following a vaginal delivery. She has inadequate local anesthesia and reports pain with placement of the suture at the perineal skin. What nerve root is responsible for this symptom?
   a. T4-6
   b. T6-8
   c. T8-10
   d. L2-4
   e. S2-S4

2. A G1P0 woman is interested in nonpharmacologic analgesia for her labor. What method is least likely to be effective treatment for the pain during labor?
   a. Continuous support person (e.g., doula)
   b. Acupuncture
   c. Immersion in water
   d. Sterile water injection
   e. Hypnosis

3. A G3P2 woman with history of spinal surgery is unable to receive neuraxial anesthesia for labor. She desires a systemic opioid for pain control. Based on its metabolism and half-life, which intravenous opioid would have the lowest risk of neonatal respiratory depression at birth?
   a. Morphine
   b. Hydromorphone
   c. Fentanyl
   d. Remifentanil
   e. Meperidine

4. A 24-year-old healthy G1P0 woman receives a combined spinal-epidural (CSE) for analgesia during active labor. While she is positioned flat on her back, she is noted to have a blood pressure of 80/50. In addition to an intravenous fluid bolus, what additional treatment should be initiated for her hypotension?
   a. Left uterine displacement
   b. Dextrose infusion
   c. Ephedrine bolus
   d. Phenylephrine drip

5. During an uncomplicated cesarean section, a woman complains of numbness and weakness in her hands. She is breathing normally and has a normal oxygen saturation. What is the most likely cause of this symptom?
   a. High spinal including levels C3-C5
   b. Anesthesia has reached levels C6-C8
   c. Nerve injury following neuraxial anesthesia
   d. Local anesthetic allergy
   e. Local anesthetic toxicity

6. A woman with HELLP syndrome and thrombocytopenia undergoes a cesarean section for delivery. What complication is she most likely to develop if she receives neuraxial anesthesia for her surgery?
   a. Epidural hematoma
   b. Epidural abscess
   c. Persistent back pain
   d. Serious neurologic injury
   e. Unrecognized spinal catheter

7. A healthy woman undergoes a spontaneous vaginal delivery with epidural analgesia. One day postpartum she develops a headache which is more severe when sitting up or standing and is improved when lying flat. She has no other neurologic symptoms and her vital signs are stable. What is the most likely diagnosis?

   a. Migraine

   b. Pneumocephalus

   c. Intracranial hemorrhage

   d. Spinal headache

   e. Cortical vein thrombosis

8. What is the relationship between epidural analgesia and cesarean section?

   a. Epidural analgesia increases the risk of cesarean section.

   b. Epidural analgesia decreases the risk of cesarean section.

   c. Epidural analgesia does not change the risk of cesarean section.

   d. Epidural analgesia changes the risk of cesarean section in primigravid women.

   e. Epidural analgesia changes the risk of cesarean section in early labor (<4 cm).

9. Which anesthetic technique can reduce the risk of aspiration of gastric contents during a rapid sequence intubation?

   a. Left lateral tilt position

   b. Preoxygenation

   c. Anesthesia induction with ketamine

   d. Cricoid pressure

   e. Early extubation

10. A 35-year-old G3P3 undergoes a scheduled, uncomplicated repeat cesarean section. She has an anaphylactic allergy to ibuprofen. As part of her enhanced surgical recovery, what medication should be used on a scheduled basis to minimize her postoperative opioid requirement?

   a. Midazolam

   b. Ketamine

   c. Gabapentin

   d. Acetaminophen

   e. Aspirin

ANSWERS

1. Answer: e

(see *Gabbe's Obstetrics* 8e: ch16)

The sensory fibers of sacral nerves 2, 3, and 4 (i.e., the pudendal nerves) transmit painful impulses from the perineum to the spinal cord during the second stage and during any perineal repair.

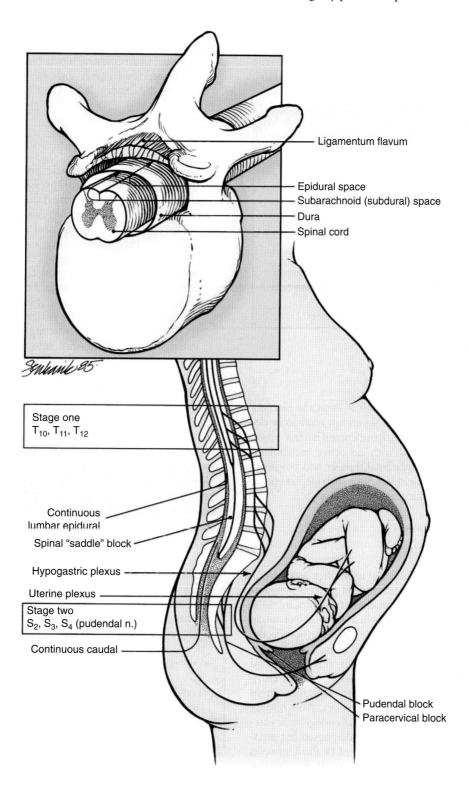

Ligamentum flavum

Epidural space
Subarachnoid (subdural) space
Dura
Spinal cord

Stage one
T_{10}, T_{11}, T_{12}

Continuous lumbar epidural

Spinal "saddle" block

Hypogastric plexus

Uterine plexus

Stage two
S_2, S_3, S_4 (pudendal n.)

Continuous caudal

Pudendal block
Paracervical block

2. Answer: d

(see *Gabbe's Obstetrics* 8e: ch16)

Psychoprophylaxis including hypnosis, breathing, gentle massage, and support person participation can decrease the perception of pain during uterine contractions. Acupuncture has been shown in some studies to alleviate labor pain and reduce use of both epidural analgesia and parenteral opioids. Laboring in water may be beneficial and delay the need for epidural analgesia. Intradermal sterile water injections are unlikely to be effective (Table 16.1).

TABLE 16.1 Evidence for the Use of Nonpharmacologic Analgesic Techniques in Labor.

Nonpharmacologic Analgesic Techniques for Labor	Cochrane Database Systematic Reviews	Conclusion of Review
Continuous support (e.g., doula)	CD003766	Benefit
Hypnosis	CD003521	Benefit
Massage, reflexology	CD009290	Cannot determine
Acupuncture, acupressure	CD009232	Benefit
Immersion in water	CD000111	Cannot determine
Transcutaneous electrical nerve stimulation	CD007214	Cannot determine
Sterile water injection	CD009107	No benefit

3. Answer: d

(see *Gabbe's Obstetrics* 8e: ch16)

Systemic maternal opioids are known to cross the placenta and can increase the likelihood of significant respiratory depression in the newborn at birth. Remifentanil is a fast-onset, short-acting synthetic opioid with no active metabolites. Rapid metabolism reduces placental transfer and promotes neonatal clearance resulting in less respiratory depression in the newborn compared to intravenous fentanyl.

4. Answer: a

(see *Gabbe's Obstetrics* 8e: ch16)

Hypotension is defined variably but most often as a systolic blood pressure less than 80–100 mm Hg, a 0%–30% decrease from baseline, or a combination of an absolute value and percentage decrease.[1] It occurs in at least 10% of spinal or epidural blocks given during labor.[2] Hypotension occurs primarily as a result of the effects of local anesthetic agents on sympathetic fibers, which normally maintain blood vessel tone. Vasodilation results in decreased venous return of blood to the right side of the heart, with subsequent decreased cardiac output and hypotension. A secondary mechanism may be decreased maternal endogenous catecholamines following pain relief. Once diagnosed, hypotension is corrected by increasing the rate of IV fluid infusion and exaggerating left uterine displacement. If these simple measures do not suffice, a vasopressor is indicated. Either ephedrine or phenylephrine can be used to treat hypotension during neuraxial anesthesia/analgesia.[3]

5. Answer: b

(see *Gabbe's Obstetrics* 8e: ch16)

This complication occurs when the level of anesthesia rises dangerously high and results in paralysis of the respiratory muscles, including the diaphragm (C3–C5). It is the most frequent complication encountered secondary to spinal or epidural anesthesia and can result from a miscalculated dose of drug or unintentional subarachnoid injection during an epidural block. Numbness and weakness of the fingers and hands indicates that the anesthesia has reached the cervical level (C6–C8).

6. Answer: a

(see *Gabbe's Obstetrics* 8e: ch16)

One of the more dramatic and correctable forms of nerve damage follows compression of the spinal cord by a hematoma that has formed during the administration of spinal or epidural anesthesia, presumably from accidental puncture of an epidural vessel. If the condition is diagnosed early by imaging, usually with the aid of a neurologist or neurosurgeon, the hematoma can be removed by laminectomy and the problem will resolve without permanent damage. Fortunately, this is a rare complication. Nonetheless, spinal and epidural blocks are contraindicated if the patient has a coagulopathy or is pharmacologically anticoagulated. Hemolysis, elevated liver enzymes, and low platelets (HELLP) syndrome may be a particularly strong risk factor because of multifactorial sources for coagulation defects.[4] Any significant motor or sensory deficit after neuraxial anesthesia should be investigated immediately and thoroughly (Table 16.2).

TABLE 16.2 Incidence of Serious Complications Related to Neuraxial (Spinal or Epidural) Anesthesia.

Complication	Complications (N)	Incidence	95% CI
Postdural puncture headache	1647	1:144	1 : 137, 1 : 151
High neuraxial block	58	1:4336	1 : 3356, 1 : 5587
Respiratory arrest in labor suite	25	1:10,042	1 : 6172, 1 : 16,131
Unrecognized spinal catheter	14	1:15,435	1 : 9176, 1 : 25,634
Serious neurologic injury	27	1:35,923	1 : 17,805, 1 : 91,244
Epidural abscess/meningitis	4	1:62,866	1 : 25,074, 1 : 235,620
Epidural hematoma	1	1:251,463	1 : 46,090, 1 : 10,142,861

CI, Confidence interval; *N*, number of complications.
Data from D'Angelo R, Smiley RM, Riley E, Segal S: Serious complications related to obstetric anesthesia. The serious complication repository project of the Society for Obstetric Anesthesia and Perinatology. *Anesthesiology.* 2014;120:1505.

7. Answer: d

(see *Gabbe's Obstetrics* 8e: ch16)

A spinal headache occurs when, during the process of administering an epidural block, the dura is punctured with a large-bore (17 or 18 gauge) epidural needle. It is thought to be caused by loss of cerebrospinal fluid which causes the brain to settle downward when upright, stretching meninges and bridging vessels. Typically, a spinal headache is more severe in the upright position and is relieved by the supine position.

8. Answer: c

(see *Gabbe's Obstetrics* 8e: ch16)

Epidural analgesia does not increase the rate of cesarean delivery but may increase oxytocin use and the rate of instrument-assisted vaginal deliveries. In the past, significant controversy surrounded how to appropriately counsel patients regarding the effect of neuraxial analgesia on their labor course and risk of cesarean delivery. The most recent Practice Bulletin on this subject from the American College of Obstetricians and Gynecologists (ACOG) states that "Neuraxial analgesia does not appear to increase the cesarean delivery rate and, therefore, should not be withheld for that concern (Level A)."[5]

9. Answer: d

(see *Gabbe's Obstetrics* 8e: ch16)

Aspiration is a potentially fatal complication of general anesthesia and pregnant women are at high risk due to poor gastric emptying and reduced lower esophageal sphincter tone. Pressure on the cricoid is a critical part of a rapid sequence intubation, to compress the esophagus and thus prevent aspiration should regurgitation or vomiting occur.

10. Answer: d

(see *Gabbe's Obstetrics* 8e: ch16)

Enhanced recovery after surgery protocols for cesarean should include multimodal pain management using scheduled administration of nonsteroidal antiinflammatories (NSAIDs) and acetaminophen with opioids used only for breakthrough pain. In this patient with an allergy to ibuprofen, aspirin and all NSAIDs including Toradol should be avoided.

REFERENCES

1. Klöhr S, Roth R, Hofmann T, Rossaint R, Heesen M. Definitions of hypotension after spinal anaesthesia for caesarean section: literature search and application to parturients. *Acta Anaesthesiol. Scand.* 2010; 54:909-921.
2. Simmons SW, Taghizadeh N, Dennis AT, Hughes D, Cyna AM. Combined spinal-epidural versus epidural analgesia in labour. *Cochrane Database Syst Rev.* 2012;CD003401.
3. Practice guidelines for obstetric anesthesia: an updated report by the American Society of Anesthesiologists Task Force on Obstetric Anesthesia and the Society for Obstetric Anesthesia and Perinatology. *Anesthesiology.* 2016;124:270-300.
4. Moen V, Dahlgren N, Irestedt L. Severe neurological complications after central neuraxial blockades in Sweden 1990–1999. *Anesthesiology.* 2004;101:950-959.
5. Obstetric analgesia and anesthesia. Practice Bulletin No. 177. American College of Obstetricians and Gynecologists. *Obstet Gynecol.* 2017; 129:e73-89.

CHAPTER 16

17

Malpresentations

Vanita D. Jain

(See *Gabbe's Obstetrics: Normal and Problem Pregnancies*, 8e: ch17)

QUESTIONS

1. The sensitivity of Leopold maneuvers for abnormal fetal lie is:

   a. 8%

   b. 17%

   c. 28%

   d. 67%

   e. 89%

2. A 22-year-old G3P0020 presents in labor and her cervix progresses to fully dilated. When you perform her vaginal examination in preparation for delivery, you suspect a face presentation. The prognosis for successful vaginal delivery with face presentation depends on orientation of the:

   a. Occiput

   b. Brow

   c. Chin

   d. Maternal sacral promontory

3. You check a patient and note a fetal position with face presentation and mentum posterior. The patient's cervix is fully dilated and she has been pushing for 3 hours. The most appropriate next step is:

   a. Manual attempt to convert to flexed attitude

   b. Manual attempt to rotate to mentum anterior

   c. Internal podalic version with breech extraction

   d. Cesarean section

4. A 42-year-old G1P0 at 35 weeks gestation presents to the labor and delivery unit. Her cervix is fully dilated and she has been pushing for 3 hours. You go into the room to examine her and note a compound presentation. The fetal vertex is palpable but so is a fetal part. An ultrasound is performed and confirms a fetal hand. You repeat your examination to assess the hand location and now palpate a pulsating mass next to the fetal hand. The most appropriate next step is:

   a. Assess for placement of forceps

   b. Attempt to push the hand out of the way

   c. Attempt to push the pulsating mass out of the way

   d. Emergency cesarean section

5. The risk of cord prolapse with a compound presentation is:

   a. 0.5%–1%

   b. 4%–6%

   c. 11%–20%

   d. 40%–50%

6. When delivering the aftercoming head during a vaginal breech delivery, the Mauriceau-Smellie-Veit maneuver may be necessary. This involves a manual effort to maximize flexion of the vertex by applying pressure to the fetal:

   a. Mandible

   b. Maxilla

   c. Orbits

   d. Brow

7. A 27-year-old G1P0 is at her routine 36-week prenatal appointment. On Leopold maneuver, you suspect a breech presentation. Bedside ultrasound confirms this. The estimated fetal weight (EFW) is 2982 g. The fetus appears to be footling breech. The patient desires an epidural. She also desires a vaginal delivery if possible. The patient is 5 feet tall and weighs 220 pounds. After reviewing her obstetric history and assessing her pelvis you determine the most appropriate next step to be:

   a. Primary cesarean section at 39 weeks

   b. Trial of labor in the breech position at 37 weeks

   c. External cephalic version (ECV) this week in the labor and delivery unit

   d. No change to management, the breech will convert by 39 weeks spontaneously

8. A 32-year-old G2P1001 presents to your office at 39 weeks gestation and the fetus is suspected to be in the breech presentation. You perform a bedside ultrasound and note the EFW to be 3960 g, complete breech. She declines intrapartum fetal monitoring. The most appropriate next step is:

   a. Primary cesarean section at 39 weeks

   b. Induction of labor of a complete breech today

   c. Allow spontaneous labor to occur in the next few weeks, perhaps the fetus will spontaneously convert to vertex or frank breech position

   d. Transfer to maternal fetal medicine

9. A 28-year-old G1P0 presents with confirmed preterm premature rupture of the fetal membranes (PPROM) at 28 weeks and her cervix is 4 cm dilated. Despite the use of tocolytics the patient continues to labor to 7 cm. She has received one dose of betamethasone and magnesium for neuroprotection. At the time of this examination, it is noted that the fetus is footling breech. The EFW earlier that day on ultrasound was 2270 g. The patient now has a temperature of 100.2° F./38.0°C. Which of the following poses the highest risk for cesarean section?

   a. Cord prolapse with footling breech presentation

   b. EFW >2000 g

   c. A nontested pelvis; patient is a primip

   d. Concern for cerebral palsy (CP) from intraamniotic infection

10. A 32-year-old G1P0 presents to discuss her options for delivery of her dichorionic diamniotic twin gestation. She is at 36 weeks gestation. Fetus A is vertex and fetus B is breech. Fetus A measures 3230 g and fetus B measures 3120 g. You are trained and comfortable with breech extraction. You recommend:

    a. Scheduled primary cesarean section at 39 weeks

    b. Emergency cesarean section today, she is already 36 weeks with twins >3000 g

    c. ECV of twin B in the delivery room after delivery of twin A

    d. Induction of labor at 38–39 weeks, with vaginal delivery of twin A and breech extraction of twin B

11. A 29-year-old G1P0 at 37 weeks and 5 days gestation with dichorionic-diamniotic twins delivers twin A vaginally without difficulty. Twin B is breech. Using ultrasound you identify feet and start a breech extraction. As you are about to extract the head, the uterine tone increases and the cervix clamps down around the baby's neck. The most appropriate next step is to rapidly:

    a. Move to cesarean section

    b. Pull harder

    c. Administer IV nitroglycerin

    d. Cut the cervix

12. A 35-year-old G5P4004 at 35 weeks gestation presents for discussion of delivery options. Last week, your partner measured her fundal height at 39 cm. She had an ultrasound which showed the EFW to be 5150 g and the fetus is in the frank breech position. The amniotic fluid index (AFI) is 7 cm. She had an abnormal 1-hour glucose tolerance test (GTT) at 30 weeks, but then a normal 3-hour GTT at 33 weeks. In counseling for mode of delivery you recommend:

    a. Planned cesarean section at 39 weeks

    b. Offer ECV at 36–37 weeks

    c. Allow spontaneous labor and plan for breech vaginal delivery

    d. Plan induction of labor for breech vaginal delivery at 37 weeks

13. All of the following are factors predisposing to persistent occiput posterior (OP) position except:

    a. Body mass index (BMI) <30

    b. Nulliparity

    c. Macrosomia

    d. Anterior placental location

    e. Use of an epidural

14. A 35-year-old G1P0 comes to her routine prenatal care appointment at 35 weeks gestation with concerns about preventing an OP position. She states her sister had a "horrible labor and delivery experience," ending with an emergency cesarean section because "the baby stayed sunny-side up." She wants to prevent this from happening. After further questioning, you conclude that her sister's child had a persistent OP position. You recommend which of the following options to the patient?

    a. Hand/knees with pelvic rocking starting at 37 weeks

    b. Acupuncture

    c. Trendelenburg position every night

    d. Yoga

    e. No change in her current prenatal care

ANSWERS

1. Answer: c

(see *Gabbe's Obstetrics* 8e: ch17)

Diagnosis of the abnormal lie may be made by palpation using Leopold maneuvers or by vaginal examination verified by ultrasound. Although routine use of Leopold maneuvers may be helpful, Thorp and colleagues found the sensitivity of Leopold maneuvers for the detection of malpresentation to be only 28%, and the positive predictive value was only 24% compared with immediate ultrasound verification.[1]

2. Answer: c

(see *Gabbe's Obstetrics* 8e: ch17)

A face presentation is characterized by a longitudinal lie and full extension of the fetal neck and head with the occiput against the upper back (top figure). The fetal chin (mentum) is chosen as the point of designation during vaginal examination. For example, a fetus presenting by the face whose chin is in the right posterior quadrant of the maternal pelvis would be called a *right mentum posterior (RMP)* (middle figure). The labor of a face presentation must include engagement, descent, internal rotation, generally to a mentum anterior position, and delivery by flexion as the chin passes under the symphysis (bottom figure). The prognosis for labor with a face presentation depends on the orientation of the fetal chin.

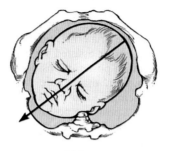

RMP

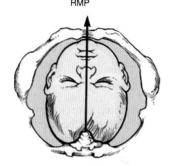

MA

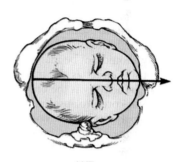

LMT

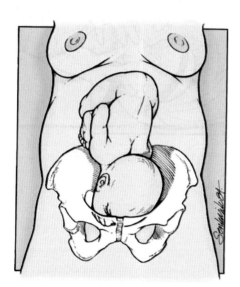

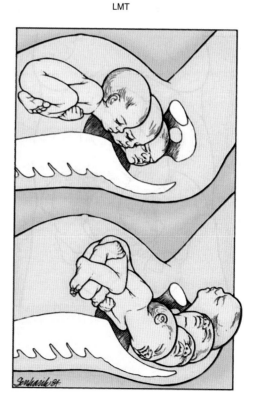

3. Answer: d

(see *Gabbe's Obstetrics* 8e: ch17)

Almost all average-sized infants presenting mentum anterior with adequate maternal pelvic dimensions will achieve spontaneous or assisted vaginal delivery. Persistence of the mentum posterior position with an infant of normal size, however, makes safe vaginal delivery less likely. Manual attempts to convert the face to a flexed attitude or to rotate a posterior position to a more favorable mentum anterior position are rarely successful and increase both maternal and fetal risks. As such, manual attempts to correct a face or brow presentation by flexing the fetal head during labor are contraindicated.

4. Answer: d

(see *Gabbe's Obstetrics* 8e: ch17)

Whenever an extremity, most commonly an upper extremity, is found prolapsed beside the main presenting fetal part, the situation is referred to as a compound presentation. The reported incidence ranges from 1 in 250 to 1 in 1500 deliveries.[2-4] The combination of an upper extremity and the vertex is the most common. Recognition late in labor is common, and as many as 50% of persisting compound presentations are not detected until the second stage. Again, although laboring is not proscribed, the prolapsed extremity should not be manipulated. However, it may spontaneously retract as the major presenting part descends. Cesarean delivery is the only appropriate clinical intervention for cord prolapse and nonreassuring fetal heart rate (FHR) patterns because both version extraction and repositioning the prolapsed extremity are associated with adverse outcome and should be avoided.

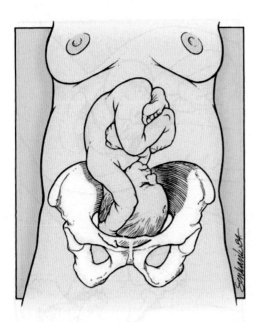

5. Answer: c

(see *Gabbe's Obstetrics* 8e: ch17)

Cord prolapse occurs in 11%–20% of cases, and it is the most frequent complication of this malpresentation. Cord prolapse probably occurs because the compound extremity splints the larger presenting part and results in an irregular fetal aggregate that incompletely fills the pelvic inlet.

6. Answer: b

(see *Gabbe's Obstetrics* 8e: ch17)

With further maternal expulsive forces alone, spontaneous controlled delivery of the fetal head often occurs. If not, delivery may be accomplished with a simple manual effort to maximize flexion of the vertex using pressure on the fetal maxilla (not the mandible), with the Mauriceau-Smellie-Veit maneuver, or using gentle downward traction along with suprapubic pressure (Credé maneuver; see figure). Although maxillary pressure facilitates flexion, the mother is still the main force affecting delivery.

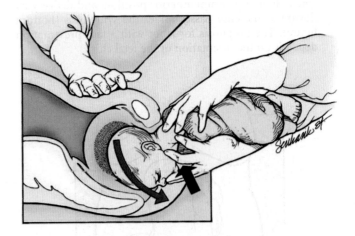

7. Answer: c

(see *Gabbe's Obstetrics* 8e: ch17)

Factors generally considered in making a decision to deliver a breech vaginally or by cesarean delivery are listed in Box 17.1. Certainly, in no case should a woman with an infant presenting as a breech be allowed to labor unless: (1) anesthesia coverage is immediately available, (2) cesarean delivery can be undertaken promptly, (3) continuous FHR monitoring is used, and (4) the delivery is attended by a pediatrician and two obstetricians, of whom at least one is experienced with vaginal breech birth. Primary cesarean section is an option, however, in this case, the patient prefers a vaginal delivery. In a trial of labor, planned vaginal delivery is associated with an increased risk of complications. It is unlikely the breech will convert spontaneously if it is already present at 36 weeks, but offering an external cephalic version (ECV) may be a reasonable option as well.

BOX 17.1   Management of Breech Presentation

A trial of labor may be considered if the following conditions are met:

- EFW is between 2000 g and 4000 g
- Presentation is a frank or incomplete breech
- Maternal pelvis is adequate
- Fetal neck and head are flexed
- Fetal monitoring is used
- Rapid cesarean delivery is possible
- Good progress is maintained in labor
- An attendant experienced in vaginal breech delivery is available
- Informed consent is possible

Cesarean delivery may be prudent if:

- EFW is <1500 g or >4000 g
- Fetus is in a footling presentation
- Parturient has a small pelvis
- Fetal neck and head are hyperextended
- Expertise in breech delivery is absent
- A nonreassuring FHR pattern is present
- Arrest of progress has occurred despite adequate contractions

EFW, Estimated fetal weight; *FHR*, fetal heart rate.

---

8. Answer: a

(see *Gabbe's Obstetrics* 8e: ch17)

As in the prior question, first assess if the patient is a candidate for vaginal delivery. Frank breech is preferred to complete breech position. The patient is declining intrapartum monitoring, which is a relative contraindication to breech delivery and induction. Allowing a spontaneous labor to occur can increase the risk of cord prolapse at the time of labor (in an uncontrolled situation). To offer a planned vaginal breech delivery the clinician must possess the necessary training and experience in the procedure. Furthermore, the relationship between the patient and the clinician should be well established, and the discussions of risks and benefits must be objective and nondirective, with accurate documentation of the discussion. If any of these factors are lacking, cesarean delivery becomes the safer choice. However, even if a clinician has made the choice that he or she will never prospectively offer a patient with breech presentation a trial of labor, the burden of responsibility to know and understand the mechanism and management of a breech delivery is not relieved. No one active in obstetrics will avoid the occasional emergency breech delivery, as such transfer to maternal fetal medicine is not recommended.

9. Answer: a

(see *Gabbe's Obstetrics* 8e: ch17)

The premature breech, the breech with a hyperextended head, and the footling breech are categories that have high rates of fetal morbidity or mortality. Complications associated with incomplete dilation and cephalic entrapment may be more frequent. For these three breech situations, in general, cesarean delivery appears to optimize fetal outcome and is therefore recommended. PPROM is associated with prematurity and chorioamnionitis, both of which have been found to be independent risk factors for the development of CP. Knowing the association of chorioamnionitis with periventricular leukomalacia (PVL), a lesion found to precede development of CP in the premature neonate, Baud and colleagues correlated the mode of delivery with PVL and subsequent CP in breech preterm deliveries.[5] They found that in the presence of chorioamnionitis, delivery by planned cesarean section was associated with a significant decrease in the incidence of PVL. Finally, the footling breech carries a prohibitively high (16%–19%) risk of cord prolapse during labor.

10. Answer: d

(see *Gabbe's Obstetrics* 8e: ch17)

The management alternatives in the case of the cephalic/breech twin pregnancy in labor include cesarean delivery, vaginal delivery of the first twin, and either attempted ECV or internal podalic version (IPV) and breech extraction of the second twin. The outcomes of another study of 136 pairs of cephalic/noncephalic twins weighing more than 1500 g allow us to conclude that breech extraction of the second twin appears to be a safe alternative to cesarean delivery.[6] A Danish retrospective evaluation of IPV for a noncephalic second twin demonstrated that, although it occurs only rarely, IPV is associated with fewer asphyxiated neonates than second twins delivered by cesarean delivery after a vaginal delivery of the first twin[7]; in addition, a trend was seen toward higher cord pH and higher Apgar scores in the IPV group. The Twin Birth Study, a multicenter randomized trial, showed that cesarean delivery of twins demonstrated no change in the rate of fetal or neonatal death or morbidity compared with vaginal delivery.[8] The authors of this study advocate that patients seek out providers who are skilled in the vaginal birth of the second twin. In the absence of a provider skilled and experienced in IPV and breech extraction, vaginal delivery of the first twin followed by external version of the second is a viable alternative, using ultrasound in the delivery room to directly visualize the fetus. Often a transient decrease in uterine activity occurs after the delivery of the first infant, which can be used to advantage in the performance of a cephalic version.

11. Answer: c

(see *Gabbe's Obstetrics* 8e: ch17)

During breech extraction, and perhaps more often with a breech extraction of a smaller twin, the fetal head can become entrapped in the cervix. In such cases, the operator's entire hand is placed in the uterus, the fetal head is cradled, and as the hand is withdrawn, the head is protected.[9] This splinting technique has also been used for the safe extraction of the breech head at the time of cesarean delivery. Head entrapment may also occur because of increased uterine tone or contractions. In this case, a uterine relaxing agent may be used, with nitroglycerin 50–200 μg IV being one of the fastest acting, safest agents in appropriately selected patients. Terbutaline or inhalational anesthesia may also be used.

12. Answer: a

(see *Gabbe's Obstetrics* 8e: ch17)

In general, reported success with ECV varies from 50%–75%, and a similar percentage of these remain vertex at the time of labor. Although many infants in breech presentation before 34 weeks gestation will convert spontaneously to a cephalic presentation, the percentage that spontaneously convert decreases as term approaches. A number of factors predict success of ECV with reliability. Successful version is reported more often in parous than in nulliparous women and more often with attempts at 37 to 39 weeks gestation than after 40 weeks. On the adverse side, factors associated with failure of ECV include obesity, deep pelvic engagement of the breech, oligohydramnios, and posterior positioning of the fetal back. In this situation it is the EFW > 5000 g and concern for shoulder dystocia if the fetus converts to vertex that is the contraindication to anything other than cesarean section.

13. Answer: a

(see *Gabbe's Obstetrics* 8e: ch17)

Factors predisposing to persistent OP position include nulliparity, BMI >30, macrosomia, the need for augmentation of labor, anterior placental location, race, pelvic architecture, and epidural analgesia.[10–13] The contribution of epidural analgesia to persistent occiput posterior has been a matter of debate.

14. Answer: e

(see *Gabbe's Obstetrics* 8e: ch17)

There are no interventions proven to be effective for the prevention of OP position before labor. A randomized trial with 2500 women demonstrated that a program of maternal hands and knees positioning with pelvic rocking from 37 weeks until delivery had no effect on the rate of persistent OP (8.1% in the treatment group versus 7.8% in the control group).[14] Though commonly recommended, the majority of randomized controlled trials have shown no effect of purposeful maternal positioning during labor for the prevention or treatment of persistent OP in the active phase or during the second stage.[15–18] None of these trials showed harm from such positioning, and some suggest improvements in maternal comfort levels.

REFERENCES

1. Thorp JM Jr, Jenkins T, Watson W. Utility of Leopold maneuvers in screening for malpresentation. *Obstet Gynecol.* 1991;78:394-396.
2. Breen JL, Wiesmeier E. Compound presentation: a survey of 131 patients. *Obstet Gynecol.* 1968;32(3):419-422.
3. Weissberg SM, O'Leary JA. Compound presentation of the fetus. *Obstet Gynecol.* 1973;41(1):60-64.
4. Quinlivan WL. Compound presentation. *Can Med Assoc J.* 1957; 76(8):633-635.
5. Ballas S, Toaff R, Jaffa AJ. Deflexion of the fetal head in breech presentation. Incidence, management, and outcome. *Obstet Gynecol.* 1978;52:653-655.
6. Gocke SE, Nageotte MP, Garite T, Towers CV, Dorcester W. Management of the nonvertex second twin: primary cesarean section, external version, or primary breech extraction. *Am J Obstet Gynecol.* 1989;161:111-114.
7. Jonsdottir F, Henriksen L, Secher NJ, Maaløe N. Does internal podalic version of the non-vertex second twin still have a place in obstetrics? A Danish national retrospective cohort study. *Acta Obstet Gynecol Scand.* 2015;94:59-64.
8. Barrett JF, Hannah ME, Hutton EK, et al. A randomized trial of planned cesarean or vaginal delivery for twin pregnancy. *New Engl J Med.* 2013;369:1295-1305.
9. Druzin ML. Atraumatic delivery in cases of malpresentation of the very low birth weight fetus at cesarean section: the splint technique. *Am J Obstet Gynecol.* 1986;154:941-942.
10. Lieberman E, Davidson K, Lee-Parritz A, Shearer E. Changes in fetal position during labor and their association with epidural analgesia. *Obstet Gynecol.* 2005;105:974-982.
11. Gardberg M, Stenwall O, Laakkonen E. Recurrent persistent occipito-posterior position in subsequent deliveries. *BJOG.* 2004; 111:170-171.
12. Cheng YW, Shaffer BL, Caughey AB. Associated factors and outcomes of persistent occiput posterior position: a retrospective cohort study from 1976 to 2001. *J Matern Fetal Neonatal Med.* 2006; 19:563-568.
13. Sizer AR, Nirmal DM. Occipitoposterior position: associated factors and obstetric outcome in nulliparas. *Obstet Gynecol.* 2000; 96:749-752.
14. Kariminia A, Chamberlain ME, Keogh J, Shea A. Randomised controlled trial of effect of hands and knees posturing on incidence of occiput posterior position at birth. *BMJ.* 2004;328:490.
15. Hunter S, Hofmeyr GJ, Kulier R. Hands and knees posture in late pregnancy or labour for fetal malposition (lateral or posterior). *Cochrane Database Syst Rev.* 2007;CD001063.
16. Stremler R, Hodnett E, Petryshen P, Stevens B, Weston J, Willan AR. Randomized controlled trial of hands-and-knees positioning for occipitoposterior position in labor. *Birth.* 2005;32:243-251.
17. Desbriere R, Blanc J, Le Dū R, et al. Is maternal posturing during labor efficient in preventing persistent occiput posterior position? A randomized controlled trial. *Am J Obstet Gynecol.* 2013;208:60. e1-8.
18. Guittier MJ, Othenin-Girard V, de Gasquet B, Irion O, Boulvain M. Maternal positioning to correct occiput posterior fetal position during the first stage of labour: a randomized controlled trial. *BJOG.* 2016;123:2199-2207.

18

Antepartum and Postpartum Hemorrhage

Audrey Merriam

(See *Gabbe's Obstetrics: Normal and Problem Pregnancies*, 8e: ch18)

QUESTIONS

1. A 38-year-old G5P4004 presents at 34 weeks gestation with vaginal bleeding. She denies any abdominal trauma. She is having some cramping. Her obstetric history is significant for four uncomplicated vaginal deliveries at home and she was planning to have a home birth with this child. She has been receiving care with a midwife in the community and has not had any ultrasounds. Fetal heart tracing is category I and she is having contractions every 5–8 minutes. On her bed you notice approximately 100 mL of bright red blood. The nurse states she has placed an intravenous cannula and drawn blood for laboratory tests. What is your next step?

   a. Commence magnesium sulfate for neuroprotection.

   b. Commence nifedipine for tocolysis.

   c. Perform a transvaginal ultrasound to evaluate for a placenta previa.

   d. Examine her cervix to see if she is in labor.

   e. Move to the operating room (OR) for delivery via cesarean section.

2. A 24-year-old G3P0020 presents at 37 weeks complaining of decreased fetal movement. She admits to using cocaine regularly throughout her pregnancy. She last used 4 hours ago. She does not have other medical problems. Her initial vital signs are temperature (T) 98.5°F, pulse 120, blood pressure (BP) 96/62, and respirations 18. She is having abdominal pain that has been worsening since she last used cocaine. The nurse is having a difficult time finding the fetal heart rate (FHR) and on a bedside ultrasound you diagnose an intrauterine fetal demise. You see a large echolucent area behind the placenta. After you inform the patient of the demise, she asks you how she should deliver now. What do you tell the patient?

   a. She will have a cesarean section because she has an abruption.

   b. She will have a vaginal delivery because the fetus is demised.

   c. The mode of delivery is up to her since she has a fetal demise.

   d. The mode of delivery will depend on laboratory evaluation and serial vital signs to determine if she is clinically stable.

   e. She will have a vaginal delivery because performing a cesarean section with an abruption could worsen a coagulopathy.

3. A 28-year-old G2P1001 presents at 36 weeks gestation with a new onset of vaginal bleeding. Her obstetric history is significant for one full-term, uncomplicated vaginal delivery. She has had regular prenatal care and her last ultrasound at 18 weeks showed a fundal placenta. Her first trimester screen results were low risk with a low Pregnancy Associated Plasma Protein A (PAPP-A) level (<0.2 Multiples of the Median (MoM)). She denies any abdominal pain, contractions, or recent trauma. Her vital signs are stable. Fetal heart tracing is category II. She is contracting once every 15–20 minutes. On speculum examination, you notice 50 mL of clot in the vault and a slow trickle of bright red blood from the cervical os, which is closed. On bedside ultrasound you confirm the fetus is cephalic and there is a fundal placenta. What is your diagnosis and recommendation for management?

   a. Suspected abruption and recommend vaginal delivery

   b. Suspected abruption and recommend cesarean delivery

   c. Suspected preterm labor and give steroids for fetal lung maturity

   d. Suspected abruption and give steroids and wait until 37 weeks for delivery

   e. Suspected preterm labor and give steroids and tocolysis

4. A 33-year-old G3P2002 has been admitted for the past 4 days after her first episode of bleeding with a placenta previa. She has not had bleeding since she was admitted and she has completed a course of antenatal steroids. The fetal tracing has always been reassuring and there are no signs of preterm labor. Prior to admission she had been receiving regular prenatal care. She is asking about going home because she is the primary caretaker for her two young children. Her mother lives with them and her husband works from home. They live about 1 hour from the closest hospital. Which of the following makes her a poor candidate for outpatient management?

   a. Placenta previa should never be managed on an outpatient basis after a bleeding episode.

   b. She does not understand the risks of a placenta previa.

   c. She is noncompliant with her care.

   d. She does not have emergency transportation to the hospital.

   e. She does not have a short commute to the hospital.

5. A 31-year-old G1P0 presents for her anatomy ultrasound at 20 weeks gestation. This pregnancy was conceived via in vitro fertilization (IVF). She has no significant medical or surgical history. On transabdominal imaging, a velamentous cord insertion is noted. She presents to labor and delivery with vaginal bleeding at 33 weeks gestation. The fetal heart tracing appears sinusoidal and there are no contractions noted on the tocometer. What is the most likely source of the vaginal bleeding?

   a. Vasa previa

   b. Placenta previa

   c. Placental abruption

   d. Preterm labor

   e. Vaginal trauma

6. A 42-year-old G5P0313 presents at 24 weeks gestation for a prenatal visit after an anatomy ultrasound demonstrated an anterior placenta previa with multiple large intraplacental vascular lacunae. Her obstetric history is significant for three preterm cesarean deliveries due to preterm labor at 34–36 weeks gestation. She is on 17-hydroxyprogesterone. Your hospital performs about 2000 deliveries a year and your blood bank currently does not have a massive transfusion protocol. You discuss your concern for placenta accreta syndrome and outline your concerns with the diagnosis and plans for delivery. What is the most important factor for minimizing her morbidity and mortality with this condition?

   a. Inform your blood bank of this patient so they can start to prepare now.

   b. Obtain an MRI to further characterize the extent of suspected placental invasion.

   c. Arrange a consultation with a placenta accreta syndrome center of excellence with a multidisciplinary team.

   d. Admit her to the hospital until delivery because of her preterm deliveries.

   e. Stop her 17-hydroxyprogesterone because she will be delivering preterm anyway due to the suspected placenta accreta syndrome diagnosis.

7. A 29-year-old G5P4004 at 37 weeks gestation has been undergoing an induction of labor for preeclampsia without severe features. During the course of her induction she developed persistent severe range BP and a headache; magnesium sulfate was initiated for seizure prophylaxis. Her cervix became fully dilated after she was on oxytocin for 20 hours and she is now beginning to push. You consider her potential hemorrhage risk after delivery. In addition to having additional uterotonic agents in the room, what steps will you take to minimize her hemorrhage risk due to uterine atony?

   a. Apply controlled cord traction and uterine massage, while awaiting placental separation and give a bolus of oxytocin after delivery but no continuous infusion because her Pitocin receptors are saturated.

   b. Apply controlled cord traction and uterine massage, while awaiting placental separation and do not give any uterotonics after delivery unless she starts bleeding.

   c. Immediately after delivery attempt a manual extraction of the placenta while initiating an oxytocin bolus followed by a continuous infusion.

   d. Have the patient brought to the OR prior to delivery and set up for a dilation and curettage (D&C) for placental removal following delivery while giving an oxytocin bolus to be followed by continuous infusion.

   e. Apply controlled cord traction and uterine massage, while awaiting placental separation and give a bolus of oxytocin followed by a continuous infusion after delivery of the infant.

8. A 25-year-old G1P1001 at 38 weeks gestation presented in labor and rapidly delivered a 3600 g male infant. Her prenatal care was only complicated by asthma requiring daily steroid inhaler use. The placenta delivered spontaneously, and a first-degree laceration was repaired, but now she is having continued vaginal bleeding. You estimate that she lost 650 mL between delivery and postpartum. The nurse was able to insert an IV cannula and gave an oxytocin bolus followed by a continuous infusion. You have also administered misoprostol 1000 µg per rectum and 1 dose of Methergine 0.2 mg intramuscularly. The nurse calls you 1 hour later because she has expressed another large clot from the uterus and the patient is bleeding again. Her vital signs are as follows: heart rate 118, BP 143/95, respirations 16. She appears pale when you walk in the room and you estimate she has lost another 200 mL. What medication do you call for next?

   a. Tranexamic acid

   b. Misoprostol

   c. Methergine

   d. Carboprost

   e. Oxytocin bolus

9. A 28-year-old G1P1001 just delivered a 4000 g infant vaginally. After delivery of the placenta, she began bleeding briskly. You administer an oxytocin bolus, administer misoprostol, carboprost, and Methergine. Anesthesia has started a 2nd IV line and you have moved to the OR to examine the patient for a laceration. You find no laceration besides the first-degree perineal laceration, which is not contributing to her blood loss. You place a tamponade balloon and it fills with 200 mL within 10 minutes. A second dose of carboprost is given, as is a dose of tranexamic acid. Anesthesia informs you they have had to start phenylephrine to keep her blood pressure at 80/50 and her pulse is now 160. They have sent a complete blood count (CBC), fibrinogen, and Prothrombin time (PT)/activated partial thromboplastin time (aPTT) but the results are not back. Upon reaching the operating room the patient's nurse informs you her total estimated blood loss (EBL) is around 2.5 liters total since delivery. What is your next step?

   a. Attempt to reposition the tamponade balloon.

   b. Call Interventional Radiology for a uterine artery embolization.

   c. Give another dose of Methergine.

   d. Proceed with laparotomy and hysterectomy for uterine atony.

   e. Place vaginal packing.

10. You are taking over call for your partner who has just completed a cesarean delivery on a G4P2022 who presented at 37 weeks gestation with the fetus in the breech presentation. Her obstetric history is significant for one prior vaginal delivery. Her cesarean delivery was complicated by a difficult delivery of the fetus due to the breech being deep in the maternal pelvis. There was a large left cervical extension, but she feels she was able to visualize the extension and the case was hemostatic at the end, without evidence of a broad ligament hematoma. The nurse calls you from post-anesthesia care unit (PACU) to state the patient is having moderate bleeding from the vagina, but her fundus is firm, and she is not passing clots. Her vital signs are normal. What is your next step?

   a. Tell the nurse to increase the oxytocin infusion.

   b. Place misoprostol rectally.

   c. Have the nurse administer Methergine.

   d. Call Interventional Radiology for a uterine artery embolization.

   e. Perform a speculum examination to see if the extension continues into the cervix or the vagina and needs repair.

11. You are rounding on the postpartum floor and see a 36-year-old G2P1011 who had a vaginal delivery of a 4250 g male infant yesterday. Her vital signs are normal except for tachycardia at 126. She states she feels a little weak and tired, she has pressure, and it hurts "down there." Your examination is unremarkable. Her postpartum day 1 hematocrit returns at 24% (from 34% on admission). Her EBL from delivery is listed as 400 mL and the nurse tells you she has a normal amount of lochia. You order a repeat CBC. The nurse calls you 2 hours later with the following vital signs: T 98.8°F, pulse 137, respirations 16, and BP 98/61. She states the lochia is unchanged, her fundus is firm, and she has started an IV fluid bolus. The patient appears pale and diaphoretic. What is your next step?

   a. Order the CBC now with blood cultures.

   b. Tell the nurse to give a dose of carboprost on your way to see the patient.

   c. Perform a digital vaginal examination to evaluate for a vaginal hematoma.

   d. Order a CT scan of the pelvis.

   e. Order an ultrasound of the uterus.

12. A 43-year-old G5P4004 presents at 40 weeks and 5 days gestation in spontaneous labor. Her obstetric history is significant for a cesarean delivery for breech presentation in her first pregnancy followed by three vaginal deliveries. She is requesting an epidural. Initial vaginal examination is 5/70/−2 and fetal heart tracing is category I. She receives the epidural and progresses in labor without issue. Her membranes rupture spontaneously and her cervix is 7/100/0. You examine the patient to place a fetal scalp electrode. You note 350 mL of bright red blood on the pad, the vaginal examination is unchanged, and the FHR is 70. When the nurse replaces the monitor, the fetal heart rate baseline is 70 bpm. What is the most likely diagnosis?

    a. Abruption

    b. Uterine rupture

    c. Vasa previa

    d. Placenta previa

    e. Placenta accreta syndrome

13. A 29-year-old G2P0010 has been undergoing an induction of labor at 39 weeks for chronic hypertension. Her BP readings have all been normal. Her history is significant for an elective termination of pregnancy at 13 weeks via dilation and evacuation. She has an uneventful vaginal delivery after a 36-hour induction of labor. The placenta delivers intact 23 minutes after the infant and a large amount of bleeding follows the delivery of the placenta. You attempt to perform a bimanual uterine massage but feel a firm mass just inside her introitus and when you push on the mass it does not move. What is your diagnosis and what are your next steps?

    a. Uterine inversion; call for assistance (nursing and anesthesia), ask for an additional IV line, relocate to the OR, and ask anesthesia to administer IV nitroglycerin.

    b. Uterine inversion; call for assistance (nursing and anesthesia), ask for an additional IV line, and move to the OR for a laparotomy.

    c. Uterine fibroid; call for assistance (nursing and anesthesia), ask for an additional IV line, and move to the OR to remove the fibroid.

    d. Placenta accreta syndrome; call for assistance (nursing and anesthesia), ask for an additional IV line, and move to the OR for a hysterectomy.

    e. Placenta accreta syndrome; call for assistance (nursing and anesthesia), ask for an additional IV line, and call Interventional Radiology for a uterine artery embolization.

14. You perform a primary cesarean delivery for a placenta previa at 37 weeks gestation. A postpartum hemorrhage secondary to uterine atony is encountered, resulting in a 1500 mL blood loss, and transfusion of two units of packed red blood cells is performed. Fifteen minutes after the transfusion is complete, the patient complains of shortness of breath and looks unwell. She has an oxygen saturation 88% on 10 L facemask, increased work of breathing, pulse 120, BP 88/54, respirations 28. On examination she has minimal lochia and her pulmonary examination has diffuse crackles. What is the most likely diagnosis?

    a. Postpartum cardiomyopathy

    b. Amniotic fluid embolism

    c. Retroperitoneal hematoma

    d. Transfusion-related acute lung injury (TRALI)

    e. Preeclampsia with severe features

15. A patient with von Willebrand disease that is not responding to Desmopressin (DDAVP) has a postpartum hemorrhage requiring a massive transfusion protocol. What is the most appropriate product to give her for blood product replacement that will decrease her chance of fluid overload?

    a. Packed red blood cells

    b. Cryoprecipitate

    c. Fresh Frozen Plasma (FFP)

    d. Platelets

    e. Albumin

16. Pregnancy is associated with all the following hemodynamic changes, **except:**

    a. Plasma volume expansion

    b. Increased fibrinogen and Factors V, VII, VIII, and X

    c. Decrease in red blood cell mass

    d. Increased cardiac output

    e. Decreased systemic vascular resistance

ANSWERS

1. Answer: c

(see *Gabbe's Obstetrics* 8e: ch18)

Although this might sound like a placental abruption—and the patient has risk factors for abruption (advanced maternal age and multiparity)—because she has not had an ultrasound, placental location has not been confirmed; an ultrasound should be performed prior to any vaginal examination to confirm there is no placenta previa. Steroids may be considered, and the patient may ultimately require a cesarean section but only after her diagnosis is confirmed.

2. Answer: d

(see *Gabbe's Obstetrics* 8e: ch18)

At this stage of the evaluation, it is unclear if the patient is medically stable. When there is an intrauterine fetal demise due to a suspected placental abruption (risk factor: cocaine use) the mode of delivery depends on if the patient is stable. If the abruption is large enough, it could lead to hemorrhagic shock and coagulopathy in the mother, and cesarean delivery is preferred to expedite delivery. If the patient is hemodynamically stable and does not have a rapidly worsening coagulopathy, a vaginal delivery is preferred.

3. Answer: a

(see *Gabbe's Obstetrics* 8e: ch18)

The most likely diagnosis is abruption, given the closed cervix and infrequent contractions. A low PAPP-A is also a risk factor for abruption. Given her gestational age, delivery is recommended, due to the increased risk for maternal and fetal complications, with expectant management and relatively reassuring neonatal outcomes with delivery at this gestational age. Delivery should not be delayed for steroid administration, and tocolysis should not be used in the setting of vaginal bleeding or suspected preterm labor over 34 weeks gestation.

4. Answer: e

(see *Gabbe's Obstetrics* 8e: ch18)

One of the four criteria for outpatient management of placenta previa is having a short commute to the hospital. Even though the patient understands the risks, is compliant, and has transportation back to the hospital from her husband and mother, the distance to the closest hospital makes her a poor candidate for outpatient management.

5. Answer: a

(see *Gabbe's Obstetrics* 8e: ch18)

Although the incidence is low, factors that should increase concern for vasa previa include velamentous cord insertion, bilobed or succenturiate-lobed placentas, assisted reproductive technology, multiple gestations, and history of second-trimester placenta previa or low-lying placenta. Because vaginal bleeding associated with vasa previa is fetal in origin, it will lead to nonreassuring fetal heart tracings and fetal anemia if the vessels are compromised.

6. Answer: c

(see *Gabbe's Obstetrics* 8e: ch18)

Ultrasound is the preferred imaging modality for placenta accreta syndrome, and MRI should only be used as an adjunct in certain cases. Delivery preparation includes consultation at a placenta accreta spectrum (PAS) center of excellence where multidisciplinary teams skilled in management of these conditions exist, including, but not limited to, maternal-fetal medicine specialists, anesthesiologists, advanced pelvic surgeons, urologists and/or general surgeons, blood conservation teams, interventional radiologists, neonatologists, and nursing teams. Additionally, blood banks at these centers should be equipped with a massive transfusion protocol.

7. Answer: e

(see *Gabbe's Obstetrics* 8e: ch18)

Three preventive methods for atonic postpartum hemorrhage are: (1) active management of the third stage of labor (controlled cord traction, uterine massage, and administration of uterotonic therapy), (2) allowing spontaneous placental separation, and (3) prolonged postpartum oxytocin infusion following delivery.

8. Answer: a

(see *Gabbe's Obstetrics* 8e: ch18)

Tranexamic acid is an intravenous antifibrinolytic drug that has been used for the prevention and treatment of hemorrhage. A large randomized trial demonstrated decreased need for laparotomy and maternal death when administered within 3 hours of the bleeding onset.

9. **Answer: d**

(see *Gabbe's Obstetrics* 8e: ch18)

Given the patient is hemodynamically unstable and has been given all uterotonic and coagulation agents without success, the next step is laparotomy and hysterectomy to treat her uterine atony with hemodynamic instability. The patient is too unstable to proceed to Interventional Radiology for uterine artery embolization. Methergine should not be redosed sooner than 2 hours from the last dose.

10. **Answer: e**

(see *Gabbe's Obstetrics* 8e: ch18)

Genital tract lacerations may occur with both vaginal and cesarean deliveries. These lacerations involve the maternal soft tissue structures, and fetal malpresentation is a risk factor. For diagnosis it is best to evaluate the lower genital tract superiorly from the cervix and progress inferiorly to the vagina, perineum, and vulva. Adequate exposure and retraction are essential for identification of many of these lacerations.

11. **Answer: c**

(see *Gabbe's Obstetrics* 8e: ch18)

Genital tract lacerations are the second leading cause of postpartum hemorrhage. Risk factors include fetal macrosomia. Vaginal hematomas result from delivery-related soft tissue often accumulating above the pelvic diaphragm and protruding into the vaginal-rectal. Depending on the extent of the bleeding, vaginal hematomas may or may not require surgical drainage.

12. **Answer: b**

(see *Gabbe's Obstetrics* 8e: ch18)

Strong risk factors for uterine rupture include prior uterine rupture, previous fundal or vertical hysterotomy due to cesarean delivery or myomectomy, induction of labor, and trial of labor after cesarean section (TOLAC) with increasing maternal age and parity. Clinical findings can include sudden development of a category II or III fetal heart tracing, a loss of fetal station, acute vaginal bleeding, abdominal pain, change in uterine shape, cessation of contractions, hematuria (if extension into the bladder has occurred), and signs of hemodynamic instability.

13. **Answer: a**

(see *Gabbe's Obstetrics* 8e: ch18)

Risk factors for uterine inversion include fetal macrosomia, rapid or prolonged labor and delivery, nulliparity, retained placenta, and placenta accreta syndrome.[1] It can present with brisk vaginal bleeding and inability to palpate the fundus abdominally. Diagnosis is made clinically with bimanual examination, during which the uterine fundus is palpated in the lower uterine segment or within the vagina. This complication necessitates rapid intervention to control bleeding. Moving to the OR is recommended. The uterus and cervix should initially be relaxed with intravenous nitroglycerin (50–500 µg), a tocolytic agent (magnesium sulfate or β-mimetic), or an inhaled anesthetic prior to moving to laparotomy.

14. **Answer: d**

(see *Gabbe's Obstetrics* 8e: ch18)

Transfusion-related acute lung injury (TRALI) is a rare lung injury from blood-product administration. The hallmark sign is sudden onset of hypoxemic respiratory insufficiency during or within 6 hours of blood-product administration. Additional findings include noncardiogenic pulmonary edema, hypotension, fever, tachypnea, tachycardia, and cyanosis. Given the proximity to transfusion, this is the most likely cause of the patient's symptoms.

15. **Answer: b**

(see *Gabbe's Obstetrics* 8e: ch18)

Cryoprecipitate is indicated for patients with coagulopathy and concerns of volume overload, fibrinogen deficiency, factor VIII deficiency, and von Willebrand disease. Each unit of cryoprecipitate should raise the fibrinogen level by 10 mg/dL and, unlike FFP, each unit of cryoprecipitate provides minimal volume (5–15 mL), so it is an ineffective agent for volume resuscitation.

16. Answer: c

(see *Gabbe's Obstetrics* 8e: ch18)

Pregnancy is associated with an increase in red blood cell mass of 20%–30% by term. Plasma volume begins to increase early in the first trimester and reaches its peak of 40%–50% by 30 weeks gestation. Cardiac output begins to increase in the second trimester and can be expected to reach levels of 30%–50% above nonpregnant levels, due to increases in stroke volume and heart rate. Systemic vascular resistance falls during pregnancy due to hormonal and postural related changes from the gravid uterus, which allows for maintenance of a normal blood pressure in the setting of increased plasma volume and cardiac output. Fibrinogen and many procoagulant factors (V, VII, VIII, X, XII) increase in pregnancy, contributing to the hypercoagulable nature of pregnancy.

REFERENCES

1. Coad SL, Dahlgren LS, Hutcheon JA. Risks and consequences of puerperal uterine inversion in the United States, 2004 through 2013. *Am J Obstet Gynecol.* 2017;217(3):377.e1-177.Epub 2017 May 15.

19

Cesarean Delivery

Rini Banerjee Ratan

(See *Gabbe's Obstetrics: Normal and Problem Pregnancies*, 8e: ch19)

QUESTIONS

1. Which of the following obstetrician/gynecologists is considered the "father" of the modern cesarean delivery (CD) for popularizing the Pfannenstiel skin incision and lower segment uterine incision?
   a. Hermann Johannes Pfannenstiel
   b. Ferdinand Adolf Kehrer
   c. Max Sänger
   d. J. Marion Sims
   e. John Martin Munro Kerr

2. A 27-year-old G2P1 at 39 weeks gestation is admitted to the labor and delivery unit for a scheduled elective repeat CD. Her past obstetric history is notable for one prior CD at term for arrest of dilation. Her pregnancy has been uncomplicated. Fetal heart rate (FHR) tracing is category I. She has no known allergies to medication. At what point should prophylactic preoperative antibiotics be administered?
   a. 30 minutes after skin incision
   b. Immediately after the umbilical cord is clamped
   c. At the time of uterine incision
   d. 60 minutes before skin incision
   e. Prophylactic antibiotics are not indicated for scheduled elective CDs

3. Which of the following is the most common indication for CD?
   a. Cephalopelvic disproportion (CPD)
   b. Prior CD
   c. Nonreassuring FHR pattern
   d. Fetal malpresentation
   e. Placenta previa

4. A 24-year-old G1P0 at 36 weeks gestation presents to her obstetrician's office for a routine prenatal visit. Her pregnancy has been uncomplicated thus far. She asks if a CD can be performed prior to the onset of labor as she is very worried that she will not be able to tolerate the pain associated with childbirth. She would like to have two children to complete her family. Which of the following is the most appropriate initial response to this patient?
   a. Advise against nonmedically indicated CD because of the association with increasing number of CDs and increasing risk of abnormal placentation.
   b. Inform her that perinatal mortality is several times higher with a planned CD at 39 weeks gestation compared with labor and vaginal birth.
   c. Provide reassurance that adequate maternal pain relief will be provided in labor.
   d. Schedule CD on maternal request at 38 weeks gestation.
   e. Schedule CD on physician request at 38 weeks gestation.

5. Which of the following terms best describes a CD wound?
   a. Clean
   b. Clean-contaminated
   c. Contaminated
   d. Dirty

6. A 32-year-old G1P0 at 41 weeks gestation is admitted to the labor and delivery unit in spontaneous labor. She remains in labor for 24 hours, but does not progress beyond 6 cm dilation. CD for arrest of dilation is advised. The FHR tracing has been category I throughout labor. She has no known allergies to medication. Which of the following should be administered as preoperative antibiotic prophylaxis?
   a. Azithromycin
   b. Azithromycin and cefazolin
   c. Cefazolin
   d. Cefazolin and clindamycin
   e. Clindamycin
   f. Clindamycin and gentamicin

7. A 36-year-old G1P0 at 40 weeks gestation is admitted to the labor and delivery unit in spontaneous labor. Estimated fetal weight is 3600 g. She progresses to full dilation and pushes for 3 hours, but the fetal vertex does not descend below 0 station. The FHR tracing is category I. CD for arrest of descent is performed. Intraoperatively, the vertex is found to be wedged into the maternal pelvis, and the head cannot be delivered easily, even after extension of the uterine incision. Which of the following is the most appropriate maneuver to perform next to facilitate delivery?

   a. Apply short Simpson forceps.

   b. Employ vacuum extraction.

   c. Apply fundal pressure.

   d. Reverse breech extraction.

   e. Inflate fetal pillow.

8. A 35-year-old G2P1 at 39 weeks gestation is admitted to the labor and delivery unit for scheduled elective repeat CD. Her past obstetric history is notable for one prior CD at term. Of note, the patient's body mass index (BMI) is 45. Her antepartum course has been otherwise uncomplicated. A low transverse CD via Pfannenstiel skin incision is planned. Which of the following steps should be taken intraoperatively to reduce her risk of wound complication?

   a. Closure of the parietal peritoneum

   b. Reapproximation of the rectus muscles

   c. Closure of the subcutaneous tissue

   d. Prophylactic wound drainage

   e. Staple closure of the skin incision

9. A 38-year-old G3P2 at 39 weeks gestation is admitted to the labor and delivery unit for scheduled elective repeat CD. Her past obstetric history is notable for two prior CDs at term. Each of her pregnancies has been complicated by significant hyperemesis gravidarum, and she does not desire future fertility. Informed consent for permanent sterilization was obtained 2 months ago. A low transverse CD via Pfannenstiel skin incision is planned. She requests that the most effective form of tubal ligation be performed at the time of delivery. Which of the following sterilization procedures should be performed at the time of CD?

   a. Modified Pomeroy

   b. Parkland

   c. Uchida

   d. Irving

10. A 21-year-old G1P1 presents to the emergency department with worsening pain and drainage from her incision over the past 12 hours. She underwent primary CD 6 days ago and was discharged 2 days ago in good condition. Her BMI is 43. She appears uncomfortable. Her temperature is 38.3°C (101°F). Blood pressure is 100/60 and pulse is 104. The skin around the incision is discolored and purulent drainage is noted. Upon gentle probing with a cotton swab, the entire length of the incision opens. The fascia appears intact, but the patient states that she cannot really feel the cotton swab touching her skin. Which of the following is the most appropriate next step in management?

    a. Wound debridement under general anesthesia

    b. Initiation of oral cephalexin therapy

    c. Vacuum-assisted closure of the wound

    d. Bedside irrigation, followed by reclosure of the wound with staples

    e. Initiation of intravenous, full-dose heparin therapy

11. A 33-year-old G2P2 admitted to the inpatient postpartum service reports increasing abdominal pain and foul-smelling vaginal discharge for the past day. She underwent repeat low transverse CD the previous day, after undergoing an unsuccessful trial of labor after cesarean (TOLAC). She was in labor for 36 hours after rupture of membranes. Her intrapartum course was complicated by chorioamnionitis, for which she received ampicillin and gentamicin while in labor. Her BMI is 28. She appears comfortable. Her temperature is 38.6°C (101.5°F). Blood pressure is 110/70 and pulse is 96. Exquisite fundal tenderness is noted on examination. No rebound or guarding are present. The incision appears clean, dry, and intact. Which of the following is the most appropriate next step in management?

    a. Initiation of oral cephalexin

    b. Suction dilatation and curettage

    c. Initiation of intravenous full dose heparin

    d. Irrigation and debridement of the wound at bedside

    e. Initiation of parenteral gentamicin and clindamycin

ANSWERS

1. Answer: e

(see *Gabbe's Obstetrics* 8e: ch19)

Between 1890 and 1925, more and more surgeons began using transverse incisions of the uterus. John Martin Munro Kerr (1868–1960), a professor of Midwifery at the University of Glasgow, popularized the Pfannenstiel skin incision and lower segment uterine incision and is considered the "father" of the modern CD.

2. Answer: d

(see *Gabbe's Obstetrics* 8e: ch19)

Prophylactic preoperative antibiotics are of clear benefit in reducing the frequency of postcesarean endomyometritis and wound infection in both emergent and planned CDs.[1] Prophylactic antibiotics should be given approximately 30–60 minutes before the skin incision to allow for adequate tissue concentrations; pharmacokinetic studies of cefazolin demonstrate that adequate concentration in maternal and amniotic fluid samples are attained 30 minutes after administration.[2–4] The preferred agent for prophylaxis is either a first-generation cephalosporin (e.g., cefazolin) or ampicillin.[5–8]

3. Answer: a

(see *Gabbe's Obstetrics* 8e: ch19)

The most common current indications are, in order of frequency, (1) failure to progress, also called CPD or dystocia (about 30%); (2) prior CD (30%); (3) nonreassuring FHR patterns (10%–20%); and (4) fetal malpresentation (5%–10%).

4. Answer: c

(see *Gabbe's Obstetrics* 8e: ch19)

Occasionally CD is performed on maternal request because of a fear of excessive pain and fear of damage to the vagina and perineum. Fear of childbirth is present in about 3%–8% of women, who should be reassured of the ability to receive adequate maternal pain relief in labor.

5. Answer: b

(see *Gabbe's Obstetrics* 8e: ch19)

Incision-site preparation is accomplished in the operating room through application of a surgical scrub. CD wounds are considered to be clean-contaminated. Chlorhexidine-alcohol scrub has been associated with a lower incidence of wound infection compared with povidone-iodine scrub.[9]

6. Answer: b

(see *Gabbe's Obstetrics* 8e: ch19)

The preferred agent for prophylaxis is either a first-generation cephalosporin (e.g., cefazolin) or ampicillin.[5–8] For women who have an anaphylactic allergic reaction to penicillin, either metronidazole or clindamycin and gentamicin can be used. No apparent advantage has been shown with more broad-spectrum antibiotic prophylaxis (e.g., azithromycin or metronidazole), except for women in labor or with rupture of membranes (e.g., preoperative azithromycin should be added to cefazolin in these women).[10]

7. Answer: d

(see *Gabbe's Obstetrics* 8e: ch19)

When the vertex is wedged in the maternal pelvis, usually in advanced second-stage arrest, reverse breech extraction (the "pull" method) has been associated with shorter operating time, less extension of the uterine incision, and postpartum endometritis compared with vaginal displacement of the presenting part upward,[11] but the evidence is insufficient to make a strong recommendation. Another method is the fetal pillow,[12] but this has been insufficiently studied to make a strong recommendation. Vacuum extraction or short Simpson forceps should in general be avoided because they are rarely necessary if the previously mentioned steps are taken.

8. Answer: c

(see *Gabbe's Obstetrics* 8e: ch19)

The parietal and visceral peritoneum are not reapproximated because spontaneous closure will occur within days, and nonclosure has been associated in several randomized controlled trials with less operative time, less fever, reduced hospital stay, and less need for analgesia compared with closure.[13] Rectus muscle reapproximation among women undergoing primary CD is associated with significant increase in the postoperative pain and analgesic requirements,[14] and is therefore not recommended. Closure of the subcutaneous tissue of at least 2 cm with sutures is associated with fewer wound complications—such as a hematoma, seroma, wound infection, or wound separation—compared with no closure.[15] Prophylactic wound drainage is not associated with benefits and should therefore not be performed routinely.[16–18] The transverse cesarean skin incision should be closed with subcuticular suture, rather than staples, because suture closure decreases the risks of wound complications by 57% (from 10.6% to 4.9%) and specifically wound separation (from 7.4% to 1.6%).[19,20]

9. Answer: d

(see *Gabbe's Obstetrics* 8e: ch19)

Irving first reported his sterilization technique in 1924 with a modification in 1950. A window is created in the mesosalpinx and the fallopian tube is doubly ligated, as in the Parkland procedure. The fallopian tube is then transected about 4 cm from the uterotubal portion; the two free ends of the ligation stitch on the proximal tubal segment are held long. The proximal portion of the fallopian tube is dissected free from the mesosalpinx and is then buried into an incision in the myometrium of the posterior uterine wall, near the uterotubal junction. This is accomplished by first creating a tunnel about 2 cm in length, with a mosquito clamp in the uterine wall. The two free ends of the ligation stitch on the proximal tubal segment are then brought deep into the myometrial tunnel and are brought out through the uterine serosa. Traction is then placed on the sutures to draw the proximal tubal stump into the myometrial tunnel; tying the free sutures fixes the tube in that location. No treatment of the distal tubal stump is necessary, but some choose to bury the segment in the mesosalpinx. Although this technique is slightly more complicated than the others, it has the lowest failure rate.

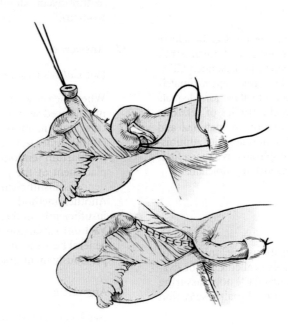

10. Answer: a

(see *Gabbe's Obstetrics* 8e: ch19)

Extreme wound discoloration, extensive infection, gangrene, bullae, or anesthesia of the surrounding tissue should prompt consideration of necrotizing fasciitis, a life-threatening surgical emergency that has been reported to develop in 1 in 2500 women undergoing primary CD. In these cases, the wound should be debrided under general anesthesia.

11. Answer: a

(see *Gabbe's Obstetrics* 8e: ch19)

Postcesarean endomyometritis remains the most common complication of CD. The diagnosis of postpartum endomyometritis is based on fever (100.4° F/38 degrees Celsius or more) with either fundal tenderness or foul-smelling discharge in the absence of any other source. The presence of chorioamnionitis, prolonged labor, and ruptured membranes should prompt early treatment in suspected cases. Parenteral antibiotics that use a regimen directed against possible anaerobic infection are the preferred therapeutic agents. A regimen of clindamycin and an aminoglycoside such as gentamicin is associated with improved safety and efficacy compared with other regimens.

REFERENCES

1. Robson MS. Can we reduce the caesarean section rate? *Best Pract Res Clin Obstet Gynaecol.* 2001;15:179-194.
2. Mackeen AD, Packard RE, Ota E, Berghella V, Baxter JK. Timing of intravenous prophylactic antibiotics for preventing postpartum infectious morbidity in women undergoing cesarean delivery. *Cochrane Database Syst Rev.* 2014;(12):CD009516.
3. Fiore MT, Pearlman MD, Chapman RL, Bhatt-Mehta V, Faix RG. Maternal and transplacental pharmacokinetics of cefazolin. *Obstet Gynecol.* 2001;98(6):1075-1079.
4. Elkomy MH, Sultan P, Drover DR, Epshtein E, Galinkin JL, Carvalho B. Pharmacokinetics of prophylactic cefazolin in parturients undergoing cesarean delivery. *Antimicrob Agents Chemother.* 2014;58(6):3504-3513.
5. Ziogos E, Tsiodras S, Matalliotakis I, Giamarellou H, Kanellakopoulou K. Ampicillin/sulbactam versus cefuroxime as antimicrobial prophylaxis for cesarean delivery: a randomized study. *BMC Infect Dis.* 2010;10:341.
6. Alekwe LO, Kuti O, Orji EO, Ogunniyi SO. Comparison of ceftriaxone versus triple drug regimen in the prevention of cesarean section infectious morbidities. *J Matern Fetal Neonatal Med.* 2008;21(9):638-642.
7. Rudge MV, Atallah AN, Peraçoli JC, Tristão Ada R, Mendonça Neto M. Randomized controlled trial on prevention of postcesarean infection using penicillin and cephalothin in Brazil. *Acta Obstet Gynecol Scand.* 2006;85(8):945-948.
8. Mackeen AD, Packard RE, Ota E, Speer L. Antibiotic regimens for postpartum endometritis. *Cochrane Database Syst Rev.* 2015;(2):CD001067.
9. Darouiche RO, Wall MJ Jr, Itani KM, et al. Chlorhexidine-alcohol versus povidone-iodine for surgical-site antisepsis. *N Engl J Med.* 2010;362(1):18-26.
10. Tita AT, Szychowski JM, Boggess K, et al. Adjunctive azithromycin prophylaxis for cesarean delivery. *N Engl J Med.* 2016 Sep 29;375(13):1231-1241.
11. Fasubaa OB, Ezechi OC, Orji EO, et al. Delivery of the impacted head of the fetus at caesarean section after prolonged obstructed labour: a randomised comparative study of two methods. *J Obstet Gynaecol.* 2002;22(4):375-378.
12. Seal SL, Dey A, Barman SC, Kamilya G, Mukherji J, Onwude JL. Randomized controlled trial of elevation of the fetal head with a fetal pillow during cesarean delivery at full cervical dilatation. *Int J Gynaecol Obstet.* 2016;133(2):178-182.
13. Bamigboye AA, Hofmeyr GJ. Closure versus non-closure of the peritoneum at caesarean section: short- and long-term outcomes. *Cochrane Database Syst Rev.* 2014;(8):CD000163.
14. Omran EF, Meshaal H, Hassan SM, Dieb AS, Nabil H, Saad H. The effect of rectus muscle re-approximation at cesarean delivery on pain perceived after operation: a randomized control trial. *J Matern Fetal Neonatal Med.* 2019;32 (19):3238-3243.
15. Anderson ER, Gates S. Techniques and materials for closure of the abdominal wall in caesarean section. *Cochrane Database Syst Rev.* 2004;(4):CD004663.
16. Gates S, Anderson ER. Wound drainage for caesarean section. *Cochrane Database Syst Rev.* 2005;(1):CD004549.
17. Hellums EK, Lin MG, Ramsey PS. Prophylactic subcutaneous drainage for prevention of wound complications after cesarean delivery–a meta analysis. *Am J Obstet Gynecol.* 2007;197(3):229-235.
18. CAESAR study collaborative group. Caesarean section surgical techniques: a randomised factorial trial (CAESAR). *BJOG.* 2010;117(11):1366-1376.
19. Mackeen AD, Khalifeh A, Fleisher J, et al. Suture compared with staple skin closure after cesarean delivery: a randomized controlled trial. *Obstet Gynecol.* 2014;123(6):1169-1175.
20. Mackeen AD, Berghella V, Larsen ML. Techniques and materials for skin closure in caesarean section. *Cochrane Database Syst Rev.* 2012;(9):CD003577.

20

Vaginal Birth After Cesarean Delivery (VBAC)

Thaddeus P. Waters

(See *Gabbe's Obstetrics: Normal and Problem Pregnancies,* 8e: ch20)

QUESTIONS

1. A 32-year-old G2P1 at 38 weeks gestation is diagnosed with preeclampsia without severe features. Her prior obstetric history is significant for a previous low cesarean delivery for breech presentation. The fetal tracing is category I and the estimated fetal weight is 3150 g. The patient desires a trial of labor in this pregnancy. The most appropriate counseling for this patient would be:

   a. Induction of labor does not affect the frequency of complications, including uterine rupture.

   b. The risk of uterine rupture is similar with all methods of induction.

   c. Repeat cesarean delivery is the preferred option for delivery.

   d. A trial of labor is appropriate but with avoidance of prostaglandin E1.

   e. A cervical examination is needed to make a final recommendation.

2. A 27-year-old G3P2 with two prior low transverse cesarean deliveries presents at 36 weeks gestation in active labor. The patient desires a trial of labor after cesarean (TOLAC). The most consistent sign suggestive of uterine rupture would be:

   a. Maternal vaginal bleeding

   b. Recurrent fetal decelerations

   c. A change in fetal station

   d. Uterine tachysystole

3. A 41-year-old G3P2002 at 36 weeks and 4 days presents to the labor and delivery unit complaining of leakage of fluid. Her obstetric history is significant for a postterm low transverse cesarean section due to nonreassuring fetal heart rate and a full-term elective repeat cesarean delivery. Her pregnancy has been complicated by maternal obesity with BMI 40 kg/m² and a large for gestational age fetus at 34 weeks (3000 g). On examination, she is confirmed to have ruptured membranes. Her cervix is 3–4 cm dilated, 90% effaced, and −1 station. Non-stress test (NST) is category I, and she is contracting every 10 minutes. Which of the following is the most accurate statement regarding contraindications to a TOLAC in this patient?

   a. BMI ≥40 kg/m²

   b. Inability to adequately monitor the fetus

   c. History of two previous cesarean sections

   d. Large for gestational age fetus

   e. She has no contraindications for TOLAC

4. A 31-year-old G2P1001 at 36 weeks gestation presents for a routine prenatal visit. She would like to discuss her options for a TOLAC. Her obstetric history is significant for a full-term low transverse cesarean delivery due to cephalopelvic disproportion. The operative report documents a single layer closure. That pregnancy was also complicated by Insulin dependent gestational diabetes and the infant weighed 4200 g. Her 2-hour oral glucose tolerance test (OGTT) was normal at her 6-week postpartum visit. She had an abnormal 1-hour GTT but normal 3-hour GTT this pregnancy. Her fetus was appropriate for gestational age at her growth ultrasound last week, with the estimated fetal weight at 40%. Her vaginal examination today is 1 cm dilated, thick, −3 station. Which of the following statements is incorrect?

   a. It is unclear if a single layer closure technique increases the risk for uterine rupture.

   b. Labor augmentation with oxytocin has been demonstrated to be safe at all infusion rates.

   c. Induction of labor with misoprostol (prostaglandin E1) is contraindicated.

   d. Estimated fetal weight >4000 g has a higher risk for failed vaginal birth after cesarean (VBAC).

   e. Nonreassuring fetal heart rate (FHR) patterns have consistently been reported to be the most common finding with uterine rupture.

5. A 30-year-old G2P1001 with one prior term cesarean delivery (documented as low transverse cesarean section [LTCS]) wishes to discuss her chance of success of a TOLAC. Which of the following factors are not a part of the clinically available assessment tools developed from the National Institutes of Health (NIH) that estimate the chance of success of a TOLAC?

   a. Maternal age

   b. BMI

   c. Prior fetal weight at delivery

   d. Maternal race

   e. Indication for prior cesarean listed as arrest of dilatation

6. The risk of uterine rupture is related to several factors except:

   a. Type of prior uterine incision

   b. Location of prior uterine incision

   c. History of unknown incision type

   d. Number of prior cesarean deliveries

   e. Time interval since last cesarean delivery

ANSWERS

1. **Answer: d**

   (see *Gabbe's Obstetrics* 8e: ch20)

   At present, based on the limited data that do exist, American College of Obstetricians and Gynecologists (ACOG) suggests that misoprostol (prostaglandin E1) not be used for third-trimester cervical ripening or labor induction in women who have had a cesarean delivery and that it is difficult to make definitive recommendations regarding the use of prostaglandin E2. Prostaglandins may be used for induction with a scarred uterus in the setting of fetal demise prior to 28 weeks gestation, as the risk of uterine rupture in this setting is low.

2. **Answer: b**

   (see *Gabbe's Obstetrics* 8e: ch20)

   Studies that have examined FHR patterns before uterine rupture consistently report that nonreassuring signs, particularly prolonged decelerations or bradycardia, are the most common finding accompanying uterine rupture.

3. **Answer: e**

   (see *Gabbe's Obstetrics* 8e: ch20)

   The following are selection criteria suggested by ACOG[1] for identifying candidates for TOLAC: one or two previous low transverse cesarean deliveries, clinically adequate pelvis, and no other uterine scars or previous rupture. Conversely, a TOLAC is contraindicated in women at high risk for uterine rupture. A TOLAC should *not* be attempted in the following circumstances: previous classical or T-shaped incision or extensive transfundal uterine surgery, previous uterine rupture, and medical or obstetric complications that preclude vaginal delivery.

4. **Answer: b**

   (see *Gabbe's Obstetrics* 8e: ch20)

   Cahill and colleagues reported a dose-response relationship between maximal oxytocin dose and the risk for rupture among women who attempt TOLAC. A limitation of this report is that it includes both women undergoing induction and those receiving oxytocin augmentation. At their maximal dose of oxytocin (>20 mU/min), these authors noted the risk for uterine rupture to be 2.07%. From these data, it appears that oxytocin may be used in women undergoing TOLAC, although higher infusion rates should be used with caution.

5. **Answer: c**

   (see *Gabbe's Obstetrics* 8e: ch20)

   Grobman and colleagues[2] developed a model based on factors that could be assessed at the first prenatal visit. These included: maternal age, BMI, race and ethnicity, prior vaginal delivery, prior VBAC, and a recurrent indication for the cesarean delivery. After development and internal validation of the model, it was found to be accurate and discriminating, and subsequently has been validated in populations other than that in which it was developed. The calculator is available online at https://mfmunetwork.bsc.gwu.edu/PublicBSC/MFMU/VGBirthCalc/vagbirth.html.

6. **Answer: c**

   (see *Gabbe's Obstetrics* 8e: ch20)

   The large multicenter Maternal-Fetal Medicine Units Network (MFMU) Network Study reported a 0.69% frequency of uterine rupture, with 124 symptomatic ruptures occurring in 17,898 women undergoing TOLAC.[3] The rate of uterine rupture depends both on the type and location of the previous uterine incision. Women with an unknown incision type do not appear to be at increased risk for uterine rupture. Women with a prior low vertical uterine incision are not at significantly increased risk for rupture compared with women with a prior low transverse incision.

REFERENCES

1. Committee on Practice Bulletins-Obstetrics. Practice Bulletin No. 184: Vaginal birth after cesarean delivery. *Obstet Gynecol.* 2017; 130(5): e217-e233.

2. Grobman WA, Lai Y, Landon MB, Spong CY, Leveno KJ, Rouse DJ, Varner MW, Moawad AH, Caritis SN, Harper M, Wapner RJ, Sorokin Y, Miodovnik M, Carpenter M, O'Sullivan MJ, Sibai BM, Langer O, Thorp JM, Ramin SM, Mercer BM; National Institute of Child Health and Human Development (NICHD) Maternal-Fetal Medicine Units Network (MFMU), "Development of a nomogram for prediction of vaginal birth after cesarean delivery," Obstetrics and Gynecology, volume 109, pages 806-12, 2007.

3. Landon MB, Hauth JC, Leveno KJ, et al. Maternal and perinatal outcomes associated with a trial of labor after prior cesarean delivery. *N Engl J Med.* 2004;351:2581-2589.

21

Placenta Accreta

Rini Banerjee Ratan

(See *Gabbe's Obstetrics: Normal and Problem Pregnancies*, 8e: ch21)

QUESTIONS

1. A 34-year-old G3P2 at 39 weeks gestation undergoes a tertiary cesarean delivery. Intraoperatively, the placenta is noted to invade the full thickness of the myometrium down to the uterine serosa, extending into the bladder. An emergent cesarean hysterectomy is required to control profuse bleeding. The uterine specimen is sent for pathologic evaluation. Which of the following is the most likely pathologic diagnosis?

   a. Placenta accreta

   b. Placenta increta

   c. Placenta percreta

   d. Placenta adherenta

2. What is the single most important risk factor for placenta accreta spectrum (PAS) disorders?

   a. Prior cesarean delivery

   b. Placenta previa

   c. Prior endometrial ablation

   d. Prior uterine curettage

   e. Adenomyosis

3. Which of the following findings on grey-scale ultrasound are most indicative of PAS?

   a. Myometrial thickening

   b. Marked hypoechoic retroplacental (clear) space

   c. Subplacental hypovascularization on color Doppler imaging

   d. Large or irregular intraplacental lacunae

4. A 29-year-old G4P3 at 32 weeks gestation presents to the labor and delivery unit with vaginal bleeding. She has a known placenta previa and a history of three prior cesarean deliveries. Upon arrival, she is noted to have approximately 100 mL of blood in the vaginal vault, but no active ongoing bleeding. An ultrasound is performed and shows significant myometrial thinning and other sonographic signs consistent with PAS. Betamethasone is administered. Which of the following is the most appropriate recommendation regarding delivery?

   a. Proceed with delivery now

   b. Planned delivery at 34–35 weeks gestation

   c. Proceed with delivery after fetal lung maturity is documented

   d. Planned delivery at 39 weeks gestation

   e. Proceed with delivery after the 48-hour course of betamethasone is complete

5. A 38-year-old G3P2 at 33 weeks gestation presents to the labor and delivery unit with painful uterine contractions and vaginal bleeding. She has a history of two prior cesarean deliveries. An anterior placenta with suspected placenta accreta was seen on antenatal ultrasound. Upon initial evaluation, the patient is noted to have profuse vaginal bleeding. Fetal heart rate is category II with recurrent variable decelerations and minimal variability. The decision is made to proceed with emergent cesarean delivery. Which of the following is the most appropriate intraoperative management?

   a. Proceed with general anesthesia

   b. Placement of ureteral stents prior to initiation of surgical procedure

   c. Perform transverse hysterotomy in the lower uterine segment

   d. Prophylactic ligation of the internal iliac artery

   e. Conservative management in which placenta is left in situ

6. A 41-year-old G2P1 at 39 weeks gestation presents to the labor and delivery unit for scheduled elective repeat cesarean delivery. Her antepartum course has been uncomplicated. Intraoperatively, massive hemorrhage is encountered after the placenta is manually removed, and the patient undergoes emergent peripartum hysterectomy. She remains hemodynamically stable throughout the case and is transferred to the recovery room for close observation postoperatively. Which of the following is the most likely reason for this patient to require surgical reexploration?

a. Evacuation of pelvic abscess

b. Repair of unrecognized injury to the ureter

c. Resection of small bowel obstruction

d. Repair of unrecognized operative injury to the bladder

e. Control of ongoing bleeding

ANSWERS

1. Answer: c

(see *Gabbe's Obstetrics* 8e: ch21)

Placenta accreta has been divided by pathologists into different grades according to the depth of placental tissue penetration into the uterine wall. These grades are as follows: "placenta accreta," when the villi simply adhere to the myometrium; "placenta increta," when the villi invade the myometrium; and "placenta percreta," when the villi invade the full thickness of the myometrium down to and beyond the uterine serosa into surrounding pelvic organs and vessels.

2. Answer: b

(see *Gabbe's Obstetrics* 8e: ch21)

The single most important risk factor for PAS disorders, found in around half of all cases, is a placenta previa. The risk of PAS increases with both the number of prior cesarean deliveries (CDs) and the presence of a placenta previa. The risk increases from about 4% in women presenting with a placenta previa and no previous history of CD to 50%–67% in women with previa and with ≥3 prior CDs.[1]

3. Answer: d

(see *Gabbe's Obstetrics* 8e: ch21)

The main gray-scale ultrasound features indicative of PAS are myometrial thinning, loss of hypoechoic retroplacental (clear) space, and numerous large or irregular intraplacental lacunae, creating a "moth-eaten" appearance of the placenta.

4. Answer: b

(see *Gabbe's Obstetrics* 8e: ch21)

Clinical factors such as prenatal bleeding episodes, placental position (i.e., low-lying versus central previa), and evidence of large invasive accreta areas should be considered when determining the timing of administration of antenatal corticosteroids and the optimal gestational age for delivery in women with PAS. A decision analysis suggests that planned delivery at 34–35 weeks of gestation without confirmation of fetal lung maturity is associated with optimal maternal and fetal outcomes.[2]

5. Answer: a

(see *Gabbe's Obstetrics* 8e: ch21)

Regional anesthesia may limit the ability to manipulate abdominal contents for retractor placement; thus, general anesthesia may be preferable for cases with a high risk of requiring a hysterectomy. After identification of placental location, the uterine incision site (hysterotomy) should be chosen, preferably away from the placenta. This may require a fundal or even posterior uterine wall incision. The use of ancillary procedures, such as prophylactic ligation of the internal iliac artery, is of little benefit because of extensive collateral circulation. Data on the use of ureteral stents to reduce the risk of ureteral injury are limited, and further evaluation is required before considering routine use for all women with PAS. Conservative management in PAS is not recommended in women presenting with major bleeding, as it is unlikely to be successful and risks delaying definitive treatment and increasing morbidity and mortality.

6. Answer: e

(see *Gabbe's Obstetrics* 8e: ch21)

Postoperatively, febrile complications and bowel dysfunction are relatively frequent. Reoperation is required in up to a third of women who undergo peripartum hysterectomy.[3,4] Among women who require reexploration, the control of ongoing bleeding is responsible for approximately three-quarters of cases. The remainder of procedures are for the repair of operative injuries, mainly of the genitourinary tract.

REFERENCES

1. Jauniaux E, Jurkovic D. Placenta accreta: pathogenesis of a 20th century iatrogenic uterine disease. *Placenta*. 2012;33:244–251.
2. Robinson BK, Grobman WA. Effectiveness of timing strategies for delivery of individuals with placenta previa and accreta. *Obstet Gynecol*. 2010;116:835–842.
3. Wright JD, Bonanno C, Shah M, Gaddipati S, Devine P. Peripartum hysterectomy. *Obstet Gynecol*. 2010;116:429–434.
4. Grace Tan SE, Jobling TW, Wallace EM, McNeilage LJ, Manolitsas T, Hodges RJ. Surgical management of placenta accreta: a 10-year experience. *Acta Obstet Gynecol Scand*. 2013;92:445–450.

Postpartum Care

22

Patient Safety and Quality Measurement in Obstetrical Care

Vanita D. Jain

(See *Gabbe's Obstetrics: Normal and Problem Pregnancies*, 8e: ch22)

QUESTIONS

1. In the study by Geller and colleagues examining cases of morbidity and mortality, how is a "preventable event" defined?

a. An event that could have been avoided by the health-care provider

b. An event that could have been avoided by delay in diagnosis

c. An event that could have been avoided by the system

d. An event that could have been avoided by the patient

e. All of the above were included in the definition

2. Literature exists that multiple contributors are involved in the occurrence of adverse obstetric events. However, which of the following appears to be consistently noted as a potential predominant etiology?

a. Provider error with patient assessment of illness

b. Resident training systems without appropriate supervision

c. Communication and systems issues

d. Competency of the covering attending physician

3. When discussing approaches to improve obstetric safety in a labor and delivery unit, all the following key components are required except:

a. Individual concerns

b. Group levels

c. Structural concerns

d. Global evaluation

4. Various examples of simulation training are described in the chapter on Patient Safety and Quality. In particular, simulation training has been shown to improve execution of action for all of the following obstetric complications except:

a. Shoulder dystocia

b. Eclampsia management

c. Postpartum hemorrhage management

d. Breech delivery

e. Performing a postpartum tubal ligation

5. You are interested in performing a research project on patient safety and quality. You are examining complications post-cesarean delivery. Which of the following is an example of a patient safety measure?

a. Degree of maternal care optimization

b. Degree of neonatal care optimization

c. Rate of retained surgical sponge "sponges" post–cesarean section

d. Measurement of a reduction in professional liability claims

6. You seek to design a study exploring the rate of neonatal hypoglycemia after steroid administration at your institution. This is an example of which type of quality measure?

a. Structural

b. Outcome

c. Process

d. Access

e. Patient experience

7. Which of the following would be an example of a patient safety and quality project that would assess a "process" measure?

    a. A retrospective chart analysis of the frequency of preterm birth in your institution

    b. Analyzing the number of board-certified Maternal Fetal Medicine (MFM) physicians on staff compared with adverse outcomes

    c. The frequency of group B *Streptococcus* (GBS)–positive women who receive timely and appropriate antibiotics prior to delivery

    d. The rate of elective episiotomy at the time of spontaneous vaginal delivery (SVD)

8. Checklists and protocols are an important part of quality and safety. All of the following statements are correct, except:

    a. Protocols are mandatory items for completion to lead the user to a predetermined outcome.

    b. Checklists are a list of action items arranged in a manner to allow the user to record the presence (or absence) of the individual items listed to ensure that all are considered or completed.

    c. Examples of successful use of checklists include central catheter line placement in the intensive care unit and administration of oxytocin on labor and delivery.

    d. The existence of a checklist on a labor and delivery unit will always result in improvement in care

9. You are very interested in the Perinatal Collaborative in your state and are looking for a project that relates to obstetric quality. When trying to identify a primary outcome to study, what criteria determine whether an obstetrical quality measure is a good one?

    a. A balance between maternal and neonatal outcomes

    b. Can be affected by a change in behavior within the hospital

    c. Be affordable to use not just in your hospital but across the state

    d. Be reproducible

    e. All of the above

10. You are designing a retrospective cohort study focusing on quality improvement within your hospital. You will be collecting data through a chart review. Your hospital utilizes an electronic medical record (EMR) for all charts after the year 2010 but paper charts for the years prior to such. Your study spans the years calendar years 1/2000 until 12/2019. As you are reviewing the patient charts, you realize that one of the advantages of an EMR is:

    a. The lack of clinical detail documented by the physician, makes your chart review go faster

    b. The time spent by physicians in documenting visits appears extensive as opposed to paper charts with brief and often illegible handwriting

    c. The ability to link inpatient and outpatient information

    d. The use of quick text or drop-downs

ANSWERS

1. **Answer: e**

   (see *Gabbe's Obstetrics* 8e: ch22)

   In their study, morbid and mortal events were often found to be preventable, and a *preventable event* was defined as one that could have been avoided by any action on the part of the health-care provider (e.g., mismanagement of patients, failure or delay in diagnosis), the system (e.g., failure in communication), or the patient (e.g., noncompliance).

2. **Answer: c**

   (see *Gabbe's Obstetrics* 8e: ch22)

   Despite the many factors that have been implicated in the occurrence of preventable adverse events, it is worth noting that communication and "systems" issues that transcend simple individual error have consistently been found to be predominant etiologies in the occurrence of these events. *Systems issues* is a term that refers to problems that stem not from one individual's actions but from the interconnected relationships of people and institutional policies.

3. **Answer: d**

   (see *Gabbe's Obstetrics* 8e: ch22)

   The potential need for a multifaceted approach is further suggested by the different levels within an organization at which these factors can manifest. Specifically, key components required for the prevention of adverse events occur at (1) the individual level, such as the level of education or training provided to workers; (2) the group level, as with team effectiveness and communication; and (3) the structural level, like the standardization of processes within an organization.

4. Answer: e

(see *Gabbe's Obstetrics* 8e: ch22)

Although simulation may have benefits for any type of obstetric procedure (e.g., vaginal delivery), it has often been studied in events such as shoulder dystocia and eclampsia. In these occurrences, simulation may be particularly helpful not only for the novice but even for experienced professionals, who can maintain their skills in managing unpredictable and uncommon events. Postpartum hemorrhage (PPH) and breech delivery are examples of uncommon events that lend themselves well to simulation training/practice.

5. Answer: c

(see *Gabbe's Obstetrics* 8e: ch22)

Measurement is required to understand whether safe care is being provided and whether changes in approaches to patient safety are actually improving the quality of care. Examples of *patient safety measures* are rates of retained surgical sponge or wrong-site surgery. A *quality measure* assesses the degree to which maternal and neonatal care is optimized.

Quality vs. Safety

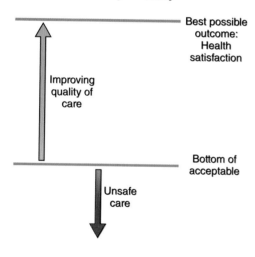

6. Answer: b

(see *Gabbe's Obstetrics* 8e: ch22)

Outcome measures, as indicated by their name, reflect patient outcomes. An example of an outcome measure would be the frequency of maternal mortality or neonatal hypoglycemia. Because obstetricians generally treat healthy women, adverse outcomes in obstetrics are relatively uncommon. Consequently, the usefulness of many outcome measures, such as maternal mortality, may be limited because most hospitals have few or none of these outcomes to measure. Furthermore, if outcomes measures are to be maximally useful and reflective of the actual care provided at a given institution, they need to reflect outcomes that the institution can actually affect and should be risk-adjusted to account for differences in patients that could materially affect the outcome of interest.

7. Answer: c

(see *Gabbe's Obstetrics* 8e: ch22)

Process measures reflect practices that physicians or hospitals actually use in their care of patients. An example of a process measure is the frequency with which women known to be GBS-positive receive appropriate antibiotics. If a process measure were to conceivably be an adequate reflection of quality of care, there should be evidence that the process is related to improved outcomes. The most central advantage of a process measure is that it gives direct insight into desired actions within the health-care system.

8. Answer: d

(see *Gabbe's Obstetrics* 8e: ch22)

These approaches have taken the form of *protocols*, mandatory items for completion to lead the user to a predetermined outcome, and *checklists*, a list of action items or criteria arranged in a systematic manner that allow the user to record the presence or absence of the individual items listed to ensure that all are considered or completed. Although both are concerned with standardization, checklists provide explicit lists of items, actions thought to act as a cognitive aid due to grouping related items in an organized fashion to improve recall performance. Nevertheless, a word of caution regarding checklists and protocols is warranted: The mere existence of one of these on a unit cannot be assumed to automatically result in improved care.

9. Answer: e

(see *Gabbe's Obstetrics* 8e: ch22)

A good measure should (1) balance maternal and neonatal outcomes—that is, it should not reflect improved care for one member of the mother-child dyad while embodying markedly worse care for the other; (2) have the potential to be altered by behaviors within the health-care system of interest; (3) be affordable and applicable for use on a larger scale; (4) be acceptable to stakeholders as a meaningful marker of quality; and (5) be reliable and reproducible.

10. Answer: c

(see *Gabbe's Obstetrics* 8e: ch22)

Paper-based medical records in particular are hard to obtain in a uniform manner for a population and are expensive to collect and abstract. Increasingly, EMRs have been used to provide the data for quality measures. These data are easy to collect within an institution and have clinical detail. However, because many different types of EMR systems exist, collating medical records information from many sources can be time intensive. EMRs have the advantage of being able to link outpatient and inpatient information, something that is very difficult to do with administrative data or paper-based medical records. EMRs, however, have been shown to increase work for the physician, with regard to documentation. The use of quick texts was developed to help with this situation but sometimes can result in documentation errors due to copy/pasting or inappropriate use of these "dot-phrases."

23

The Neonate

Eva K. Pressman

(See *Gabbe's Obstetrics: Normal and Problem Pregnancies*, 8e: ch23)

QUESTIONS

1. A 26-year-old G2P0101 comes to the labor and delivery unit at 31 weeks gestation with contractions every 3 minutes and light vaginal bleeding. She is placed on the fetal monitor, confirming the frequency of uterine contractions and a fetal heart rate (FHR) of 140 beats per minute, with moderate variability and accelerations but no decelerations. Ultrasound confirms vertex presentation and a posterior mid placenta. Cervical examination reveals that her cervix is 4 cm dilated, 80% effaced, and the vertex is at 0 station. She is started on multiple medications to curtail her labor and improve neonatal outcome should she deliver early. Which of the following medications will have the greatest effect on fetal surfactant production and improve neonatal respiratory status if the infant is born preterm?

   a. Betamethasone

   b. Magnesium sulfate

   c. Penicillin

   d. Nifedipine

   e. Terbutaline

2. Which of the following is part of the transition from fetal to neonatal circulation?

   a. An increase in pulmonary vascular resistance (PVR)

   b. A rise in left atrial pressure

   c. A decrease in systemic blood pressure

   d. Dilation of the ductus arteriosus

   e. Opening of the foramen ovale

3. A 29-year-old G3P2002 has a spontaneous vaginal delivery of a 3500-g male neonate at 39 weeks gestation. The tracing leading up to delivery had good variability and no decelerations. The delivery occurs after 40 minutes of pushing and over the course of two contractions. Just prior to delivery, there is a large gush of blood, and tracing the FHR becomes difficult to trace, but the infant is delivered within the next minute. There is no change in the maternal blood pressure or respiratory function. The infant is initially cyanotic and has poor tone, but with drying, stimulation, and supplemental blow-by oxygen, the infant does well and has Apgar scores of 6 at 1 minute and 9 at 5 minutes. What is the most likely cause of the infant's initial color and tone?

   a. Acute interruption of umbilical cord blood flow

   b. Chronic uteroplacental insufficiency

   c. Failure to execute a proper resuscitation

   d. Maternal hypotension or hypoxia

   e. Premature placental separation

4. A 32-year-old G2P0010 comes to the labor and delivery unit at 38 weeks gestation in active labor and progresses to a spontaneous vaginal delivery of a male infant without complications. After delivery, clamping of the umbilical cord is delayed by 60 seconds. Which of the following outcomes is due to delayed cord clamping?

   a. More rapid neonatal transition to extrauterine life

   b. Greater transfusion of blood from the placenta

   c. Lower risk of neonatal jaundice

   d. Improved neonatal outcomes in the setting of placental abruption

   e. Inability to place the infant skin to skin with the mother

5. A 25-year-old G1P0 undergoes a vacuum-assisted vaginal delivery due to a prolonged second stage. After delivery, examination of the infant's scalp reveals swelling over the parietal bone that does not cross the suture lines. What is the most likely diagnosis?

   a. Caput succenedum

   b. Cephalohematoma

   c. Subgaleal hemorrhage

   d. Subdural hemorrhage

   e. Depressed skull fracture

6. A 32-year-old G2P1001 undergoes a primary cesarean section at 27 weeks gestation for breech presentation and active preterm labor. The infant is placed on a radiant warmer that was preheated and dried with warm blankets but not wrapped. What is the biggest source of heat loss for this infant?

   a. Convection

   b. Conduction

   c. Evaporation

   d. Radiation

   e. Respiration

7. Which of the following is not a contraindication to breastfeeding?

   a. Maternal chemotherapy

   b. Maternal HIV infection

   c. Maternal marijuana use

   d. Neonatal galactosemia

   e. Neonatal phenylketonuria

8. A 37-year-old G2P0010 undergoes induction of labor at 34 weeks gestation for a pregnancy complicated by insulin-dependent pregestational diabetes and preeclampsia with severe features. After reaching full dilation, she pushes for 45 minutes with recurrent severe variable decelerations and has a vaginal delivery of a 1550-g male infant with Apgar scores of 4 and 7 at 1 and 5 minutes, respectively. The infant is taken to the neonatal intensive care unit (NICU) for observation and is noted to have a blood glucose of 35 mg/dl at 2 hours of life. Which of the following is not a risk factor for this infant's blood glucose level?

   a. Growth restriction

   b. Maternal diabetes

   c. Perinatal stress

   d. Preeclampsia

   e. Prematurity

9. A 27-year-old G2P0101 presents in active preterm labor at 28 weeks. Despite treatment with nifedipine, magnesium sulfate, and betamethasone, she proceeds to a vaginal delivery of a 1200-g male infant who is admitted to the NICU. On day 3 of life, the infant develops abdominal distension and bloody stools. Which of the following radiographic findings are not consistent with the diagnosis?

   a. Biliary free air

   b. Bowel wall edema

   c. Double bubble

   d. Free peritoneal air

   e. Pneumatosis intestinalis

10. A 36-year-old G1P0 has a spontaneous vaginal delivery of a 3700-g female infant with Apgar scores of 8 and 9 and no delivery complications. The mother's blood type is AB+. On day 2 of life, the infant is noted to have yellow sclera and orange skin. The infant has been exclusively breastfed and has been feeding every 4–5 hours. Laboratory tests reveal a total bilirubin of 15 mg/dl and a hemoglobin level of 19 g/dl. The infant's blood type is A−. What is the most likely etiology of the clinical findings?

    a. ABO incompatibility

    b. Dehydration

    c. Gastrointestinal obstruction

    d. Glucose-6-phosphate dehydrogenase (G6PD) deficiency

    e. Hereditary spherocytosis

11. A 7-day-old female infant is brought to the emergency department with lethargy. The infant delivered at home after an uncomplicated term pregnancy and did well until today, breastfeeding well every 2–3 hours. Head ultrasound shows a large unilateral intraventricular hemorrhage. What is the most likely cause of the clinical findings?

    a. Bacterial colonization of the gastrointestinal (GI) tract

    b. Biliary atresia

    c. Hyperbilirubinemia

    d. Dehydration

    e. Vitamin K deficiency

12. A 3650-g male infant develops cyanosis, grunting, nasal flaring, retracting, and tachypnea 2 hours after a scheduled cesarean birth for breech presentation. The pregnancy was uncomplicated and clear amniotic fluid was noted upon rupture of membranes on entry into the uterus. The chest radiograph shows prominent perihilar streaking and fluid in the interlobar fissures. What is the most likely diagnosis?

    a. Congenital pneumonia

    b. Meconium aspiration

    c. Respiratory distress syndrome (RDS)

    d. Spontaneous pneumothorax

    e. Transient tachypnea

ANSWERS

1. Answer: a

(see *Gabbe's Obstetrics* 8e: ch23)

Glucocorticoids are the most important and are used clinically to augment the synthesis of surfactant and accelerate morphologic development. Pregnant women with anticipated preterm delivery have received corticosteroid treatment since 1972. Numerous controlled trials have since been performed. Based on a metaanalysis, a significant reduction of about 50% in the incidence of RDS is seen in infants born to mothers who received antenatal corticosteroids, irrespective of sex, race, or ethnicity.

2. Answer: b

(see *Gabbe's Obstetrics* 8e: ch23)

With delivery, a variety of factors interact to decrease PVR acutely; these include mechanical ventilation, increased oxygen tension, and the production of endothelium-derived relaxing factor or nitric oxide. With the increase in pulmonary flow, left atrial return increases with a rise in left atrial pressure (Table 23.1). In addition, with the removal of the placenta, inferior vena cava (IVC) return to the right atrium is diminished. The foramen ovale is a flap valve, and when left atrial pressure increases over that on the right side, the opening is functionally closed. With occlusion of the umbilical cord, the low-resistance placental circulation is interrupted, which causes an increase in systemic pressure. Ductal closure occurs in two phases: constriction and anatomic occlusion. Initially, the muscular wall constricts, followed by permanent closure achieved by endothelial destruction, subintimal proliferation, and connective tissue formation.

TABLE 23.1 **Differences Between Fetal and Neonatal Blood Pressures in the Cardiac Circulation**		
	Fetal (mm Hg)	**Neonatal (mm Hg)**
Right atrium	4	5
Right ventricle	65/10	40/5
Pulmonary artery	65/40	40/25
Left atrium	3	7
Left ventricle	60/7	70/10
Aorta	60/40	70/45

From Nelson NM. Respiration and circulation after birth. In Smith CA, Nelson NM (eds): The Physiology of the Newborn Infant, 4th ed; 1976:117. Courtesy of Charles C Thomas Publisher, Ltd., Springfield, Illinois.

3. Answer: e

(see *Gabbe's Obstetrics* 8e: ch23)

Even normal infants may experience some limitation of oxygenation (asphyxia) during the birth process. A variety of circumstances can exaggerate this problem and can result in respiratory depression in the infant, including (1) acute interruption of umbilical blood flow, as occurs during cord compression; (2) premature placental separation; (3) maternal hypotension or hypoxia; (4) any of the above-mentioned problems superimposed on chronic uteroplacental insufficiency; and (5) failure to execute a proper resuscitation. Other contributing factors include anesthetics and analgesics used in the mother, mode and difficulty of delivery, maternal health, and prematurity.

4. Answer: b

(see *Gabbe's Obstetrics* 8e: ch23)

According to the Neonatal Resuscitation Program, the optimal timing for cord clamping for most vigorous term and preterm newborns should be between 30 and 60 seconds. During the period between birth and clamping of the cord, the initial steps of resuscitation should be commenced. This includes thermoregulation, which for a term newborn may include placing the baby skin to skin on the mother's chest or abdomen. Historically, clamping and cutting of the umbilical cord took place within seconds; however, it has been found that delaying this separation of the newborn from the placental circulation for 30 to 60 seconds results in (1) a more gradual perinatal transition after birth, (2) transfusion of placental blood to the newborn, and (3) a variety of improved outcomes. This practice is now endorsed for preterm births by the American College of Obstetricians and Gynecologists, although specific patient populations and situations require further study. In cases where there has been a disruption of the placental circulation, like abruption, previa with bleeding, and cord avulsion, the cord should be clamped immediately after birth.

5. Answer: b

(see *Gabbe's Obstetrics* 8e: ch23)

A caput succedaneum is superficial hemorrhagic edema resulting from pressure applied to the scalp and skull during delivery. On physical examination, this boggy and diffuse swelling crosses suture lines and rarely needs intervention. A cephalohematoma occurs in 0.2% to 2.5% of live births. Caused by rupture of blood vessels that traverse from the skull to the periosteum, the bleeding is subperiosteal and is therefore limited by suture lines; the most common site of bleeding is over the parietal bones. Associations include prolonged or difficult labor and mechanical trauma from operative vaginal delivery. Linear skull fractures beneath the hematoma have been reported in 5.4% of cases but are of no major consequence except in the unlikely event that a leptomeningeal cyst develops. Most cephalohematomas are reabsorbed in 2 weeks to 3 months. Subgaleal bleeds, which are not limited by suture lines, can occur in association with vacuum extraction alone—especially with multiple pop-offs and prolonged traction—in combination with the use of forceps or with difficult forceps deliveries, and they can result in life-threatening anemia, hypotension, or consumptive coagulopathy. Depressed skull fractures are also seen in neonates, but most do not require surgical elevations. With improvements in obstetric care, subdural hemorrhages fortunately are now rare. Three major varieties of subdural bleeds have been described: (1) posterior fossa hematomas due to tentorial laceration with rupture of the straight sinus, vein of Galen, or transverse sinus or due to occipital osteodiastasis (a separation between the squamous and lateral portions of the occipital bone); (2) falx laceration, with rupture of the inferior sagittal sinus; and (3) rupture of the superficial cerebral veins. The clinical symptoms are related to the location of bleeding.

6. Answer: c

(see *Gabbe's Obstetrics* 8e: ch23)

Radiant heat loss, heat transfer from a warmer to a cooler object that is not in contact, depends on the temperature gradient between the objects. Heat loss by convection to the surrounding gaseous environment depends on air speed and temperature. Conduction, heat loss to a contacting cooler object, is minimal in most circumstances. Heat loss by evaporation is cooling secondary to water loss at the rate of 0.6 cal/g water evaporated and is affected by relative humidity, air speed, exposed surface area, and skin permeability. In infants in excessively warm environments, such as those under overhead radiant heat sources, or in very immature infants with thin, permeable skin, evaporative losses increase considerably.

7. Answer: c

(see *Gabbe's Obstetrics* 8e: ch23)

Few contraindications to breastfeeding exist. Infants with galactosemia should not ingest lactose-containing milk. Infants with other inborn errors of metabolism such as phenylketonuria may ingest some human milk with close monitoring of the amount. Most medications do not contraindicate breastfeeding, but a few exceptions do exist. The Academy of Breastfeeding Medicine and the American Academy of Pediatrics (AAP) have written policy statements guiding clinicians on breastfeeding and use of breast milk in drug-dependent women. Relative contraindications to breastfeeding and use of maternal breast milk include positive maternal toxicology screen for substances other than marijuana at delivery, absence of prenatal care, and no plan for postpartum substance abuse treatment and chronic alcohol use. Transmission of some viral infections via breast milk is a concern as well. Mothers who are HIV-positive should not breastfeed if safe and effective alternatives to breast milk are available.

8. Answer: d

(see *Gabbe's Obstetrics* 8e: ch23)

Infants at risk for low blood glucose concentrations and in whom glucose should be monitored include preterm infants, small for gestational age (SGA) infants, hyperinsulinemic infants (infant of a diabetic mother [IDM]), large for gestational age (LGA) infants, and infants with perinatal stress or asphyxia. As in term babies, blood glucose drops after birth in preterm babies, but they are less able to mount a counterregulatory response. In addition, the presence of respiratory distress, hypothermia, and other factors can increase glucose demand and exacerbate hypoglycemia. SGA infants are at risk for hypoglycemia resulting from rapidly utilized glycogen stores and impaired gluconeogenesis and ketogenesis. Hyperinsulinemia occurs in IDMs.

9. Answer: c

(see *Gabbe's Obstetrics* 8e: ch23)

Necrotizing enterocolitis (NEC) is the most common acquired GI emergency in the NICU. This disorder predominantly affects premature infants, with higher incidences present with decreasing gestational age. Clinically, the spectrum of disease varies from a mild GI disturbance to a rapid fulminant course characterized by intestinal gangrene, perforation, sepsis, and shock. The hallmark symptoms are abdominal distension, ileus, delayed gastric emptying, and bloody stools. The radiographic findings are bowel wall edema, pneumatosis intestinalis, biliary free air, and free peritoneal air.

10. **Answer: b**

(see *Gabbe's Obstetrics* 8e: ch23)

The most common problem encountered in a term nursery population is jaundice. "Jaundice" is the visible manifestation of elevated serum concentrations of bilirubin. Neonatal hyperbilirubinemia occurs when the normal pathways of bilirubin metabolism and excretion are altered. Red blood cells (RBC), Reticuloendothelium system (RE system).

The normal destruction of circulating red cells accounts for about 75% of the newborn's daily bilirubin production. Feto-maternal blood group incompatibilities—ABO, Rh, and other minor antibodies—are the most common cause of hemolysis in the neonatal period. Other causes of hemolysis include genetic disorders: specifically, hereditary spherocytosis and nonspherocytic hemolytic anemias, such as G6PD deficiency. The majority of neonatal jaundice necessitating treatment is not caused by increased production of bilirubin (hemolysis, etc.), but rather decreased excretion of bilirubin. A strong association exists between breastfeeding and neonatal hyperbilirubinemia. Breastfed infants as a whole have higher bilirubin levels over the first 3 to 5 days of life than their formula-fed counterparts. Suggested mechanisms for breastfeeding-associated jaundice include decreased early caloric intake, inhibitors of bilirubin conjugation in breast milk, and increased intestinal reabsorption of bilirubin. In some patients, overlap is considerable in these described syndromes. This jaundice is early onset, occurring in the first 2–4 days of life, and associated with evidence of poor intake, excessive weight loss, and dehydration. This early jaundice is responsive to increased frequency of breastfeeding.

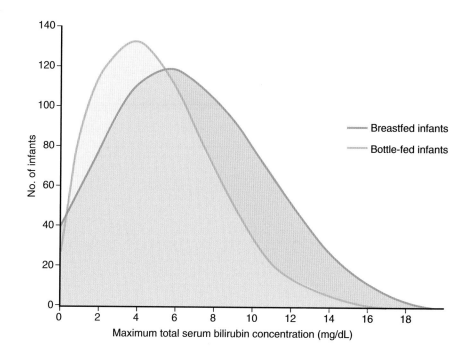

11. **Answer: e**

(see *Gabbe's Obstetrics* 8e: ch23)

Vitamin K is an essential cofactor for the carboxylation process of factors II, VII, IX, and X. Poor placental transfer of vitamin K, inadequate dietary intake especially in breastfed infants, and insufficient colonic bacterial colonization at birth place newborns at risk for vitamin K deficient bleeding (VKDB). Classic VKDB occurs between 2 and 7 days of life and is primarily secondary to inadequate dietary intake of vitamin K. Late VKDB arises after day 8, peaking at 3–8 weeks, and usually presents in exclusively breastfed infants who either did not receive vitamin K at birth, were given oral vitamin K, or had a condition (biliary atresion, cystic fibrosis, etc.) that impairs intestinal absorption of vitamin K.

12. **Answer: e**

(see *Gabbe's Obstetrics* 8e: ch23)

The presentation of respiratory distress is among the most common symptom complexes seen in the newborn and may be secondary to both noncardiopulmonary and cardiopulmonary etiologies. The syndrome of transient tachypnea presents as respiratory distress in nonasphyxiated term infants or slightly preterm infants. The clinical features include various combinations of cyanosis, grunting, nasal flaring, retracting, and tachypnea during the first hours after birth. The chest radiograph is the key to the diagnosis, with prominent perihilar streaking and fluid in the interlobar fissures. The symptoms generally subside in 12 to 24 hours, although they can persist longer. The preferred explanation for the clinical features is delayed reabsorption of fetal lung fluid. Transient tachypnea is seen more commonly in infants delivered by elective cesarean section.

24

Postpartum Care and Long-Term Health Considerations

Vanita D. Jain

(See *Gabbe's Obstetrics: Normal and Problem Pregnancies* 8e: ch24)

QUESTIONS

1. A 17-year-old G1P1001 calls the office on postpartum day 12 concerned about her bleeding. She is brought into the office and her examination is normal with no evidence of acute hemorrhage. What is the next appropriate step?

a. MRI

b. Reassurance

c. CT-angiogram

d. Pelvic ultrasound

e. Dilation and curettage

2. A 22-year-old G3P3003 comes in for her postpartum visit. She is interested in contraception. She is breastfeeding and says that she read on the internet this is adequate for contraception. You counsel her that if she is exclusively breastfeeding, on demand, with no scheduling, pumping or formula supplementation, then the likelihood of ovulation in the first 6 months is approximately:

a. 1%

b. 1%–5%

c. 10%

d. 20%

3. A 40-year-old G1P0101 presents for her second postpartum visit. She is very concerned that it has been 7 weeks and she has not lost any weight. You review that for most women, postpartum weight loss does not typically occur rapidly. She is interested in options for weight loss. You counsel that which of the following methods is the most effective:

a. High-intensity interval training

b. Exclusive breastfeeding

c. Diet and moderate exercise in combination

d. Strength training alone

4. A 26-year-old G1P1001 is in the hospital on postpartum day 2 from her uncomplicated vaginal delivery. She is ready to go home. Her blood type is A+. In discussing and preparing her paperwork, which of the following is also recommended?

a. Prescription for oxycontin for pain management

b. Administration of RhoGAM

c. Administration of her tetanus, diphtheria, pertussis vaccine if not given during pregnancy

d. HIV testing prior to discharge

5. The nurse from the postpartum floor calls you to see a patient with a fever. The patient is a 19-year-old G1P1001 postoperative day 1 following low transverse cesarean delivery for arrest of descent. Her temperature is 102.2F/39°C. The most common cause of postpartum fever is:

a. Urinary tract infection

b. Pneumonia

c. Mastitis

d. Endometritis

e. Wound cellulitis

6. A 29-year-old G2P2002 presents to you for preconception counseling. She would like her intrauterine device (IUD) removed and is excited to attempt to conceive. She would like to get pregnant immediately, preferably next month. She had her last child 3 months ago. It was an uncomplicated full-term vaginal delivery. In counseling about family planning, you discuss that short interpregnancy intervals, especially those <18 months, are significantly associated with all of the following risks except:

a. Low birth weight

b. Preterm delivery

c. Neonatal/infant death

d. Preeclampsia

7. A 32-year-old G2P2002 is about to be discharged from the hospital after a normal uncomplicated vaginal delivery. You review postpartum contraception options with her. During counseling, she states she would like the method that is the most reliable. When counseling, you explain the most effective postpartum birth control option for her is:

a. levonorgestrel-intrauterine device (LNG-IUD)

b. Combined oral contraceptives

c. Condoms

d. Depo (DMPA)

8. A 32-year-old G5P4105 presents for her postpartum visit. She wishes to discuss her contraceptive options. She is not interested in future childbearing, but she is interested in reliable, safe, and permanent sterilization. Which of the following statements is true?

a. The risks of the procedure include risk of lung injury.

b. Failure of the sterilization can be identified by β-hCG levels immediately post procedure.

c. The rate of regret for woman over the age of 30 is 30%.

d. The rate of regret for woman over the age of 30 is 5%.

9. A 17-year-old G1P1001 presents to the office for evaluation. She recently experienced a stillbirth at 22 weeks. She reports her mood is "ok" and she has returned to school. It has been about 14 weeks since delivery. When questioned more about her mood, she reports she feels sad when she sees babies at the playground, has general all over body aches, sleeps a lot, and still feels tired. She is also very anxious about her upcoming examinations and passing to obtain her General Education Diploma (GED) on time. You are concerned for postpartum depression, but also plan to obtain what laboratory tests?

a. β-hCG

b. Thyroid stimulating hormone (TSH), Free Thyroxine 4 (FT4)

c. Follicle stimulating hormone (FSH), Luteinizing hormone (LH)

d. Cortisol levels

10. You are seeing a 29-year-old G3P2012 in the hospital on postpartum day 2. She is interested in obtaining the single rod implant and would like it placed prior to discharge. She is breastfeeding her child and anticipates breastfeeding for at least 6 months as she did with her first. When counseling about the pros/cons of this method, all of the following statements are true except:

a. The implant contains etonogestrel, which acts primarily to inhibit ovulation.

b. The bleeding patterns for this device are unpredictable.

c. The implant is effective for up to 3 years.

d. The implant can cause a decrease in breast milk volume and production.

ANSWERS

1. Answer: b

(see *Gabbe's Obstetrics* 8e: ch24)

Postpartum uterine discharge or lochia begins as a flow of blood lasting several hours, rapidly diminishing to a reddish brown discharge through the third or fourth day postpartum. This is followed by a transition to a mucopurulent, somewhat malodorous discharge, called *lochia serosa*, requiring a change of several perineal pads per day. The median duration of lochia serosa is 22 to 27 days.[1,2] However, 10% to 15% of women will have lochia serosa at the time of the 6-week postpartum examination. In most patients, the lochia serosa is followed by a yellow-white discharge, called *lochia alba*. Breastfeeding or the use of oral contraceptive agents does not affect the duration of lochia. Frequently, there is a sudden but transient increase in uterine bleeding between 7 and 14 days postpartum. This corresponds to the slough of the eschar over the site of placental attachment. The patient should be reassured and return in 4 weeks for her routine postpartum check-up.

2. Answer: b

(see *Gabbe's Obstetrics* 8e: ch24)

Most women who breastfeed their infants have amenorrhea for extended periods of time, often until the infant is weaned. Several studies, using a variety of methods to indicate ovulation, have demonstrated that ovulation occurs as early as 27 days after delivery, with the mean time being about 70 to 75 days in nonlactating women.[3] Among women who are breastfeeding their infants, the mean time to ovulation is about 6 months. The duration of anovulation depends on the frequency of breastfeeding, the duration of each feed, and the proportion of supplementary feeds.[4] The likelihood of ovulation within the first 6 months postpartum, in a woman exclusively breastfeeding, is 1% to 5%.

3. Answer: c

(see *Gabbe's Obstetrics* 8e: ch24)

The immediate loss of 10 to 13 pounds can be attributed to the delivery of the infant, placenta, and amniotic fluid, and to blood loss. However, most women will not manifest that loss until one to two weeks after delivery because of fluid retention immediately after delivery. For most women, weight loss postpartum does not tend to compensate for weight gain during gestation. By 6 weeks postpartum, only 28% of women will have returned to their prepregnant weight. The remainder of any weight loss occurs from 6 weeks postpartum until 6 months after delivery, with most weight loss concentrated in the first 3 months. Breastfeeding has relatively little effect on postpartum weight loss. With a program of diet and exercise, weight loss of about 0.5 kg/week between 4 and 14 weeks postpartum in breastfeeding, overweight women did not affect the growth of their infants.[5] Similarly, aerobic exercise has no adverse effect on lactation, provided adequate hydration is maintained. A Cochrane Review analyzed literature on weight-loss programs. The analysis found that diet and diet plus exercise were most effective for postpartum weight loss.

4. Answer: c

(see *Gabbe's Obstetrics* 8e: ch24)

Before discharge, women should be offered any vaccines that may be necessary to protect immunity. MMR (measles, mumps, and rubella) vaccine is given to rubella nonimmune mothers. Hepatitis B, Tdap (tetanus, diphtheria, and pertussis), MMR, and influenza are the four most common vaccines given. All are safe with breastfeeding.[6] As recommended in 2012 by the Centers for Disease Control and Prevention, Tdap should be administered during pregnancy to all pregnant women, regardless of the interval since the last Tdap.[7] If Tdap was not given during pregnancy, it should be given immediately postpartum. The varicella vaccine should be initiated postpartum in those with a negative varicella titer.

5. Answer: d

(see *Gabbe's Obstetrics* 8e: ch24)

Although the standard definition of postpartum febrile morbidity is a temperature of 38°C (100.4°F) or higher on any two of the first 10 days after delivery, exclusive of the first 24 hours, most clinicians do not wait two full days to begin evaluation and treatment of patients who develop a fever in the puerperium. The most common cause of postpartum fever is endometritis, which occurs after vaginal delivery in about 2% of patients and after cesarean delivery in about 10% to 15%. The differential diagnosis includes urinary tract infection, lower genital tract infection, wound infections, pulmonary infections, thrombophlebitis, and mastitis.

6. Answer: d

(see *Gabbe's Obstetrics* 8e: ch24)

Finding out about a woman's intentions regarding future pregnancies can help to guide shared decision-making regarding contraceptive options between the patient and the health-care provider. Postpartum contraception use can decrease unintended pregnancy and provide women with a method to control the timing of their pregnancies. Women should be advised to avoid interpregnancy intervals shorter than 6 months. A recent metaanalysis found that birth intervals shorter than 18 months are significantly associated with small-for-gestational-age infants, preterm birth, and death in the first year of life.[8] The ideal timing of family planning advice and education about contraception has not been determined.

7. Answer: a

(see *Gabbe's Obstetrics* 8e: ch24)

Long-acting reversible contraception (LARC) methods, which include IUDs and the contraceptive implant, are the most effective reversible methods available to women, with failure rates less than 1%. LARC methods can be placed immediately postpartum or at an interval time. If IUDs are placed postpartum, the best practice is to place the device within 10 minutes of placental delivery. Insertion of an IUD is not recommended if intrauterine infection is present. Devices placed immediately postpartum have a slightly increased risk for expulsion, up to 20%. Depot medroxyprogesterone acetate (DMPA) is an injectable progestin-only contraceptive given every 3 months. It has a typical use failure rate of 6%. Combined hormonal contraception includes oral, transdermal, and vaginal estrogen and progestin containing contraception. All of these methods having a typical use failure rate of 9%. The typical use failure rate for condoms is 17% but can be as low as 2%, depending on the age and motivation of the population studied.

8. Answer: d

(see *Gabbe's Obstetrics* 8e: ch24)

The 10-year failure rate of postpartum partial salpingectomy is 0.75%. The risks of tubal ligation procedures, whether performed in the puerperium or as an interval procedure, include the short-term problems of anesthetic accidents; injury to bowel, bladder, or blood vessels; and infection. The overall risk for complication with female sterilization is 1.6%. Independent risk factors for complications are general anesthesia, diabetes, previous abdominal/pelvic surgery, and obesity. There are one to two deaths per 100,000 procedures, most often attributed to anesthesia. For women >30 years old, risk for regret was 5.9%. In contrast, women ≤30 years old had a risk of regret of 20.3%.

9. Answer: b

(see *Gabbe's Obstetrics* 8e: ch24)

The psychological reactions experienced following childbirth include the common, relatively mild, physiologic, and transient "baby blues" (50% to 70% of women, resolution by 10–14 days postpartum), true depression (8% to 20% of women), and frank puerperal psychosis (0.14% to 0.26%). Overall, anxiety is the most common emotional symptom in the puerperium. Puerperal thyroid disease will often present with symptoms that include mild dysphoria; consequently, thyroid function studies are suggested in the evaluation of patients with suspected postpartum depression that occurs 2 to 3 months after delivery.

10. Answer: d

(see *Gabbe's Obstetrics* 8e: ch24)

The contraceptive implant contains etonogestrel and acts primarily by inhibiting ovulation. The implant is usually placed in the inner aspect of the nondominant arm. The implant also causes changes to bleeding patterns, with irregular spotting or bleeding or amenorrhea. The bleeding patterns for this device are more unpredictable. The implant is Food and Drug Administration (FDA) approved for use up to 3 years. The use of the single-rod implant in postpartum women does not result in changes in milk volume, milk constituents, or infant growth rates. While package labeling advises initiating the implant at 6 weeks postpartum, clinical experience and limited randomized trial data with immediate postpartum initiation are reassuring and may be in the patient's best interest for the prevention of a rapid repeat pregnancy. Gurtcheff et al randomized women to receive the implant 1 to 2 days postpartum versus 4 to 8 weeks postpartum and found that there was no difference between groups in time to lactogenesis stage II, lactation failure, use of formula supplementation, and milk composition at 6 weeks.[9]

REFERENCES

1. Oppenheimer LS, Sheriff EA, Goodman JDS, et al. The duration of lochia. *Br J Obstet Gynaecol*. 1986;93:754.
2. Visness CM, Kennedy KI, Ramos R. The duration and character of postpartum bleeding among breast-feeding women. *Obstet Gynecol*. 1997;89:159.
3. Perex A, Uela P, Masnick GS, et al. First ovulation after childbirth: the effect of breast feeding. *Am J Obstet Gynecol*. 1972;114:1041.
4. Gray RH, Campbell ON, Apelo R, et al. Risk of ovulation during lactation. *Lancet*. 1990;335:25.
5. Lovelady CA, Garner KE, Thoreno KL, et al. The effect of weight loss in overweight, lactating women on the growth of their infants. *N Engl J Med*. 2000;342:449.
6. Bohlke K, Galil K, Jackson L, et al. Postpartum varicella vaccination: Is the vaccine virus excreted in breast milk? *Obstet Gynecol*. 2003;102:970.
7. Center for Disease Control and Prevention (CDC). Updated recommendations for use of tetanus toxoid, reduced diphtheria toxoid, and acellular pertussis vaccine (Tdap) in pregnant women. Advisory Committee on Immunization Practices 2012. *MMWR Morb Mortal Wkly Rep*. 2013; 62:131–135.
8. Kozuki N, Lee ACC, Silveira MF, et al. The association of birth intervals with small-for-gestational-age, preterm and neonatal and infant mortality: a meta-analysis. *BMC Public Health*. 2013;13 (Suppl 3):S3.
9. Gurtcheff SE, Turok DK, Stoddard G, Murphy PA, Gibson M, Jones KP. Lactogenesis after early postpartum use of the contraceptive implant: a randomized controlled trial. *Obstet Gynecol*. 2011; 117:1114-21.

SECTION V

Complicated Pregnancy

25

Lactation and Breastfeeding

Rini Banerjee Ratan

(See *Gabbe's Obstetrics: Normal and Problem Pregnancies*, 8e: ch25)

QUESTIONS

1. The World Health Organization (WHO), American College of Obstetricians and Gynecologists (ACOG) and the American Academy of Pediatrics (AAP) recommend which of the following regarding infant feeding?

   a. Exclusive breastfeeding for the first 3 months

   b. Exclusive breastfeeding for the first 6 months

   c. Exclusive breastfeeding for the first 12 months

   d. Exclusive breastfeeding for the first 6 months and continued breastfeeding at least through 12 months

   e. Exclusive breastfeeding for the first 12 months and continued breastfeeding at least through 18 months

2. A 25-year-old G1P0 gives birth to a healthy 3250-g male infant at term. She underwent reduction mammoplasty at age 18. She would like to breastfeed her newborn infant. This patient is most likely to encounter difficulty breastfeeding her newborn if the incision from her previous breast surgery disrupted which of the following structures?

   a. Lateral cutaneous branch of 4th intercostal nerve

   b. Lactiferous ducts in the tail of Spence

   c. Pectoralis fascia

   d. Perforating branches of internal thoracic artery

   e. Anterior axillary lymph nodes

3. A 19-year-old G1P1 presents to her obstetrician's office with a painful, swollen 5-cm mass in her right axilla. She underwent normal spontaneous vaginal delivery of a healthy female infant at term 4 days ago. She was discharged to home on postpartum day 2. She has been exclusively breastfeeding her infant since delivery. She is afebrile and well appearing. A 5-cm tender, round, firm mass is palpable in the right axilla. Both breasts appear engorged and symmetric. No erythema, exudate, or induration is present. Milk is expressed from both nipples. Which of the following is the most appropriate next step in management?

   a. Ultrasound of the right breast

   b. Diagnostic mammogram of the right breast

   c. Fine-needle aspiration of the mass

   d. Ice and symptomatic therapy for 48 hours

   e. Oral antibiotic regimen for 7 days

4. Which of the following statements regarding colostrum versus mature breast milk is most accurate?

   a. Colostrum has more protein than milk.

   b. Colostrum contains fewer secretory immunoglobulins than milk.

   c. Colostrum has less lactose than milk.

   d. Colostrum has a higher fat content than milk.

   e. The volume of colostrum produced is higher than that of milk.

5. Which hormone is the major promoter of milk synthesis?

   a. Oxytocin

   b. Prolactin

   c. Human placental lactogen

   d. Progesterone

   e. Estrogen

6. A 27-year-old G1P1 presents to her obstetrician's office for routine postpartum visit. She underwent primary cesarean delivery of a healthy male infant at term 6 weeks ago. An etonorgestrel implant was placed prior to discharge for long-acting reversible contraception. She notes that her milk supply is diminishing. She is nursing her infant every 2–3 hours during the day, for at least 20 minutes on each breast. Her partner feeds the infant formula overnight so that she can get some sleep. On examination, both breasts appear symmetric. No masses, axillary lymphadenopathy, or skin changes are present. Milk is expressed from both nipples. Which of the following is the most likely cause of her inadequate milk supply?

a. History of caesarean delivery

b. Etonogestrel implant

c. Inadequate duration of nursing on each breast

d. Nursing infant too often during the day

e. Lack of night nursing

7. Which of the following health benefits are associated with longer duration of breastfeeding?

a. Less premenopausal breast cancer

b. Lower rates of ovarian cancer

c. Decreased rates of cardiovascular disease

d. Lower incidence of type 2 diabetes mellitus

e. All of the above

8. A 36-year-old G1P1 presents to her obstetrician's office for routine postpartum visit. She underwent normal vaginal delivery of a healthy male infant at term 8 weeks ago. She has been nursing her infant every 2–3 hours day and night since birth. She will return to paid work next month, and her infant will transition to day care. She would like to continue breastfeeding her infant for at least 1 year. Which of the following strategies is most likely to result in the longest duration of breastfeeding after returning to work?

a. Formula feed the infant at daycare and feed directly from the breast at home

b. Pump at work and feed directly from the breast when at home

c. Pump at work and bottle feed breast milk only at daycare and at home

d. Formula feed the infant during the day and feed directly from the breast only at night

9. A 39-year-old G3P3 presents to her physician's office with concern about a lump in her right breast that has been present for at least 4 weeks. She noticed the lump while breastfeeding her youngest child, who is now 6 months old. She has made multiple efforts to massage, express, and drain the breast in that area, but the lump has persisted. On examination, a firm, fixed 1.5-cm mass is palpable in the upper outer quadrant of the right breast. The breasts appear symmetric. No axillary lymphadenopathy or skin changes are present. Milk is expressed from both nipples. Ultrasound shows a 1.5-cm solid mass in the right breast. Which of the following is the most appropriate next step in management?

a. MRI of the right breast

b. Diagnostic mammogram of the right breast

c. Fine-needle aspiration of the mass

d. Tomosynthesis (3-D mammography) of the right breast

10. A 23-year-old G1P1 presents to her obstetrician's office with a fever, malaise, and pain in her left breast for the past day. She underwent normal vaginal delivery of a healthy female infant at term 4 weeks ago. She has been breastfeeding her infant since delivery. Her temperature is 38.5°C/101.3 degrees Fahrenheit. A localized area of erythema, tenderness, induration, and calor is present over the medial aspect of the left breast. Milk is expressed from both nipples. Antibiotic therapy is recommended. Which of the following is the most appropriate recommendation regarding infant feeding at this time?

a. Discontinue breastfeeding until antibiotic therapy is completed.

b. Continue breastfeeding on the uninfected breast only.

c. Continue breastfeeding; initiate nursing on the uninfected breast first.

d. Pump and dump breast milk until antibiotic therapy is completed.

e. Discontinue breastfeeding altogether.

11. A 23-year-old G2P2 is seen in the hospital 12 hours after giving birth to a healthy male infant at term. She has been breastfeeding her newborn and would like to continue nursing when she goes home, but she stopped nursing her first child after 3 months because of painful, cracked nipples. On examination, the breasts appear symmetric. No erythema, exudate, or induration is present. Colostrum is expressed from both nipples. Which of the following is the most appropriate recommendation for this patient to prevent the development of cracked nipples?

a. Wash breasts with clean water and allow to air dry.

b. Wash breasts with antibacterial soap and gently towel dry.

c. Express colostrum and apply to nipples after every feeding.

d. Apply lanolin ointment to nipples after every feeding.

e. Clean nipples and areolae with alcohol after every feeding.

12. Which of the following recommendations regarding nutrition during lactation is correct?

   a. Folic acid intake should be increased by 20%.

   b. Breastfeeding women should consume an additional 1000 kcal/day.

   c. Most vitamins and minerals should be increased by 50%.

   d. Nursing mothers should drink at least 1 L of extra fluid every day.

   e. Infants who are breastfed should not receive vitamin D supplementation.

ANSWERS

1. **Answer: d**

   (see *Gabbe's Obstetrics* 8e: ch25)

   Breastfeeding and breast milk are the global standard for optimal infant feeding. The World Health Organization, the US Surgeon General, the Center for Disease Control and Prevention, the AAP, the ACOG, the American Academy of Family Practice, and the Academy of Breastfeeding Medicine have endorsed this recommendation for over two decades. They recommend exclusive breastfeeding for the first 6 months and continued breastfeeding at least through 12 months with subsequent weaning as a mutual decision by the mother and infant dyad in the subsequent months and years.

2. **Answer: a**

   (see *Gabbe's Obstetrics* 8e: ch25)

   While innervation patterns vary significantly among individuals, it is generally agreed upon that the nipple-areola complex (NAC) is most commonly innervated by the lateral and anterior cutaneous branches of the 3rd, 4th, and 5th intercostal nerves; the 4th lateral cutaneous branch is the most common anatomic pattern. The nerve travels deeply within the pectoralis fascia, exits through the central breast parenchyma, and reaches the nipple at its posterior surface. Incisions, like in this case, that disrupt the base of the breast or periareolar incisions that disrupt superficial nerve courses or retroareolar innervation and ductal tissue have the greatest potential to negatively affect future breastfeeding.

3. **Answer: d**

   (see *Gabbe's Obstetrics* 8e: ch25)

   All mammals, including humans, have the potential to develop mammary tissue (glandular or nipple tissue) anywhere along the milk line, also called the galactic band. The milk line extends from the axilla and inner upper arm down the abdomen along the midclavicular line to the upper lateral mons and upper inner thigh. The most common site for accessory breast tissue is the axilla. These women may present at 2 to 5 days postpartum, at initiation of galactogenesis (lactogenesis II), with painful enlargements in the axilla. Ice and symptomatic therapy for 24 to 48 hours is sufficient treatment.

4. **Answer: a**

   (see *Gabbe's Obstetrics* 8e: ch25)

   Until lactogenesis stage II has fully developed, the breasts secrete colostrum, which differs from mature milk in volume and constituents. Colostrum has more protein, especially secretory immunoglobulins, and more lactose; it also has a lower fat content than mature milk.

5. **Answer: b**

   (see *Gabbe's Obstetrics* 8e: ch25)

   Prolactin appears to be the single most important galactopoietic hormone because selective inhibition of prolactin secretion by bromocriptine disrupts lactogenesis; oxytocin appears to be the major galactokinetic hormone.

6. **Answer: e**

   (see *Gabbe's Obstetrics* 8e: ch25)

   A frequency of nursing greater than eight feedings per 24 hours, night nursing, and a duration of nursing longer than 15 minutes are needed to maintain adequate prolactin levels and milk supply. Milk production is reduced by an autocrine pathway through a protein that inhibits milk production by the alveolar cells and by distension and pressure against the alveolar cells. Thus, frequent breast drainage is essential to maintain lactation.

7. **Answer: e**

   (see *Gabbe's Obstetrics* 8e: ch25)

   Greater intensity and duration of breastfeeding are also associated with health benefits for the mother, including faster postpartum involution, less premenopausal breast cancer, less ovarian cancer, lower rates of cardiovascular disease, and less incidence type 2 diabetes mellitus.

8. Answer: b

(see *Gabbe's Obstetrics* 8e: ch25)

Among employed women in the US, 23% return to work by 10 days postpartum.[1] One-third returned to work within 3 months of birth, and two-thirds returned within 6 months. The strategies used to continue breastfeeding in the first month after the mother returned to work included to (1) feed directly from the breast (31.3%), (2) pump and feed directly from the breast (9.4%), (3) pump only and bottle feed breast milk only (43.4%), and (4) neither pump nor feed directly during the day. Directly breastfeeding and a pump-and-feed strategy resulted in the longest durations of breastfeeding after returning to work. The Centers of Disease Control and Prevention has developed a website to help the woman and employer to support the breastfeeding dyad.

9. Answer: c

(see *Gabbe's Obstetrics* 8e: ch25)

A needle aspiration of the mass is the mainstay of diagnosis. Many obstetricians refer the patient to a breast radiologist for consultation and management. Fine-needle aspiration biopsy appears to have the same accuracy in pregnancy and lactation as in the nonpregnant, nonlactating woman. Ultrasound is an accurate method of determining the cystic nature of a breast mass in lactating women. Mammography is more difficult to interpret during lactation. Young breasts are generally more dense, and the massive increase in functioning glands may obscure small cancers. In general, mammography or MRI are secondary diagnostic modalities to ultrasonography.

10. Answer: c

(see *Gabbe's Obstetrics* 8e: ch25)

Mastitis occurs most frequently in the first 2 to 4 weeks postpartum. Risk factors include maternal fatigue, poor nursing technique, nipple trauma, rapid reduction in nursing frequency, constrictive clothing, and epidemic *Staphylococcus aureus*. The most common organisms associated with mastitis are *S. aureus*, which includes methicillin-resistant *S. aureus*, *Staphylococcus epidermidis*, streptococci, and occasionally gram-negative rods. A practical case definition of mastitis is an infectious process of the breast characterized by high fever (>38.5°C), localized erythema, tenderness, induration, and palpable heat over the area.[118] Antibiotic therapy should not be delayed in acutely ill patients who meet the previously mentioned case definition. Box 25.1. describes the management of mastitis.

BOX 25.1   The Management of Mastitis

1. Breast support.
2. An appropriate intake of fluids.
3. Assessment of nursing technique.
4. Nursing initiated on the uninfected side first to establish let-down
5. The infected side emptied by nursing with each feeding (occasionally, a breast pump helps to ensure complete drainage).
6. Dicloxacillin 500 mg every 6 hours for 10–14 days. Cephalexin or clindamycin may be used in patients allergic to penicillin.
7. Analgesia with a nonsteroidal antiinflammatory drug, such as ibuprofen.

---

11. Answer: a

(see *Gabbe's Obstetrics* 8e: ch25)

Washing with harsh soaps; buffing the nipple with a towel; and using alcohol, benzoin, or other drying agents are not helpful and may increase the incidence of cracking. Normally, the breast is washed with clean water and should be left to air dry. Trials involving application of breast cream or expression of colostrum have not shown a reduction in nipple trauma or sensitivity when compared with untreated nipples.[2]

12. Answer: d

(see *Gabbe's Obstetrics* 8e: ch25)

The mother must consume an extra about 480 kcal/day unless stored energy is used.[3] In lactation, most vitamins and minerals should be increased 20% to 30% over nonpregnant requirements. However, folic acid should be doubled. The mother should drink at least 1 L of extra fluid every day to make up for the fluid lost through breastfeeding. The breastfeeding infant should receive vitamin D_3 shortly after birth in doses of 10–20 g/day (400–800 IU/day).

REFERENCES

1. Klerman JA, Daley K, Pozniak A. *Family and Medical Leave in 2012: Technical Report*. Cambridge, MA; 2014.
2. Dennis CL, Jackson K, Watson J. Interventions for treating painful nipples among breastfeeding women [review]. *Cochrane Database Syst Rev*. 2014;12:CD007366.
3. Butte NF, Wong WW, Hopkinson JM. Energy requirements of lactating women derived from doubly labeled water and milk energy output. *J Nutr*. 2001;131(1):53–58.

REFERENCES

26

Pregnancy as a Window to Maternal and Child Health

Anthony Sciscione

(see *Gabbe's Obstetrics: Normal and Problem Pregnancies*, 8e: ch26)

QUESTIONS

1. A 41-year-old G2P1001 presents for a prenatal visit at 36 weeks gestation. Her prenatal care has been uneventful except for the diagnosis of gestational diabetes, which is well controlled with metformin. You discuss arranging a date for induction of labor and she asks, "what is my risk of developing type 2 diabetes?" You state that her risk is increased and appears to be between 15% and 50% within the first 5 years of delivery and is how high at 20+ years?

   a. 30%

   b. 40%

   c. 50%

   d. 60%

   e. 70%

2. A 19-year-old nulliparous woman at 26 weeks gestation presents to the labor and delivery unit with severe range blood pressures and a headache. Her medical history and her prenatal course have been unremarkable. Her laboratory tests return with severe thrombocytopenia but are otherwise normal. A sonogram reveals a fetus in the first percentile for estimated fetal weight with reverse diastolic flow in the umbilical artery. The fetal heart rate is category II with repetitive late decelerations. It is decided to move to delivery. You counsel her at her 6-week postpartum visit that her history of preeclampsia with severe features places her at an increased lifetime risk of:

   a. Cardiovascular morbidity and mortality

   b. Type 2 diabetes

   c. Renal failure

   d. Idiopathic thrombocytopenia purpura

   e. Liver failure

3. What is the "Barker hypothesis?"

   a. Maternal origins of fetal disease

   b. Fetal origins of adult disease

   c. Maternal and fetal diseases are unrelated

   d. Paternal origins of fetal disease

   e. Environmental toxins are the origins of fetal diseases

4. A 21-year-old woman had an uncomplicated vaginal delivery. Her postpartum course has been uncomplicated. She is having difficulty with breastfeeding and a lactation consultant is helping her. You counsel the patient that longer breastfeeding has been associated with:

   a. Higher risk of breast cancer

   b. Higher risk of cardiovascular disease

   c. Lower risk of cardiovascular disease

   d. Lower risk of uterine cancer

5. A 31-year-old G1P0 woman presents for her 6-week postpartum visit after an uncomplicated vaginal delivery. Her body mass index prior to pregnancy was 28 but she gained 50 pounds during pregnancy. Her weight at the postpartum reveals an increase of 10 pounds or approximately 4.5 kg. You discuss postpartum weight reduction and counsel her that the risk of type 2 diabetes doubles with each _____ kg increase in postpartum weight.

   a. 2.5

   b. 3.5

   c. 4.5

   d. 5.5

   e. 6.5

ANSWERS

1. Answer: e

(see *Gabbe's Obstetrics* 8e: ch26)

One recent estimate suggests a 7.4-fold increased lifetime risk in women with Gestational Diabetes Mellitus (GDM).[1] A review of 28 studies[2] has demonstrated a rapid increase in the incidence of type 2 diabetes in the first 5 years after delivery (17%–50%) and a more gradual plateau thereafter to approximately 70% at 20+ years. The variability in these estimates is a function of the different populations studied, as well as the various definitions of GDM and type 2 diabetes used.

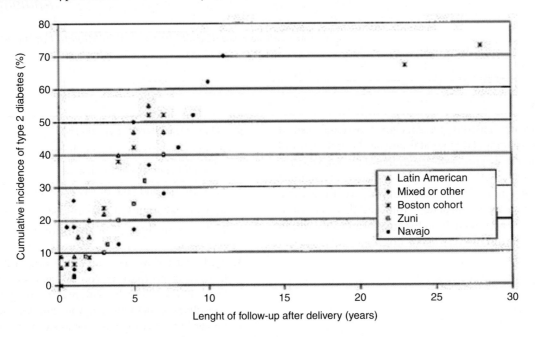

2. Answer: a

(see *Gabbe's Obstetrics* 8e: ch26)

Although mechanisms underlying the association between hypertensive diseases of pregnancy and chronic cardiometabolic disease are not well understood, there is an ever-growing body of evidence that these women comprise a high-risk population for early cardiovascular morbidity and mortality.

3. Answer: b

(see *Gabbe's Obstetrics* 8e: ch26)

Fetal Growth Restriction (FGR) is also associated with adverse long-term health outcomes for the affected offspring. David Barker, an epidemiologist, was among the first to report on this association. He noticed that the highest rates of ischemic heart disease in the UK were seen among the poorest geographic areas and lowest income groups. This demographic also had the most marked differences in infant mortality at the time the affected individuals were born. He hypothesized that impaired prenatal and early postnatal growth were important risk factors for ischemic heart disease later in life. To test his hypothesis, he reviewed midwifery records and death records for individuals born in parts of the UK from 1911 to 1930 and found that men with the lowest weights at birth and at 1 year of life had the highest death rates from ischemic heart disease.[3] The "Barker hypothesis," that there are fetal origins of adult disease, has since been tested for a multitude of prenatal exposures and adult outcomes, with substantial observational evidence supporting the hypothesis.

4. Answer: c

(see *Gabbe's Obstetrics* 8e: ch26)

The benefits of breastfeeding extend to populations beyond women and children exposed to gestational diabetes. Because longer duration of breastfeeding has been shown to be protective against cardiovascular disease later in life, and because many of the pregnancy complications reviewed earlier are associated with later cardiovascular disease, lactation support may serve as an important form of secondary prevention for cardiovascular disease in at-risk women.

5. Answer: c

(see *Gabbe's Obstetrics* 8e: ch26)

Maternal preconception weight, including interpregnancy weight gain, has been increasing over the past several decades. In turn, weight loss offers the single best protection against the development of type 2 diabetes of any long-term management strategy. The Diabetes Prevention Program demonstrated that the relative risk reduction for the development of type 2 diabetes decreases by 16% for each kilogram of weight loss.[4] Conversely, postpartum weight gain increases the risk for development of type 2 diabetes. Peters and associates demonstrated a doubling in risk for development of type 2 diabetes with every 4.5 kg weight gained after delivery.[5]

REFERENCES

1. Bellamy L, Casas JP, Hingorani AD, Williams D. Type 2 diabetes mellitus after gestational diabetes: a systematic review and meta-analysis. *Lancet.* 2009;373(9677):1773-1779.
2. Kim C, Newton KM, Knopp RH. Gestational diabetes and the incidence of type 2 diabetes: a systematic review. *Diabetes Care.* 2002;25(10):1862-1868.
3. Barker DJ, Winter PD, Osmond C, Margetts B, Simmonds SJ. Weight in infancy and death from ischaemic heart disease. *Lancet.* 1989;2(8663):577-580.
4. Hamman RF, Wing RR, Edelstein SL, et al. Effect of weight loss with lifestyle intervention on risk of diabetes. *Diabetes Care.* 2006; 29(9):2102-2107.
5. Peters RK, Kjos SL, Xiang A, Buchanan TA. Long-term diabetogenic effect of single pregnancy in women with previous gestational diabetes mellitus. *Lancet.* 1996;347(8996):227-30.

27

Antepartum Fetal Evaluation

Eva K. Pressman

(see *Gabbe's Obstetrics: Normal and Problem Pregnancies*, 8e: ch27)

QUESTIONS

1. A 26-year-old G2P0101 comes to the labor and delivery unit at 35 weeks gestation reporting no fetal movement for the last 8 hours. Her pregnancy has been uncomplicated and she has no medical conditions. Ultrasound at 20 weeks gestation showed normal fetal anatomy. She is placed on the fetal monitor and no fetal heart rate (FHR) is identified. Maternal blood pressure (BP) is 132/78 and pulse is 96. Ultrasound confirms a fetal demise, normal fetal growth and amniotic fluid volume, and a normal appearing placenta. What is the most likely cause of the fetal demise?

a. Congenital malformation

b. Maternal hypertension

c. No identifiable cause

d. Placental abruption

e. Umbilical cord abnormality

2. A 32-year-old G2P0010 comes to the office at 32 weeks gestation reporting decreased fetal movement for several days. She has not experienced abdominal pain or vaginal bleeding. Her medical history includes type 1 diabetes diagnosed at the age of 11. She has had difficulty controlling her blood glucose, with most values between 160 and 200 mg/dL. Ultrasound at 20 weeks gestation showed normal fetal anatomy but resolution of the fetal heart and spine was limited. No fetal heart rate is identified by Doppler. Maternal BP is 142/80 and pulse is 86. Ultrasound confirms a fetal demise, fetal growth at the 90th percentile, an increased amniotic fluid volume, and a normal-appearing placenta. What is the most likely etiology of the fetal demise?

a. Congenital anomalies

b. Placental abruption

c. Placental insufficiency

d. Preterm delivery

e. Unexplained fetal death

3. A 29-year-old G3P2002 comes to the office at 18 weeks gestation for a routine prenatal visit. She undergoes second trimester maternal serum screening for aneuploidy and open fetal defects and is found to have an elevated maternal serum alphafetoprotein at 2.5 multiples of the median for gestational age. Ultrasound shows no evidence of fetal anomalies. For which of the following pregnancy complications is she at an increased risk?

a. Closed neural tube defect

b. Fetal macrosomia

c. Intrauterine demise

d. Polyhydramnios

e. Postdates pregnancy

4. A 32-year-old G2P1001 with chronic hypertension comes to the office at 32 weeks. Her BP is 140/92 on a stable dose of labetalol 400 mg twice daily and her fundal height measures 31 cm. Which of the following tests would be most reassuring regarding fetal well-being?

a. A biophysical profile shows normal fluid but no fetal movement, tone, or breathing.

b. A contraction stress test (CST) shows no accelerations or decelerations.

c. A nonstress test (NST) shows one acceleration in 40 minutes.

d. The patient reports one fetal movement in the last 8 hours.

e. Vibroacoustic stimulation (VAS) does not lead to an FHR acceleration.

5. A 27-year-old G1P0 at 36 weeks gestation comes to the labor and delivery unit with decreased fetal movement. She has type 1 diabetes that has been well controlled. After 20 minutes, her NST is nonreactive and a CST is performed. The figure shows the results. What is the most appropriate interpretation of this tracing?

a. A negative, nonreactive CST

b. A negative, reactive CST

c. A positive, nonreactive CST

d. A positive, reactive CST

e. An unsatisfactory CST

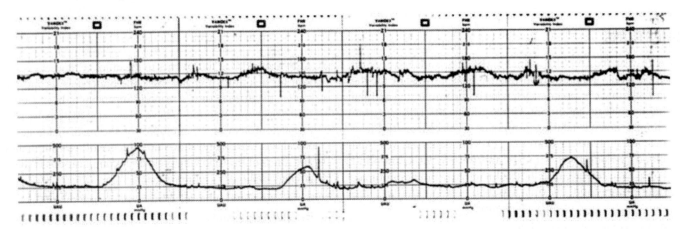

6. A 37-year-old G2P0010 comes to the labor and delivery unit at 34 weeks gestation with a pregnancy complicated by preeclampsia without severe features. Her BP is 150/90. She has the NST displayed in the figure. Ultrasound shows normal fetal growth, normal amniotic fluid, and good fetal tone, movement, and breathing. What is the most likely outcome for this pregnancy within the next week?

a. Fetal demise

b. Fetal growth restriction

c. Severe neurologic impairment

d. Neonatal hypoglycemia

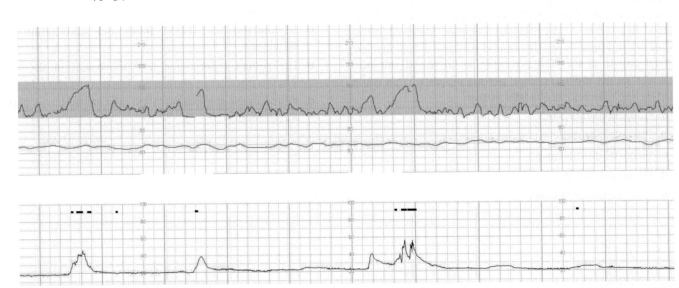

7. A 27-year-old G2P1001 comes to the labor and delivery unit with intermittent abdominal pain at 38 weeks. She reports one episode of vomiting last night and normal bowel movements. Her medical history is significant for hypothyroidism, for which she takes levothyroxine. Her pulse is 116, BP is 110/70, and temperature is 37.9°C. On examination, she has diffuse abdominal tenderness in the midline and her cervix is 1 cm dilated and 50% effaced and the presenting fetal part is not engaged in the maternal pelvis. The FHR tracing is shown in the figure. Which of the following is the most likely diagnosis?

a. Chorioamnionitis

b. Fetal arrhythmia

c. Maternal dehydration

d. Maternal hyperthyroisim

e. Placental insufficiency

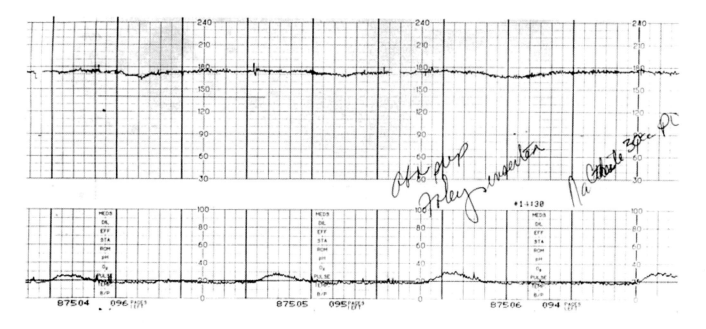

8. A 36-year-old G1P0 comes to the labor and delivery unit at 37 weeks reporting decreased fetal movement. Her pregnancy has been complicated by gestational diabetes. This initially controlled with diet, however recent blood glucose levels have been elevated. Insulin therapy was recommended 2 weeks ago but the patient declined this therapy. A NST is done and does not show any accelerations or decelerations. Ultrasound is performed showing normal amniotic fluid volume, evidence of normal fetal tone but no fetal movement or fetal breathing. The fetus is in a breech presentation. Due to immediate concern for fetal well-being, a cesarean delivery is performed. What is the most likely value of the umbilical cord arterial pH?

a. 6.2

b. 6.4

c. 6.9

d. 7.3

e. 7.4

9. The use of Doppler ultrasound of the umbilical artery has been associated with which of the following pregnancy outcomes?

a. Decreased perinatal deaths in low-risk pregnancies

b. Decreased rates of cesarean delivery

c. Increased incidence of fetal acidosis

d. Increased utilization of induction of labor

e. No effect on outcomes of high-risk pregnancies

10. The gestational age at which to initiate testing has not been clearly defined for most high-risk conditions. Which of the following is decreased by initiating testing earlier in gestation?

a. Cesarean delivery rate

b. Cost of health care

c. Maternal anxiety

d. Preterm birth rate

e. Rate of fetal demise

11. Which of the following underlying maternal medical or fetal conditions or pregnancy complications is least likely to benefit from antenatal testing?

    a. Chronic placental abruption

    b. Fetal growth restriction

    c. Fetal skeletal dysplasia

    d. Maternal hypertension

    e. Maternal sickle cell disease

12. A 37-year-old G1P0 comes to the labor and delivery unit for an NST at 41 weeks gestation. Her pregnancy has been uncomplicated and her only medication is prenatal vitamins. The FHR tracing in the figure is obtained. The patient is asymptomatic during the NST. What is the most appropriate next step in management of this patient?

    a. Biophysical profile

    b. Cesarean delivery

    c. Discharge home

    d. Doppler of the umbilical artery

    e. Induction of labor

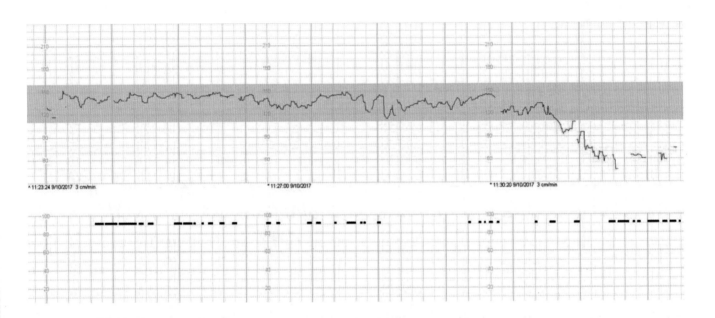

13. A 37-year-old G2P0010 comes to the labor and delivery unit at 38 weeks gestation with a diamniotic, dichorionic twin gestation for induction of labor. Her pregnancy was conceived through in vitro fertilization due to tubal disease. Her medical history includes chronic hypertension. She had negative screening for gestational diabetes and her BP has been normal on a stable dose of labetalol. Her last ultrasound at 37 weeks showed normal, concordant fetal growth and normal amniotic fluid. Both twins were in vertex presentations. Induction has been recommended due to her increased risk for perinatal mortality. Which of the following characteristics is not contributing to her risk for fetal death?

    a. Assisted reproduction

    b. Chorionicity

    c. Hypertension

    d. Maternal age

    e. Twin gestation

14. A 28-year-old G2P1000 comes to the office at 34 weeks gestation to discuss possible induction of labor. Her first pregnancy was complicated by intrauterine fetal demise at 36 weeks with no cause identified clinically, on placental pathology, or on fetal autopsy. She would like to be induced prior to 36 weeks and asks if there are any tests or treatments that would help either mature the fetus early or determine that the fetus already mature enough to prevent complications of iatrogenic prematurity. Which of the following is the most appropriate response?

a. Amniocentesis for phospholipid concentrations can determine both fetal lung and brain maturation.

b. Antenatal testing for fetal well-being is the best approach to prevent intrauterine demise and minimize the long term risks of preterm delivery.

c. Given her prior pregnancy outcome, delivery at 35 weeks is recommended without need for antenatal corticosteroids or amniocentesis.

d. Since no cause for her prior fetal loss was uncovered, there is no indication for fetal testing, amniocentesis, or preterm delivery.

e. While antenatal corticosteroids are effective in accelerating pulmonary maturity prior to 34 weeks, they are not known to be effective after 34 weeks.

ANSWERS

1. Answer: **c**

(see *Gabbe's Obstetrics* 8e: ch27)

Unspecified causes and conditions of placenta/cord/membranes are the leading classifications for fetal death utilized in a modern high-resource population at 25%–30% each, followed by maternal complications of pregnancy and congenital anomalies at 10%–15% each. In addition, fetal deaths late in gestation are more likely than earlier gestation fetal deaths to have no identifiable cause

2. Answer: **e**

(see *Gabbe's Obstetrics* 8e: ch27)

Although historically insulin-dependent diabetes has been a major risk factor for fetal death, the fetal death rate in women with optimal glycemic control now approaches that of women without diabetes. However, the relationship between glycemic control and fetal death remains uncertain. Poor glycemic control is associated with increased perinatal mortality, in large part as a result of congenital anomalies, indicated preterm deliveries, and sudden, unexplained fetal death.

3. Answer: **c**

(see *Gabbe's Obstetrics* 8e: ch27)

First- and second-trimester serum markers for aneuploidy, when abnormally low or elevated, have been associated to varying degrees with adverse perinatal outcomes, even in the absence of aneuploidy. Regarding fetal death after 24 weeks, markers of interest include first-trimester levels of pregnancy-associated plasma protein A of less than the fifth percentile (0.415 multiples of the median [MoM]); second-trimester free β-human chorionic gonadotropin, α-fetoprotein, and inhibin A of more than 2 MoM; and uterine artery pulsatility index above the 90th percentile. The sensitivity and positive predictive value of these markers for fetal death are still under investigation. The pathophysiologic link between these markers and adverse outcomes is unclear and likely variable but most plausibly involves abnormal placental attachment or function.

4. Answer: **b**

(see *Gabbe's Obstetrics* 8e: ch27)

A negative CST (no late or significant variable decelerations) has been consistently associated with good fetal outcome. Fetal movement is a more indirect indicator of fetal oxygen status and CNS function, and decreased fetal movement is noted in response to hypoxemia. However, prospective trials of this method for prevention of perinatal mortality have failed to conclusively show benefit. The most widely applied definition of a reactive NST is two accelerations of the FHR, each with a peak amplitude of 15 beats/min and total duration of 15 seconds, observed in 20 minutes of monitoring. The NST is predictive of normal fetal outcome when it is reactive. A reactive NST after VAS stimulation appears to be reliable as an indicator of fetal well-being. On a biophysical profile, fetal death is increased by 14-fold with the absence of fetal movement.

5. Answer: b

(see *Gabbe's Obstetrics* 8e: ch27)

An adequate CST requires uterine contractions of moderate intensity that last about 40 to 60 seconds, with a frequency of three in 10 minutes. These criteria were selected to approximate the stress experienced by the fetus during the first stage of labor. If uterine activity is absent or inadequate, intravenous oxytocin is begun to initiate contractions, and it is increased until adequate uterine contractions have been achieved.[1] Several methods of nipple stimulation have been used to induce adequate uterine activity, and the success rate at achieving adequate contractions and test results is comparable to that of oxytocin infusion.[1,2] The CST can be interpreted as negative (no late or significant variable decelerations), positive (late decelerations with at least 50% of contractions), or suspicious (intermittent late or variable decelerations). The presence of two or more accelerations in 20 minutes would also make the tracing reactive.

6. Answer: d

(see *Gabbe's Obstetrics* 8e: ch27)

Observations made in the mid-twentieth century that accelerations of the FHR in response to fetal activity, uterine contractions, or stimulation reflect fetal well-being formed the basis for the NST. The NST is the most widely applied technique for antepartum fetal evaluation, despite the uncertainty regarding its reliability and reproducibility as a test of fetal assessment. Most fetuses that exhibit a nonreactive NST are not compromised but simply fail to exhibit heart rate reactivity during the 40-minute period of testing.

7. Answer: a

(see *Gabbe's Obstetrics* 8e: ch27)

The most common cause of fetal tachycardia is maternal-fetal fever secondary to maternal-fetal infection such as chorioamnionitis. Other causes include chronic hypoxemia, maternal hyperthyroidism, maternal medication exposure, and fetal tachyarrhythmia. FHRs above 200 beats/min, and certainly above 220 beats/min, should increase the index of suspicion of fetal tachyarrhythmia and lead to further fetal cardiac evaluation with a targeted fetal echocardiogram. For FHRs between 160 and 180 beats/min, the presence or absence of baseline variability is an important indicator of fetal acid-base status. Fetal acidosis is more likely if baseline variability is absent.

8. Answer: c

(see *Gabbe's Obstetrics* 8e: ch27)

The use of real-time ultrasonography to assess antepartum fetal condition has enabled the obstetrician to perform an in utero physical examination and evaluate dynamic functions that reflect the integrity of the fetal CNS. The biophysical profile (BPP) correlates well with fetal acid-base status. Studies were done in patients undergoing cesarean birth before the onset of labor for severe preeclampsia, elective repeat cesarean delivery, growth restriction, breech presentation, placenta previa, and fetal macrosomia. Acidosis was defined as an umbilical cord arterial pH less than 7.20. The earliest manifestations of fetal acidosis were a nonreactive nonstress test (NST) and loss of fetal heart rate variability. With scores of 8 or more, the mean arterial pH was 7.28, and only 2 of 102 fetuses were acidotic. Nine fetuses with scores of 4 or less had a mean pH of 6.99, and all were acidotic.

9. Answer: b

(see *Gabbe's Obstetrics* 8e: ch27)

With Doppler ultrasound, information can be obtained about uteroplacental blood flow and resistance, which may be markers of fetal adaptation and reserve. This method of fetal assessment has only been demonstrated to be of value in reducing perinatal mortality and unnecessary obstetric interventions in fetuses with suspected intrauterine growth restriction (IUGR) and possibly other disorders of uteroplacental blood flow. In a 2017 Cochrane review of 19 randomized trials that included more than 10,000 high-risk women, Doppler interrogation of the umbilical artery was associated with decreased perinatal deaths (relative risk, 0.71; 95% confidence interval, 0.52–0.98) and significantly fewer inductions of labor and cesarean deliveries. Studies of low-risk pregnancies have not shown a benefit from the use of Doppler ultrasound.

10. Answer: e

(see *Gabbe's Obstetrics* 8e: ch27)

Initiating testing at 32 to 34 weeks of gestation has historically been prescribed for most high-risk pregnancies, with earlier testing recommended for cases with multiple comorbidities or particularly worrisome features. In considering the pros and cons of testing in the preterm period, it is worthwhile to return to the question of potential harms of testing, from increases in preterm birth and cesarean delivery rates to maternal anxiety and financial costs. Although no evidence exists of improved outcomes from any one testing strategy, as a counterpoint, some authors have begun to study whether the implementation of testing increases the chances of induction of labor or cesarean delivery rates. In addition, it is reasonable to question whether a program of antenatal testing contributes to maternal anxiety or other indirect costs.

11. Answer: c

(see *Gabbe's Obstetrics* 8e: ch27)

The basis for antepartum testing relies on the premise that the fetus whose oxygenation in utero is challenged will respond with a series of detectable physiologic adaptive or decompensatory signs as hypoxemia or frank metabolic academia develop. Therefore, antenatal tests should follow the changes in observable measures of fetal response to a suboptimal intrauterine environment and be used for conditions that are likely to affect in utero oxygen delivery.

12. Answer: e

(see *Gabbe's Obstetrics* 8e: ch27)

Antepartum FHR bradycardias have been observed in 1% to 2% of all NSTs, defined as an FHR of 90 beats/min or a fall in the FHR of 40 beats/min below the baseline for 60 seconds or longer. Note that this terminology is distinct from the intrapartum FHR tracing nomenclature categorizing a deceleration lasting greater than 2 but fewer than 10 minutes as a "prolonged deceleration" (Chapter 15). In a review of 121 cases, antepartum bradycardia was associated with increased perinatal morbidity and mortality, particularly antepartum fetal death, cord compression, IUGR, and fetal malformations.[3] Although about one-half of the NSTs associated with bradycardia were reactive, the incidence of a nonreassuring FHR pattern in labor that led to emergency delivery in this group was identical to that of patients who exhibited nonreactive NSTs. Clinical management decisions should be based on the finding of bradycardia, not on the presence or absence of reactivity. Bradycardia has a higher positive predictive value for fetal compromise (fetal death or fetal intolerance of labor) than does the nonreactive NST. Expectant management in the setting of a bradycardia has been associated with a perinatal mortality rate (PMR) of 25%. Therefore, preparations for delivery should be undertaken after careful consideration of gestational-age-related risks and appropriate counseling.

13. Answer: c

(see *Gabbe's Obstetrics* 8e: ch27)

The higher rate of perinatal mortality in multiple gestations compared with singletons is related both to complications unique to multiple gestations, such as twin-to-twin transfusion syndrome, and to more general complications, such as fetal abnormalities and growth restriction. Chorionicity is of paramount importance in determining fetal risk, and rates of adverse outcomes are higher among monochorionic twins. Additionally, many women who carry more than one fetus have maternal risk factors for increased perinatal mortality, including advanced maternal age and use of assisted reproductive techniques (ART), and are subject to development of complications such as preeclampsia and preterm delivery. Optimal timing of delivery between 37 and 38 weeks has been considered for twins, compared with 39 to 40 weeks among singletons, because of increased rate of late fetal death in this group.

14. Answer: b

(see *Gabbe's Obstetrics* 8e: ch27)

Available methods for evaluating fetal pulmonary maturity rely generally on either presence or quantitation of components of pulmonary surfactant in amniotic fluid. The advent of increasingly routine administration of antenatal corticosteroids for promotion of fetal lung maturity in the late preterm period between 34 and 37 weeks has decreased the frequency of fetal pulmonary maturity testing in routine clinical practice. If significant maternal or fetal risk exists, delivery should occur regardless of biochemical maturity, and if delivery could be deferred owing to the absence of pulmonary maturity, there is not a stringent indication for prompt delivery. Additionally, it is recognized that a mature fetal lung profile denoting the presence of pulmonary surfactant does not necessarily translate to maturity of other organ systems.

REFERENCES

1. Practice Bulletin. Antepartum Fetal Surveillance, Number 145. (Replaces Practice Bulletin Number 9, October 1999). American College of Obstetricians and Gynecologists. *Obstet Gynecol.* 2014; 124:182-192.
2. Devoe LD. Antenatal fetal assessment: contraction stress test, nonstress test, vibroacoustic stimulation, amniotic fluid volume, biophysical profile, and modified biophysical profile: an overview. *Semin Perinatol.* 2008;32:247.
3. Druzin ML. Fetal bradycardia during antepartum testing, further observations. *J Reprod Med.* 1989;34:47.

Amniotic Fluid Disorders

Vanita D. Jain

(see *Gabbe's Obstetrics: Normal and Problem Pregnancies*, 8e: ch28)

QUESTIONS

1. What is the gold standard for amniotic fluid volume (AFV) measurement?

   a. Inert dye injection in to amniotic cavity via amniocentesis

   b. Measurement of a four-quadrant amniotic fluid index (AFI)

   c. Measurement of a 2 × 2 cm pocket

   d. Fundal height

2. What is the main source of amniotic fluid (AF) in the human pregnancy?

   a. Fetal lungs

   b. Placenta

   c. Maternal serum and plasma

   d. Fetal urine

   e. Umbilical cord

3. You are in resident clinic and are seeing a 35-year-old G3P1102 at 35 weeks gestational age. Her fundal height measures only 27 cm. You look back at the chart and see that 2 weeks ago, the fundal height measured 31 cm. You repeat your measurement, but it is still only 27 cm. The fetal heart rate (FHR) is normal at 155 beats/min. You perform a bedside ultrasound to evaluate the AFI and note a value of 4 cm. The next best step is

   a. Obtain a history for possible preterm premature rupture of membranes (PPROM).

   b. Perform biometry.

   c. Perform a sterile speculum examination.

   d. Admit to the labor and delivery unit for induction.

4. A 29-year-old G1P0 at 21 weeks gestation presents to your office with an ultrasound report from an outside facility documenting possible "low fluid." The rupture of the membranes is ruled out. A detailed anatomy ultrasound and AFI are performed in the Maternal Fetal Medicine department and the AFI is noted to be 1.9 cm, with a single 1.9-cm vertical pocket. Which is the most important fetal organ(s) to observe for a potential cause?

   a. Kidneys

   b. Lungs

   c. Heart

   d. Liver

   e. Brain

5. Which of the following viruses is associated with polyhydramnios?

   a. HIV

   b. Varicella

   c. Parvovirus

   d. respiratory syncytial virus (RSV)

6. Which of the following has the highest risk of occurring in a pregnancy with polyhydramnios?

   a. Preterm delivery

   b. Preeclampsia

   c. Stillbirth/intrauterine fetal demise (IUFD)

   d. Macrosomia

7. A 26-year-old G1P0 at 32 weeks is noted to have a fundal height of 35 cm in the office. She is sent to maternal fetal medicine (MFM) for an ultrasound and is diagnosed with polyhydramnios and macrosomia. The amniotic fluid index (AFI) is 29 cm, with an maximum vertical pocket (MVP) of 11 cm. The rest of the anatomy appears normal. An important next step would be:

a. Request an amniocentesis for karyotype.

b. Consider gestational diabetes mellitus (GDM) screening, especially if it has been >4 weeks since she was last tested.

c. Order Toxoplasmosis, Rubella, Cytomegalovirus, and Herpes simplex virus (TORCH) titers.

d. Recommend delivery by cesarean section next week due to the risk of preterm labor.

8. A 26-year-old G1P0 presents to your office at 40 weeks and 3 days gestation. She has been feeling well and has not been interested in an elective induction. On examination, her blood pressure is normal at 110/68. The FHR is 140 beats/min. However, you notice her fundal height is only 36 cm. She reports no leaking of fluid, vaginal bleeding, or contractions. You send her to obtain a biophysical profile. You are informed that the AFI is 2 cm. The estimated fetal weight (EFW) is 3875 g, the fetus is vertex, and the NST is reactive. What is the next best step?

a. Schedule the patient for a cesarean section.

b. Ensure the patient has a return appointment next week.

c. Induction of labor.

d. Order a repeat ultrasound in 3–4 days.

ANSWERS

1. **Answer: a**

(see *Gabbe's Obstetrics* 8e: ch28)

Attempts to measure true AFV are difficult because of obvious limitations. To measure the actual volume of AF, an inert dye must be injected into the amniotic cavity via amniocentesis, and samples of AF must be obtained to determine a dilution curve. Although the dye injection technique is considered the gold standard for determining actual AFV and is compared with other methods of estimating AFV, such as ultrasound, it is impractical to utilize an invasive test to assess AFV in clinical practice.

2. **Answer: d**

(see *Gabbe's Obstetrics* 8e: ch28)

The main source of AF is fetal urination. In the human, the fetal kidneys begin to make urine before the end of the first trimester, and production of urine increases until term.

3. **Answer: b**

(see *Gabbe's Obstetrics* 8e: ch28)

In clinical practice, an MVP less than 2 cm or an AFI less than 5 cm is commonly used as criteria for the diagnosis of oligohydramnios. A not uncommon finding at the time of follow-up ultrasound is the existence of a low AFI/MVP in an otherwise normal pregnancy. Because the diagnosis of oligohydramnios has been associated with poor perinatal outcomes, many women who are at or near term are sent to the labor and delivery unit to be considered for induction solely because of a low AFI. Frequently, their cervical examination is unfavorable for induction, and an induction is attempted in spite of this; often, this ends in a cesarean delivery for failed induction. **Although the evidence for induction in the prolonged pregnancy is solid (see Chapter 29), the term or preterm patient with isolated oligohydramnios may not need immediate delivery. All cases with oligohydramnios should be evaluated for evidence of intrauterine growth restriction (IUGR) and should be followed with antepartum testing.** In this example, then, as you already have the ultrasound machine, obtaining four quick measurements for biometry is recommended as the next best immediate step. If the fetus is IUGR, this is information will guide your next steps as to where to send her—obstetric triage, the ultrasound suite for Doppler studies, or to the labor and delivery unit for induction.

4. **Answer: a**

(see *Gabbe's Obstetrics* 8e: ch28)

Visualization of the fetal kidneys and genitourinary (GU) tract (kidneys, ureters if seen, bladder) is important in establishing a cause for oligohydramnios in the mid second trimester. If the fetus is normally grown with kidneys and bladder visualized, more often than not, the amniotic membrane has ruptured prematurely (premature rupture of membranes (PROM)). If the kidneys and bladder cannot be seen, the diagnosis is most likely renal agenesis. Renal agenesis is uniformly fatal, whereas PROM can have a reasonable prognosis if it occurs after fetal viability and if infection is not present. Thus, evaluation of the GU tract will significantly impact your counseling.

5. Answer: c

(see *Gabbe's Obstetrics* 8e: ch28)
See Box 28:1: Fetal causes of polyhydramnios, parvovirus B-19

BOX 28.1 Fetal and Maternal Causes of Polyhydramnios

Fetal Conditions

Congenital anomalies
- Gastrointestinal obstruction, central nervous system abnormalities, cystic hygroma, nonimmune hydrops, sacrococcygeal teratoma, cystic adenoid malformations of lung

Aneuploidy

Genetic disorders
- Achondrogenesis type 1-B
- Muscular dystrophies
- Bartter syndrome

Twin-to-twin transfusion syndrome

Infections
- Parvovirus B-19

Placental abnormalities
- Chorioangioma

Maternal Conditions

Idiopathic

Poorly controlled diabetes mellitus

Fetomaternal hemorrhage

---

6. Answer: c (page 15, 16)

(see *Gabbe's Obstetrics* 8e: ch28)

Complications of pregnancy associated with polyhydramnios includes preterm delivery (2.7-fold increase), preeclampsia (2.7-fold increase), IUFD (7.7-fold increase), and neonatal demise (7.7-fold increase). In such cases, antenatal and maternal surveillance is warranted.

7. Answer: b

(see *Gabbe's Obstetrics* 8e: ch28)

The pregnant woman who presents with a rapidly enlarging uterus in midpregnancy, with or without preterm labor, needs to be evaluated by an ultrasound examination to measure the AFV and assess fetal anatomy. Esophageal atresia with or without tracheoesophageal fistula can present with early-onset severe polyhydramnios due to an obstruction of swallowing. Other gastrointestinal obstructions such as duodenal atresia may result in polyhydramnios. Per the vignette, the rest of the fetal anatomy is normal. Given that *no* structural defect is seen, performance of an amniocentesis is of low yield. Hydramnios is associated with a risk of preterm labor and cesarean delivery, but delivering at 33 weeks without steroids in a patient with mild hydramnios is aggressive and not recommended. Although hydramnios is associated with parvovirus, there is no indication for testing for TORCH infections. Given macrosomia and, at 32 weeks, the likelihood that her last GDM screen was at 26–28 weeks, answer b is the most reasonable next step.

8. Answer: c

(see *Gabbe's Obstetrics* 8e: ch28)

Although severe oligohydramnios has an increased PMR later in the third trimester, it is still not as high as earlier in pregnancy.[1-3] Other studies have reported similar increases in perinatal mortality associated with oligohydramnios, but most have not corrected for other underlying medical conditions.[4] Because of the increase in perinatal morbidity and mortality associated with oligohydramnios in prolonged pregnancy, delivery is recommended (see Chapter 36). Given gestational age of 40+ weeks, you should contact the patient at home and ask her to come in for an induction.

REFERENCES

1. Mercer LJ, Brown LG. Fetal outcome with oligohydramnios in the second trimester. *Obstet Gynecol.* 1986;67:840.
2. Casey BM, McIntire DD, Bloom SL, et al. Pregnancy outcomes after antepartum diagnosis of oligohydramnios at or beyond 34 weeks' gestation. *Am J Obstet Gynecol.* 2000;182:909.
3. Jeng CJ, Lee JF, Wang KG, et al. Decreased amniotic fluid index in term pregnancy. Clinical significance. *J Reprod Med.* 1992;37:789.
4. Manning FA, Hill LM, Platt LD. Qualitative amniotic fluid volume determination by ultrasound: antepartum detection of intrauterine growth retardation. *Am J Obstet Gynecol.* 1981;139:254.

CHAPTER 28

Late and Postterm Pregnancy

Alyssa Stephenson-Famy

(see *Gabbe's Obstetrics: Normal and Problem Pregnancies*, 8e: ch29)

QUESTIONS

1. What is the definition of late-term pregnancy?
   a. Before 37 0/7 weeks
   b. 37 0/7 through 38 6/7 weeks
   c. 39 0/7 through 40 6/7 weeks
   d. 41 0/7 through 41 6/7 weeks
   e. 42 0/7 weeks and beyond

2. A 23-year-old G1P0 at 40 weeks is pregnant with a fetus with anencephaly. She has not had contractions and has been counseled that she might not go into labor spontaneously. What has been hypothesized to explain the late timing of labor in anencephalic pregnancies?
   a. Persistently elevated progesterone level
   b. Lack of myometrial prostaglandin receptors
   c. Disruption of the fetal hypothalamic-pituitary-adrenal (HPA) axis
   d. Delayed cervical ripening
   e. Low serum estriol levels

3. A 36-year-old G4P3 had a last menstrual period (LMP) 7 weeks ago. She has regular periods with long cycles with intervals of 32 days in between menses, but she is certain of her date of conception. Transvaginal ultrasound shows that the fetal pole measures 8 weeks 1 day. What is the most accurate way to date her pregnancy?
   a. LMP based on 28-day cycle
   b. LMP based on 30–32-day cycle
   c. Date of conception
   d. Transvaginal ultrasound
   e. Uterine size on examination

4. A 28-year-old G1P0 at 41 0/7 weeks is admitted to the labor and delivery unit with an amniotic fluid index (AFI) of 4 cm. After starting oxytocin, the fetal heart rate tracing shows recurrent variable decelerations. What best explains the mechanism of the fetal heart rate tracing?
   a. Umbilical cord compression
   b. Fetal head compression
   c. Tight nuchal cord
   d. Uteroplacental insufficiency
   e. Rectal sphincter relaxation

5. A healthy 30-year-old woman at 36 weeks with a singleton gestation is worried about her risk of stillbirth, as a friend recently had a term fetal demise. She should be counseled that the highest risk of stillbirth occurs at which gestational age?
   a. 39 weeks
   b. 40 weeks
   c. 41 weeks
   d. 42 weeks
   e. 43 weeks

6. A 24-year-old G2P1 at 40 weeks gestation presents to clinic. She is doing well and denies contractions. On examination, the fetal heart rate is 150, maternal blood pressure is 100/60, and her cervix is closed and 50% effaced. In addition to a nonstress test, she should be scheduled for what type of antenatal testing at her next visit at 41 weeks?
   a. Umbilical artery Doppler
   b. Fetal growth ultrasound
   c. Contraction stress test
   d. Assessment of amniotic fluid

7. A 32-year-old G1P0 is 38 weeks pregnant with dichorionic twins. To minimize the risk of stillbirth, what is the most appropriate management at this time?

   a. Expectant management

   b. Antenatal testing

   c. Fetal fibronectin testing

   d. Membrane sweeping

   e. Proceed with delivery

8. A 34-year-old G3P2 is at 39 weeks gestation. She previously underwent two successful labor inductions at 41 weeks for babies that were 7–8 pounds. In this pregnancy, she is worried that the baby is much bigger than her previous two and her Leopold examination is consistent with a fetal weight of 9 pounds. Which outcome is she at greatest risk for if she has prolonged pregnancy?

   a. Glucose intolerance

   b. Fetal growth restriction

   c. Postpartum hemorrhage

   d. Neonatal postmaturity

   e. Childhood developmental delay

9. A G1P0 woman has a Bishop score of 4 at 42 0/7 weeks. What is the most appropriate recommendation for her pregnancy management?

   a. Antenatal testing

   b. Membrane sweeping

   c. Induction with prostaglandin E1 (PGE1) or prostaglandin E2 (PGE2)

   d. Induction with oxytocin

   e. Cesarean delivery

10. A healthy 20-year-old female undergoes a fetal growth ultrasound at 37 weeks. The estimated fetal weight is 4000 g (99th percentile). The predicted mean weight is 3028 g for this gestational age. To avoid delivery complications, what is the most appropriate prenatal management?

   a. Expectant management

   b. Early-term labor induction

   c. Full-term labor induction

   d. Elective cesarean section

ANSWERS

1. **Answer: d**

   (See *Gabbe's Obstetrics* 8e: ch29)

   Patients are now considered "early term" if they are 37 0/7 weeks through 38 6/7 weeks. Full term is defined as 39 0/7 weeks through 40 6/7 weeks, and late term, if they are 41 0/7 weeks through 41 6/7 weeks.

2. **Answer: c**

   (See *Gabbe's Obstetrics* 8e: ch29)

   The mechanism in human gestation is unknown but may be similar to that of other mammals. In sheep, the HPA axis is important in the timing of birth. The release of corticotrophin-releasing hormone from the fetal brain results in the secretion of adrenocorticotropic hormone from the pituitary gland and cortisol from the adrenal gland. The absence of the fetal brain in the anencephalic fetus has been hypothesized to result in dysfunction of the HPA axis that leads to prolonged gestation. Epidemiologic studies of anencephalic pregnancies have also observed prolongation of pregnancy.

3. **Answer: d**

   (See *Gabbe's Obstetrics* 8e: ch29)

   The use of ultrasound to determine the accuracy of gestational dating based on the LMP is superior to the use of LMP alone. The estimated due date (EDD) is most accurately determined if the crown rump length is measured in the first trimester with an error of plus or minus 5 to 7 days.

4. **Answer: a**

   (See *Gabbe's Obstetrics* 8e: ch29)

   The association between a reduced AFI and variable decelerations is well documented and likely related to cord compression.

5. **Answer: e**

   (See *Gabbe's Obstetrics* 8e: ch29)

   Observational studies that have evaluated the risk of perinatal mortality at each gestational week show an increased risk as gestational age advances beyond the EDD. A significant increase in fetal mortality was detected from 41 weeks gestation onward (odds ratio of 1.5, 1.8, and 2.9 at 41, 42, and 43 weeks, respectively).

6. **Answer: d**

   (See *Gabbe's Obstetrics* 8e: ch29)

   Given the increased risk of stillbirth, antenatal surveillance is recommended in the management of prolonged and postterm pregnancies. The American College of Obstetricians and Gynecologists currently recommends the initiation of fetal surveillance at 41 or beyond with assessment of amniotic fluid volume.

7. Answer: e

(See *Gabbe's Obstetrics* 8e: ch29)

The nadir of stillbirth occurs at 38 weeks for twins and 35 weeks for triplets and is unknown for quadruplets and higher order multiples. Since the nadir of stillbirth occurs at 38 weeks gestation for twins, it is reasonable accomplish delivery at the nadir of stillbirth risk.

8. Answer: c

(See *Gabbe's Obstetrics* 8e: ch29)

There is an increasing risk of maternal complications for women who deliver after the EDD. Maternal complications of prolonged pregnancies include perineal laceration, chorioamnionitis, endomyometritis, cesarean section, and postpartum hemorrhage.

9. Answer: c

(See *Gabbe's Obstetrics* 8e: ch29)

Delivery at 42 0/7 weeks is recommended and prostaglandin preparation (either PGE1 or PGE2) is recommended for the induction of the postterm pregnancy for women with a Bishop score less than 6.

10. Answer: a

(See *Gabbe's Obstetrics* 8e: ch29)

The diagnosis of fetal macrosomia by ultrasound is not precise, and early induction of labor or cesarean delivery has not been shown to reduce the morbidity associated with fetal macrosomia.

30

Fetal Growth Restriction

Vanita D. Jain

(see *Gabbe's Obstetrics: Normal and Problem Pregnancies*, 8e: ch30)

QUESTIONS

1. What is the primary fuel utilized by the fetus of all actively transported nutrients?
   a. Amino acids
   b. Glucose
   c. Insulin
   d. Potassium

2. Which of the following is the correct order of blood flow in the fetus in regard to preferential streaming?
   a. inferior vena cava (IVC)-hepatic artery (HA)-right atrium (RA)
   b. umbilical vein (UV)-IVC-RA
   c. UV-portal vein-ductus venosus (DV)-RA
   d. UV-portal vein-right portal vein-IVC-RA

3. All of the following are examples of maternal causes of fetal growth restriction except:
   a. chronic hypertension (CHTN)
   b. Type 2 diabetes
   c. Smoking
   d. Systemic lupus
   e. Trisomy 18

4. Fetal organs have the ability to regulate their individual blood flow through a process called autoregulation. This autoregulatory mechanism has been identified in which fetal organ?
   a. Gallbladder
   b. Stomach
   c. Cerebellum
   d. Myocardium

5. A 32-year-old G1P0 presents at 14 weeks gestational age based on her last menstrual period (LMP). You perform a dating ultrasound and measure the fetus to only be 11 weeks 2 days gestation. The patient is worried her baby is "too small". Which of the following is the correct next step?
   a. Change the estimated date of delivery (EDD) to dating by today's ultrasound, given a >7-day discrepancy in the first trimester.
   b. Leave the EDC by her LMP dating and confirm the patient's fears that the baby is too small.
   c. Bring the patient back in 7 days for fetal viability.
   d. Average the EDC obtained by ultrasound and that obtained by LMP to generate a new EDC.

6. Which fetal biometry parameter is the single best measurement for the detection of intrauterine growth restriction (IUGR)?
   a. Biparietal diameter (BPD)
   b. head circumference (HC)
   c. Transcerebellar diameter (TCD)
   d. abdominal circumference (AC)
   e. femur length (FL)

7. A 32-year-old G2P1 at 28 weeks gestation presents for an ultrasound after measuring size < dates in the office. As you perform the ultrasound, you note that the calculated estimated fetal weight (EFW) is <10th percentile. The patient is concerned. While providing counseling about birth weight and outcomes, what percentage of small for gestational age (SGA) fetuses are constitutionally small and not at risk for adverse outcomes?
   a. 20%
   b. 50%
   c. 70%
   d. 90%

8. A 16-year-old G1P0 presents to obstetric triage with no prior prenatal care. Her gestational age is unknown. She thinks she might be "8 or 9 months." You perform an ultrasound to obtain an EDC and check fetal growth. The EFW is 1806 g, which, if she is 36 weeks gestation, would be concerning for fetal growth restriction. What parameters can be used to help identify fetal growth restriction rather than a dating discrepancy?

   a. FL/AC ratio with amniotic fluid index (AFI)

   b. HC/AC ratio and biophysical profile (BPP)

   c. BPD/FL ratio

   d. TCD

9. A 17-year-old G2P1001 presents for her anatomy ultrasound at 22 weeks due to late entry to care. On examination, you suspect fetal growth restriction (FGR) with an EFW below the fifth percentile. She reports a definite LMP and had an early ultrasound in obstetric triage at 12 weeks confirming this EDC. You perform a detailed anatomy evaluation. What combination of factors would pose the highest risk or suspicion for aneuploidy?

   a. EFW <5th percentile alone

   b. EFW <5th percentile along with hydramnios

   c. EFW <5th percentile along with cleft lip

   d. EFW <5th percentile, congenital heart defect and hydramnios

10. A 33-year-old G2P1001 presents for routine prenatal care. Her obstetric history is complicated by her first child weighing 2300 grams at 39 weeks. This birthweight was <10th percentile. No cause was identified, and her son is doing very well now. You discuss that her history of delivering of a prior child with FGR is associated with what risk of a recurrent SGA infant?

    a. 10%

    b. 25%

    c. 50%

    d. 90%

11. A 29-year-old G3P2002 presents to the office at 28 weeks gestational age. During your evaluation, her fundal height measures only 22 cm. You order a growth ultrasound and the EFW returns at <10th percentile. You order a biophysical profile, umbilical artery Doppler, middle cerebral artery (MCA) Doppler, umbilical venous (UV) Doppler, and ductus venosus (DV) Doppler. At this gestational age, inpatient admission and possibly delivery should be considered if any of the following is noted, except:

    a. non stress test (NST) with repetitive late decelerations

    b. BPP 2/10

    c. Tricuspid regurgitation with oligohydramnios

    d. Elevated systolic/diastolic (S/D) ratio only in the umbilical artery Doppler

12. What is the earliest gestational age at which fetal Doppler studies should be applied when fetal growth restriction is identified?

    a. 18 weeks

    b. 22 weeks

    c. 24 weeks

    d. 26 weeks

    e. 28 weeks

13. A 28-year-old G2P1001 is admitted to the labor and delivery unit for observation after a diagnosis of severe IUGR below the first percentile at her ultrasound appointment at 30 weeks gestation. You are considering timing of delivery. As such, which of the following findings poses the highest risk for acidemia and stillbirth?

    a. BPP 8/10

    b. Category II fetal hearth rate (FHR) tracing

    c. absent end diastolic flow (AEDF) in the umbilical artery

    d. Category III FHR tracing, along with oligohydramnios

14. A 28-year-old G2P1001 is admitted to the labor and delivery unit for observation after diagnosis of severe IUGR below the first percentile at her ultrasound appointment at 37 weeks gestation. You are considering timing of delivery. As such, which of the following findings poses the highest risk for acidemia and stillbirth and as such you would recommend delivery today?

    a. MCA Doppler changes suggestive of brain sparing

    b. Minimal variability on the FHR tracing

    c. AFI <5 cm

    d. All of the above

15. A 35-year-old patient is admitted to the labor and delivery unit after severe IUGR below the first percentile is identified on her ultrasound in MFM. This pregnancy is complicated by invitro fertilization (IVF). The pregnancy is 24 weeks 2 days today. The AFI is 8 cm on ultrasound. The umbilical artery Doppler studies show preserved diastolic flow, the MCA Doppler flow study is normal, the DV and UV Dopplers are also normal. For which of the following indications would you recommend delivery despite anticipated poor neonatal outcomes?

    a. AEDF in the UA Doppler

    b. Abnormal MCA Doppler showing brain sparing

    c. Oligohydramnios <5 cm

    d. Severe preeclampsia

ANSWERS

1. Answer: b

(see *Gabbe's Obstetrics* 8e: ch30)

Of the actively transported primary nutrients, glucose is the predominant oxidative fuel, whereas amino acids are major contributors to protein synthesis and muscle bulk. Glucose and, to a lesser extent, amino acids drive the insulin-like growth factors axis and therefore stimulate longitudinal fetal growth.

2. Answer: c

(see *Gabbe's Obstetrics* 8e: ch30)

Near term, 18% to 25% of umbilical venous flow shunts through the DV to reach the right atrium in this high-velocity stream; 55% reaches the dominant left hepatic lobe, and 20% reaches the right liver lobes. The direction and velocity of DV blood entering the right atrium ensure preferential streaming of nutrient-rich blood to the left ventricle, myocardium, and brain, while low-nutrient venous return is distributed to the placenta for reoxygenation and waste exchange.

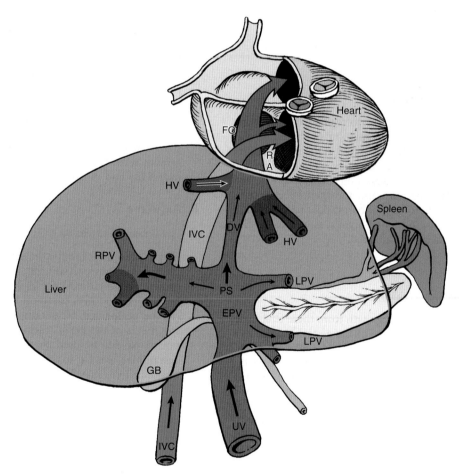

Fig. 30.1 (From Mavrides E, Moscoso G, Carvalho JS, et al. The anatomy of the umbilical, portal and hepatic venous systems in the human fetus at 14–19 weeks of gestation. *Ultrasound Obstet Gynecol.* 2001;18:598.)

3. Answer: e

(see *Gabbe's Obstetrics* 8e: ch30)

Maternal causes of FGR include vascular disease such as hypertensive disorders of pregnancy, diabetic vasculopathy, collagen vascular disease, thrombophilia, and chronic renal disease. Trisomy 18 is a fetal cause (Box 30.1).

BOX 30.1   Etiologies and Risk Factors for Intrauterine Growth Restriction

Maternal
- Hypertensive disease
- Pregestational diabetes
- Cyanotic cardiac disease
- Autoimmune disease
- Restrictive pulmonary disease
- High altitude (>10,000 feet)
- Tobacco/substance abuse
- Malabsorptive disease/malnutrition
- Multiple gestation

Fetal
- Teratogenic exposure
- Fetal infection
- Genetic disorders
- Structural abnormalities

Placental
- Primary placental disease
- Placental abruption and infarction
- Placenta previa
- Placental mosaicism

---

4. Answer: d

(see *Gabbe's Obstetrics* 8e: ch30)

Fetal organs also have the ability to regulate their individual blood flow through autoregulation. Such autoregulatory mechanisms have been identified in the myocardium, adrenal glands, spleen, liver, celiac axis, mesenteric vessels, and kidneys. These autoregulatory mechanisms are evoked at different levels of compromise and their effect is typically complementary to central blood flow redistribution by enhancing perfusion of vital organs, as long as cardiovascular homeostasis is maintained.

5. Answer: a

(see *Gabbe's Obstetrics* 8e: ch30)

Accurate estimation of fetal growth from these fetal measurements requires knowledge of the gestational age as a reference point to calculate percentile ranks. An EDC should be based on the last menstrual period when the sonographic estimate of gestational age is within the predictive error (7 days in the first, 14 days in the second, and 21 days in the third trimester). Once the EDC is set by this method or by a first-trimester ultrasound, it should not be changed because such practice interferes with the ability to diagnose FGR.

6. Answer: d

(see *Gabbe's Obstetrics* 8e: ch30)

Measurement of the biparietal diameter (BPD) alone is a poor tool for the detection of FGR. The physiologic variation in size inherent with advancing gestation is high. As a screening tool for FGR, the HC poses a similar problem as the BPD in that two-thirds of FGR fetuses with asymmetric growth pattern would be detected late. The TCD is one of the few soft tissue measurements that correlate well with gestational age, being relatively spared from the effects of mild to moderate uteroplacental dysfunction.[1] The AC is the single best measurement for the detection of FGR.[2]

7. Answer: c

(see *Gabbe's Obstetrics* 8e: ch30)

Small for gestational age is defined as a birthweight below the population 10th percentile corrected for gestational age. This definition has also been extended into the prenatal period by using an suspected estimated fetal weight (SEFW) below the 10th percentile as an indicator of FGR. Because such an approach is purely based on a weight threshold, it can only serve as a screen for the identification of the small fetus at risk for adverse outcomes. Approximately 70% of infants with a birthweight below the 10th percentile are normally grown (i.e., constitutionally small) and are not at risk for adverse outcomes because they present one end of the normal spectrum for neonatal size.[3] The remaining 30% consist of infants who are truly growth restricted and are at risk for increased perinatal morbidity and mortality.

8. Answer: a

(see *Gabbe's Obstetrics* 8e: ch30)

Oligohydramnios may be the first sign of FGR detected on ultrasonography preceding an assessment for lagging fetal growth. If gestational age is known, ultrasound assessment of fetal growth based on the HC, AC, FL, and SEFW can be performed. If gestational age is unknown, measurements of the FL/AC ratio and a single amniotic fluid pocket have to be used because they are independent of gestational age. Up to 96% of fetuses with fluid pockets less than 1 cm may be growth restricted.

9. **Answer: d**

(see *Gabbe's Obstetrics* 8e: ch30)

Trisomy 18 may present with the unusual combination of growth restriction and polyhydramnios (see Chapter 10). If the diagnosis of a lethal anomaly can be made with certainty, cesarean delivery for fetal distress is unnecessary and may be prevented (Table 30.1).

TABLE 30.1   Chromosomal Abnormalities and Intrauterine Growth Restriction.

ULTRASOUND FINDINGS PRESENT			Abnormal Karyotype
FGR	Anomaly	Hydramnios	
X			12/180 (7%)
X	X		18/57 (32%)
X		X	6/22 (27%)
X	X	X	7/15 (47%)

FGR, Intrauterine growth restriction.
From Eydoux P, Choiset, A, LePorrier, N, et al. Chromosomal prenatal diagnosis: study of 936 cases of intrauterine abnormalities after ultrasound assessment. Prenat Diagn. 1989;9:255.

10. **Answer: b**

(see *Gabbe's Obstetrics* 8e: ch30)

A history of poor pregnancy outcome is clearly correlated with the subsequent delivery of a growth-restricted infant. A prior birth of a growth-restricted infant is the obstetric factor most often associated with the subsequent birth of a growth-restricted infant. The history of delivery of a growth-restricted infant in the first pregnancy is associated with a 25% risk of delivering a second infant below the 10th percentile. After two pregnancies complicated by FGR, this risk is increased fourfold.

11. Answer: d

(see *Gabbe's Obstetrics* 8e: ch30)

In the fetal compartment, elevation of the UA Doppler index is observed when approximately 30% of the fetal villous vessels are abnormal. These studies and subsequent analyses confirm that fetal Doppler assessment based on the UA alone is no longer appropriate, particularly in the setting of early-onset FGR prior to 34 weeks. Incorporation of MCA and venous Doppler provide the best prediction of acid-base status, risk of stillbirth, and the anticipated rate of progression. In growth-restricted fetuses with an elevated Doppler index in the UA, brain sparing in the presence of normal venous Doppler parameters is typically associated with hypoxemia but a normal pH. Elevation of venous Doppler indices, either alone or in combination with umbilical venous pulsations, increases the risk for fetal acidemia. Abnormal venous Doppler parameters are the strongest Doppler predictors of stillbirth. Even among fetuses with severe arterial Doppler abnormalities (e.g., absent end diastolic velocity (AEDV) or reverse end diastolic velocity (REDV)), the risk of stillbirth is largely confined to those fetuses with abnormal venous Dopplers.[4]

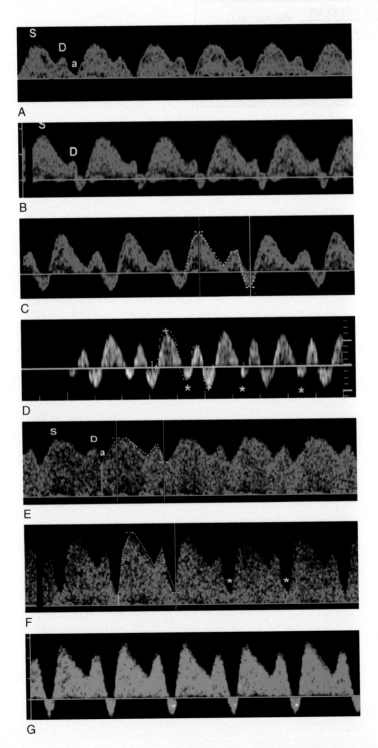

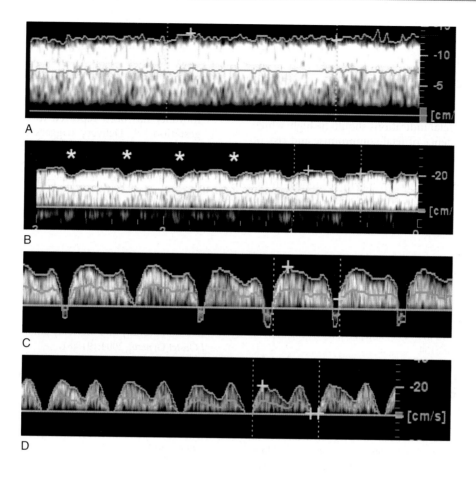

12. Answer: c, p. 58

(see *Gabbe's Obstetrics* 8e: ch30)

In general, fetal Doppler studies are indicated once intervention would be feasible for the neonate. Since fetal Doppler studies in the setting of FGR are unreliable at <24 weeks gestation, they should not be performed. In fetuses with elevated UA pulsatility index, positive end-diastolic flow, and absence of any additional abnormality, weekly BPP is performed, along with multivessel Doppler monitoring studies every 2 weeks. In fetuses with an AFI of less than 5 cm or AEDV in the umbilical artery, surveillance intervals are shortened to every 3 to 4 days. With elevation of the DV Doppler index to less than 2 SD, testing frequency is increased to every 2 to 3 days. Further escalation of the DV Doppler index may require daily testing, and inpatient admission may be prudent based on local practice.

13. Answer: d

(see *Gabbe's Obstetrics* 8e: ch30)

Delivery is typically indicated when the risk for these complications is high or there is no added benefit from prolongation of pregnancy. In the preterm growth-restricted fetus, the risk for acidemia and stillbirth is highest when repetitive late decelerations are observed in association with oligohydramnios and/or anhydramnios, when the BPP is below 6, when the DV Doppler index elevation escalates beyond 3 SDs, or when reversal of the DV a-wave is observed with accompanying umbilical venous pulsations.

14. Answer: d

(see *Gabbe's Obstetrics* 8e: ch30)

In the growth-restricted fetus beyond 37 weeks, risks of unanticipated stillbirth increase when brain sparing, loss of heart rate reactivity, or a decrease in the AFV are observed.[5] A recent study from the Washington University group[6] demonstrated that although the overall risk of stillbirth is low in fetuses beyond 37 weeks, an increase in stillbirth risk occurs with each advancing week for ongoing pregnancies. Thus, they recommend delivery of the FGR fetus at 37 to 38 weeks. The study is limited by its retrospective nature and that the growth-restricted fetuses that died in utero may not have been identified and followed with Doppler or antenatal testing.

15. **Answer: d, p. 63**

(see *Gabbe's Obstetrics* 8e: ch30)

Between 24 and 26 weeks gestation, a growth-restricted fetus is periviable, and interventions are typically undertaken for maternal conditions such as severe preeclampsia. Thresholds for fetal indications should be high, which requires strong evidence of fetal compromise and risk of stillbirth. Management is frequently individualized, and a multidisciplinary approach is helpful in stressing that outcome may be poor even with maximal support in the neonatal intensive care unit. Parents need to be aware that despite maximum management and effort, perinatal mortality exceeds 50%.[7,8] Based on retrospective studies, 29 weeks gestation may be an important milestone to reach. Gestational age appears to be the strongest predictor of infant survival until 29 weeks, and 94% of perinatal morality has been reported to occur prior to 29 weeks gestation.[7,9,10] Delivery triggers can be considered to be any one or a combination of: FHR tracing with decelerations, BPP of 4 or less, or reverse a-wave in the ductus venosus, a marker of fetal acidemia.

REFERENCES

1. Smith PA, Johansson D, Tzannatos C, et al. Prenatal measurement of the fetal cerebellum and cisterna cerebellomedullaris by ultrasound. *Prenat Diagn.* 1986;6:133.

2. Baschat AA, Weiner CP. Umbilical artery Doppler screening for detection of the small fetus in need of antepartum surveillance. *Am J Obstet Gynecol.* 2000;182:154.

3. Ott WJ. The diagnosis of altered fetal growth. *Obstet Gynecol Clin North Am.* 1988;15:237.

4. Paolini CL, Marconi AM, Ronzoni S, et al. Placental transport of leucine, phenylalanine, glycine, and proline in intrauterine growth-restricted pregnancies. *J Clin Endocrinol Metab.* 2001;86:5427.

5. Crimmins S, Desai A, Block-Abraham D, Berg C, Gembruch U, Baschat AA. A comparison of Doppler and biophysical findings between liveborn and stillborn growth-restricted fetuses. *Am J Obstet Gynecol.* 2014;211: 669.e1-669.e10.

6. Trudell AS, Cahill AG, Tuuli MG, et al. Risk of stillbirth after 37 weeks in pregnancies complicated by small-for-gestational-age fetuses. *Am J Obstet Gynecol.* 2013;208:376.e1-e7.

7. Baschat AA, Bilardo CM, Germer U, et al. Thresholds for intervention in severe early onset growth restriction. *Am J Obstet Gynecol.* 2004;191:S143.

8. Garite TJ, Clark R, Thorp JA. Intrauterine growth restriction increases morbidity and mortality among premature neonates. *Am J Obstet Gynecol.* 2004;191:481.

9. Mariari G, Hanif F, Treadwell MC, Kruger M. Gestational age at delivery and Doppler waveforms in very preterm intrauterine growth-restricted fetuses as predictors of perinatal mortality. *J Ultrasound Med.* 2007;26:555-559.

10. McIntire DD, Bloom SL, Casey BM, et al. Birth weight in relation to morbidity and mortality among newborn infants. *N Engl J Med.* 1999;340:1234.

31

Surgery During Pregnancy

Alyssa Stephenson-Famy

(see *Gabbe's Obstetrics: Normal and Problem Pregnancies*, 8e: ch31)

QUESTIONS

1. A woman at 16 weeks gestation presents with right lower quadrant abdominal pain and emesis. Her abdominal examination shows rebound and guarding. Laboratory tests demonstrate an elevated WBC count (14,000 cells/mm^3). Laparoscopy confirms the diagnosis of appendicitis. For this patient, what sign or symptom was most consistent with the diagnosis of appendicitis in pregnancy?

   a. Right lower quadrant abdominal pain

   b. Nausea and vomiting

   c. Rebound

   d. Guarding

   e. Leukocytosis

2. Ultrasound of maternal urinary system commonly shows which normal physiologic finding during pregnancy?

   a. Mild hydronephrosis

   b. Severe hydroureter

   c. Thickened bladder wall

   d. Absent ureteral jets

   e. Ureterocele

3. A woman at 8 weeks gestation is in a motor vehicle accident and requires several imaging studies to evaluate for traumatic injuries. She should be counseled that radiation exposure below which threshold has not been associated with fetal anomalies or loss?

   a. Less than 0.5 Rad (0.5 cGy or 5 mGy)

   b. Less than 1 Rad (1 cGy or 10 mGy)

   c. Less than 5 Rad (5 cGy or 50 mGy)

   d. Less than 10 Rad (10 cGy or 100 mGy)

   e. Less than 50 Rad (50 cGy or 500 mGy)

4. A woman at 6 weeks gestation presents with hematuria and right costovertebral-angle back tenderness. Her pain is intermittent but is severe when it occurs. Which imaging study carries the highest risk of ionizing radiation and should be avoided during this patient's evaluation?

   a. Ultrasound

   b. MRI

   c. Abdominopelvic radiograph

   d. Abdominopelvic CT (stone protocol)

   e. Abdominopelvic CT

5. A woman at 20 weeks gestation undergoes laparoscopic removal of an ovarian cyst which was at risk for torsion. She is required to stop eating and drinking 8 hours in advance and is given a dose of sodium citrate (30 mL) prior to the surgery. These interventions decrease the risk of which complication of general anesthesia?

   a. Aspiration

   b. Oropharyngeal edema

   c. Esophageal ulceration

   d. Gastric compression by the gravid uterus

   e. Bowel ileus

6. A woman with Crohn disease undergoes an urgent laparotomy for bowel obstruction at 32 weeks. What is the optimal maternal position on the operating room table to minimize aortocaval compression?

   a. Left-lateral tilt

   b. Right-lateral tilt

   c. Dorsal lithotomy

   d. Supine

   e. Prone

7. A 40-year-old woman is diagnosed with cholelithiasis at 10 weeks gestation. When is the safest time to undergo laparoscopic cholecystectomy for recurrent biliary colic during pregnancy?

    a. First trimester

    b. Early second trimester

    c. Late second trimester

    d. Third trimester

    e. Should be delayed indefinitely

8. A 43 year-old-woman at 18 weeks gestation is found on ultrasound to have a 7-cm adnexal mass with solid and cystic components, mural nodules, internal septations, and increased blood flow. She is scheduled to undergo a diagnostic laparoscopy. What is the optimal insufflation pressure during surgery?

    a. 5–10 mm CO_2

    b. 10–15 mm CO_2

    c. 20–30 mm CO_2

    d. Manage CO_2 insufflation pressure by use of capnography

    e. There is no safe CO_2 insufflation pressure in pregnancy

9. A 30-year-old woman becomes pregnant 1 year after a Roux-en-Y gastric bypass. What vitamin deficiency is she most likely to develop during pregnancy?

    a. Vitamin B_6

    b. Vitamin B_{12}

    c. Vitamin A

    d. Vitamin E

    e. Vitamin K

ANSWERS

1. **Answer: a**

    (See *Gabbe's Obstetrics* 8e: ch31)

    Despite the progressive upward displacement of the appendix in pregnancy, the most consistent and reliable symptom in pregnant women with appendicitis remains right lower quadrant pain. Many other classic signs and symptoms of appendicitis—such as nausea, vomiting, and leukocytosis—may be normal findings in pregnancy. Similarly, physical examination findings of rebound and guarding may not be reliable indicators of intraperitoneal inflammation in pregnancy.

2. **Answer: a**

    (See *Gabbe's Obstetrics* 8e: ch31)

    Some anatomic changes related to the growing uterus may confound the interpretation of diagnostic imaging. For example, mild to moderate upper urinary tract dilation is often a normal finding in pregnancy secondary to compression of the distal ureters by the uterus and progesterone-induced smooth muscle relaxation.

3. **Answer: c**

    (See *Gabbe's Obstetrics* 8e: ch31)

    Overall, the use of diagnostic radiation in pregnant women requires adequate patient counseling to allay concerns of fetal harm and to balance any small potential risk against the need to arrive at an accurate and timely diagnosis. Per American College of Obstetricians and Gynecologists (ACOG), women should be counseled that X-ray exposure to less than 5 Rad (50 mGy) has not been associated with an increase in fetal anomalies or pregnancy loss.

4. **Answer: e**

(See *Gabbe's Obstetrics* 8e: ch31)

Overall, the safety and versatility of ultrasonography makes it the first-line diagnostic tool during pregnancy whenever appropriate to address the clinical question at hand. There are numerous advantages to MRI use during pregnancy. Like ultrasound, MRI does not use ionizing radiation, and no harmful effects to the mother or fetus have been reported. The highest dose of ionizing radiation is an abdominopelvic CT scan (2.5–3.5 cGy) (Table 31.1).

TABLE 31.1 Estimated Fetal Exposure to Radiation from Common Diagnostic Radiologic Studies.

Radiologic Study	Estimated Fetal Dose (cGy)[a]
Chest radiograph (posteroanterior, lateral)	0.0002
Abdominal radiograph	0.1–0.3
Head CT	0.0005
Chest CT	0.002–0.02
Abdominal CT	0.4–0.8
Abdominopelvic CT	2.5–3.5
Abdominopelvic CT (stone protocol)	1
Ventilation scan	0.007–0.05
Perfusion scan	0.04
Intravenous pyelography	0.6–1.0
Bone scan	0.3–0.5
Positron emission scan	1.0–1.5
Thyroid scan	0.01–0.02
Mammography	0.007–0.02
Small bowel series	0.7
Barium enema	0.7

[a]Fetal dose can vary significantly based on a number of patient and imaging parameters. If necessary, more precise estimates can be obtained through consultation with a radiation safety officer or radiation physicist.

5. **Answer: a**

(See *Gabbe's Obstetrics* 8e: ch31)

There is an increased risk for aspiration in pregnant women who undergo general anesthesia because of prolonged gastric emptying time and decreased tone at the gastroesophageal junction, due to progesterone. Strategies to decrease the risk for aspiration include preoperative fasting, antacid prophylaxis (e.g., 30 mL of sodium citrate), and airway protection.

6. **Answer: a**

(See *Gabbe's Obstetrics* 8e: ch31)

Aortocaval compression by the gravid uterus in the supine position in the latter half of pregnancy leads to a decreased preload and cardiac output, with a resultant decrease in uterine and placental perfusion. Pregnant women who undergo a surgical procedure should be positioned with a lateral tilt to relieve some of this compression by displacing the gravid uterus to the side.

7. **Answer: b**

(see *Gabbe's Obstetrics* 8e: ch31)

Surgery in the first trimester is avoided due to risks of teratogenicity with anesthesia. In the late-second and third trimester, intraoperative visibility may be more challenging and there is an increased risk for preterm birth. Therefore, the early second trimester is considered the optimal time for elective surgery that cannot be safely deferred until after the pregnancy.

8. Answer: b

(see *Gabbe's Obstetrics* 8e: ch31)

Fortunately, most adnexal masses encountered in pregnancy are benign and spontaneously resolve during the course of pregnancy. In fact, rates of spontaneous resolution have been reported to be as high as 72%–96%. Although most adnexal masses encountered in pregnancy are benign, the rare possibility of malignancy should not be discounted. In fact, between 1%–3% of masses removed in pregnancy are found to be malignant. When laparoscopy is indicated, abdominal insufflation pressures should be kept below 15 mm Hg whenever possible. CO_2 insufflation of 10–15 mm Hg can be safely used for laparoscopy in the pregnant patient. Intraabdominal pressure should be sufficient to allow for adequate visualization (Box 31.1).

9. Answer: b

(see *Gabbe's Obstetrics* 8e: ch31)

Bariatric surgery is an increasingly common and effective treatment for obesity and has been associated with a significant improvement in overall health and a reduction in adverse pregnancy outcomes. As a result of the surgery, there is reduced absorptive capacity of the stomach and proximal small bowel, which often leads to deficiencies in several essential nutrients, including iron, vitamins B_{12} and D, folate, and calcium.

> **BOX 31.1 Relevant Guidelines for Laparoscopy in Pregnancy From the Society of American Gastrointestinal and Endoscopic Surgeons**
>
> - Diagnostic laparoscopy is safe and effective when used selectively in the workup and treatment of acute abdominal processes in pregnancy.
> - Laparoscopic treatment of acute abdominal processes has the same indications in pregnant and nonpregnant patients.
> - Laparoscopy can be safely performed during any trimester of pregnancy.
> - Gravid patients should be placed in the left lateral recumbent position to minimize compression of the vena cava and the aorta.
> - Initial access can be safely accomplished with open (Hassan), Veress needle, or optical trocar technique if the location is adjusted according to fundal height, previous incisions, and experience of the surgeon.
> - CO_2 insufflation of 10–15 mm Hg can be safely used for laparoscopy in the pregnant patient. Intraabdominal pressure should be sufficient to allow for adequate visualization.
> - Intraoperative CO_2 monitoring by capnography should be used during laparoscopy in the pregnant patient.
> - Intraoperative and postoperative pneumatic compression devices and early postoperative ambulation are recommended prophylaxis for deep venous thrombosis in the gravid patient.
> - Laparoscopic cholecystectomy is the treatment of choice in the pregnant patient with gallbladder disease, regardless of trimester.
> - Laparoscopic appendectomy may be performed safely in pregnant patients with suspicion of appendicitis.
> - Laparoscopic adrenalectomy, nephrectomy, and splenectomy are safe procedures in pregnant patients when indicated, and standard precautions are taken.
> - Laparoscopy is safe and effective treatment in gravid patients with symptomatic adnexal cystic masses. Observation is acceptable for all other adnexal cystic lesions, provided ultrasound is not worrisome for malignancy and tumor markers are normal. Initial observation is warranted for most adnexal cystic lesions smaller than 6 cm.
> - Laparoscopy is recommended for both diagnosis and treatment of adnexal torsion unless clinical severity warrants laparotomy.
> - Fetal heart monitoring should occur before and after operation in the setting of urgent abdominal surgery during pregnancy.
> - Obstetric consultation can be obtained before and after operation, based on the acuteness of the patient's disease, gestational age, and availability of the consultant.
> - Tocolytics should not be used prophylactically but should be considered perioperatively, in coordination with obstetric consultation, when signs of preterm labor are present.
>
> From Yumi H. Guidelines for diagnosis, treatment, and use of laparoscopy for surgical problems during pregnancy: this statement was reviewed and approved by the Board of Governors of the Society of American Gastrointestinal and Endoscopic Surgeons (SAGES), September 2007. It was prepared by the SAGES Guidelines Committee. *Surg Endosc.* 2008;22:849-861.

32

Trauma in Pregnancy

Audrey Merriam

(see *Gabbe's Obstetrics: Normal and Problem Pregnancies*, 8e: ch32)

QUESTIONS

1. An 18-year-old G1P0 at 30 weeks gestation presents for a prenatal visit. She says that she has stopped wearing her seatbelt in the car because it has become uncomfortable with her growing abdomen and she feels like she cannot breathe when it is on. What do you tell her about this practice?

 a. It is fine that she is not wearing her seatbelt because it is safer for pregnant women to not wear a seatbelt if they get in a car accident.

 b. It is fine that she does not wear her seatbelt if she is not on the highway. If she is traveling at 55 mph or over she should wear her seatbelt.

 c. She should wear her seatbelt at all times in the car and the lap part of the belt should go across her abdomen at the level of her umbilicus.

 d. She should wear her seatbelt at all times in the car but she should put the shoulder strap under her arm and breasts rather than across her collarbone.

 e. She should wear her seatbelt at all times in the car and the lap part of the belt should go across her hips and upper thighs, underneath her abdomen.

2. A 17-year-old G1P0 presents for her first prenatal visit at 16 weeks gestation. She has no significant medical or surgical history. She just moved out of her parents' house and in with the father of the baby, who has guns in the home. She had found a job cleaning houses and is happy about the pregnancy and living away from home because her parents were "always in her business." During the examination you lift her shirt to assess fetal heart tones and notice large bruises on her abdomen in different stages of healing. She says that she is just clumsy at work. What is the most likely cause?

 a. Intimate partner violence (IPV)

 b. Gestational thrombocytopenia

 c. Intravenous drug use

 d. Multiple sclerosis with bruising from multiple falls

 e. Hemophilia A

3. A 34-year-old G2P1001 at 26 weeks gestation has fallen off a second-story balcony. She is en route to the hospital and the emergency medical technicians (EMTs) call the hospital for advice on care. She is conscious but appears confused. You learn she has two 18-gauge IV cannulas in, she is on a backboard with a left tilt (with a towel under the board), and she has a cervical collar on. You are concerned because your neonatal intensive care unit (NICU) only accepts infants 32 weeks and above, but the EMT tells you she is concerned about the woman's level of consciousness and the large laceration on her forehead. She is now having a bradyarrhythmia on the electrocardiogram (EKG) in the ambulance. What do you advise the EMT?

 a. Go to the hospital with a level IV NICU that is a further 10 minutes down the highway.

 b. Bring the patient to the emergency department, not the labor floor.

 c. The patient should not be strapped to a backboard while pregnant.

 d. Tell them to listen to the fetal heart with a stethoscope.

 e. Do not administer a shock if the patient goes into cardiac arrest because it will harm the fetus.

4. A 26-year-old G3P1011 at 26 weeks gestation presents after a minor motor vehicle accident at 6:00 p.m. She had a rear-end collision with the car in front of her. She was driving 20 mph at the time of the collision. Her airbag deployed. She is not complaining of any abdominal pain, contractions, or vaginal bleeding. Your physical examination is unremarkable and there is no bruising on her abdomen. You order appropriate laboratory tests. The fetal heart tracing is category I. She has had eight contractions in the hour on the monitor. She is asking when she can return home because she feels fine. What is your response?

   a. Since her labs are normal and she is only at 26 weeks gestation she can leave now.

   b. She can leave after 4 hours of monitoring total if the fetal heart rate remains reactive.

   c. Since she is contracting every 10 minutes, 24 hours of monitoring is recommended.

   d. She can leave at 10:00 p.m., which is 4 hours from the accident, if the fetal tracing remains normal.

   e. She must stay for 48 hours to receive a full course of betamethasone.

5. A 22-year-old woman is brought to the emergency department after being struck by a motor vehicle while she was crossing the street. She is unconscious and is unaccompanied on arrival. She is visibly pregnant and ultrasound biometry reveals a gestational age of 20 weeks and a fetal heart rate at 160 bpm. The trauma team would like to image her head, chest, abdomen, and pelvis to assess for injuries and fractures. They ask you for advice on the optimal imaging modality given the patient is pregnant. What is your response?

   a. Ultrasound of her abdomen followed by MRI with gadolinium of her head, chest, abdomen, and pelvis

   b. Ultrasound of her abdomen followed by CT with IV contrast of her head, chest, abdomen, and pelvis

   c. Ultrasound of her abdomen followed by MRI of her head and chest only

   d. Ultrasound of her abdomen followed by CT of her head and chest only

   e. CT of her head and chest followed by MRI of her abdomen and pelvis, both with contrast

6. Which adverse pregnancy outcome has the highest risk after abdominal trauma in pregnancy?

   a. Abruption

   b. Stillbirth

   c. Fetal bone fractures

   d. Preterm labor

   e. Preterm premature rupture of membranes

ANSWERS

1. **Answer: e**

   (see *Gabbe's Obstetrics* 8e: ch32)

   There is evidence that restraint use reduces maternal and fetal morbidity and mortality in car crashes and American College of Obstetricians and Gynecologists (ACOG) recommends seatbelt use in pregnancy. The National Highway and Traffic Safety Administration recommends pregnant women wear their seatbelts with the shoulder harness portion over the collarbone, between the breasts and the lap, belt portion under the abdomen, as low as possible on the hips, and across the upper thighs.

2. **Answer: a**

   (see *Gabbe's Obstetrics* 8e: ch32)

   Incidence of IPV ranges from 6%–22% during pregnancy. Risk factors for IPV include African American and Native American ethnicity and lower socioeconomic status. Patients who present with a vague or inconsistent history of trauma should raise suspicion. The abdomen is the most common target for assault.

3. **Answer: b**

   (see *Gabbe's Obstetrics* 8e: ch32)

   Guidelines for emergency medical personnel include displacing the uterus from the inferior vena cava (IVC) by positioning the mother in a lateral decubitus position, and a towel may be placed under the spine immobilization board to do this. A pregnant trauma victim should be transported to the closest facility rather than a designated trauma center because of concerns for maternal survival. Regardless of gestational age, all pregnant women with serious injuries should be evaluated in the emergency department first, with maternal well-being prioritized and fetal evaluation occurring simultaneously with maternal evaluation and treatment.

4. Answer: c

(see *Gabbe's Obstetrics* 8e: ch32)

After abdominal trauma, if contractions are noted at least every 15 minutes, even if no other signs or symptoms of abruption are present, 24 hours of monitoring is recommended, due to the risk for delayed placental abruption. Delayed abruption is unlikely to occur if contraction frequency is more than every 10 minutes with normal fetal heart rate activity. This level of monitoring is recommended from viability (23–24 weeks gestation).

5. Answer: b

(see *Gabbe's Obstetrics* 8e: ch32)

Guidelines support the use of ultrasound as the initial modality but recommend the use of CT as the preferred method of evaluation when visceral injuries or injuries of the chest, aorta, mediastinum, spine, bones, bowel, or bladder are suspected. IV contrast should be used, because the use of iodinated contrast agents during pregnancy is preferable to the patient receiving repetitive CT studies because of the suboptimal imaging.

6. Answer: a

(see *Gabbe's Obstetrics* 8e: ch32)

Fetal death certificate review calculates the rate of fetal death from maternal trauma at 2.3 per 100,000 live births, and placental abruption was the leading contributing factor.

33

Early Pregnancy Loss

Rini Banerjee Ratan

(see *Gabbe's Obstetrics: Normal and Problem Pregnancies*, 8e: ch33)

QUESTIONS

1. How many women with clinically recognized pregnancies will suffer a pregnancy loss?

   a. 1%–2%

   b. 5%–7%

   c. 10%–15%

   d. 20%–30%

   e. 50%–70%

2. A 24-year-old G1P0 at 8 weeks gestation presents to her obstetrician's office with vaginal bleeding. Ultrasound shows an early pregnancy failure. The patient undergoes surgical evacuation of the uterus and the products of conception are sent for pathologic evaluation. Which of the following is the most likely etiology for this patient's pregnancy loss?

   a. Autosomal trisomy

   b. Nonmosaic triploidy

   c. Structural anomalies

   d. Sex chromosomal polysomy

   e. Tetraploidy

3. When do most clinical pregnancy losses occur?

   a. Before 6 weeks

   b. Before 8 weeks

   c. Between 10–12 weeks

   d. After 12 weeks

   e. After 16 weeks

4. A 35-year-old G1P0 at 36 weeks gestation presents to the labor and delivery unit because she has not felt her baby move for the past 12 hours. Her pregnancy has been uncomplicated thus far. She is otherwise healthy. A fetal heart beat cannot be detected using a Doppler transducer. Bedside ultrasound confirms an intrauterine fetal demise. Biometry shows an appropriately grown fetus. Which of the following laboratory tests should be performed to help determine the etiology of this patient's stillbirth?

   a. Antinuclear antibodies

   b. Rubella titer

   c. Cytomegalovirus immunoglobulin M (IgM) and immunoglobulin G (IgG)

   d. Lupus anticoagulant (LAC)

   e. Herpes simplex virus serologies

5. Approximately what percentage of stillbirths are caused by genetic factors?

   a. 5%

   b. 10%

   c. 25%

   d. 50%

   e. 75%

6. A 28-year-old G3P0030 presents to her physician's office for evaluation of recurrent pregnancy loss. She has had three first-trimester miscarriages over the past 4 years. She is otherwise healthy. She reports regular monthly menses. She and her male partner have sexual intercourse 2–3 times weekly, and they have not had difficulty conceiving. Her partner has had a normal semen analysis. Which of the following is the most appropriate next step in maternal evaluation?

   a. Fasting insulin level

   b. Thyroid studies

   c. Hereditary thrombophilia screening

   d. Luteal phase progesterone level

   e. Karyotype

7. A 31-year-old G2P0010 presents to her physician's office for preconceptual counseling. She has had two miscarriages in the past 2 years, both before 10 weeks gestation. She reports regular monthly menses. She was recently diagnosed with depression and has been taking fluoxetine daily. She has no other medical problems. She drinks two to three glasses of wine during the week. She drinks one cup of coffee every morning. She smokes a half-pack of cigarettes daily. She weighs 120 lb (54 kg), is 5′5″ tall, and her BMI is 20. Which of the following interventions is most likely to reduce her risk of miscarriage?

   a. Discontinuing fluoxetine

   b. Decreasing alcohol intake

   c. Switching to decaffeinated coffee in the morning

   d. Smoking cessation

   e. Weight gain of 5–10 lb

8. A 38-year-old G3P0030 presents to her physician's office for a follow-up visit after undergoing dilatation and curettage for her third early pregnancy loss 4 months ago. Laboratory testing done at that time and again 1 week ago showed markedly elevated anticardiolipin antibodies (aCL) and anti-β2-glycoprotein antibodies (aβ2GPI). She is otherwise healthy and would like to become pregnant again as soon as possible. Which of the following interventions in a future pregnancy is most likely to reduce her risk of recurrent miscarriage?

   a. Low-dose aspirin and heparin

   b. Metformin

   c. Low-molecular-weight heparin

   d. Progesterone

   e. Human chorionic gonadotropin supplementation

9. A 32-year-old G2P0020 presents to her physician's office for evaluation of recurrent pregnancy loss. She has had two miscarriages over the past 3 years—one at 16 weeks and the other at 18 weeks. She is otherwise healthy. Maternal laboratory testing has been within normal limits. She reports regular monthly menses. She has not had difficulty conceiving. Transvaginal 3-dimensional ultrasonography is ordered. Which of the following findings is the most likely etiology of her recurrent miscarriages?

   a. Submucosal leiomyoma

   b. Subseptate uterus

   c. Arcuate uterus

   d. Intramural leiomyoma

   e. Bicornuate uterus

   f. Subserosal leiomyoma

10. A 27-year-old G3P1021 presents to her physician's office for preconceptual counseling. Her first pregnancy ended in a first-trimester spontaneous abortion. She subsequently had a full-term normal spontaneous vaginal delivery of a healthy male infant. She then had another first-trimester miscarriage. She and her partner are otherwise healthy. What is her risk of recurrence for spontaneous abortion in a future pregnancy?

   a. 2%

   b. 5%

   c. 10%

   d. 25%

   e. 30%

ANSWERS

1. Answer: **c**

(see *Gabbe's Obstetrics* 8e: ch33)

About 50%–70% of spontaneous conceptions are lost before completion of the first trimester, most before implantation or during the first month after the last menstrual period. These losses are often not recognized as conceptions. Of clinically recognized pregnancies, 10%–15% are lost.

2. Answer: **a**

(see *Gabbe's Obstetrics* 8e: ch33)

Autosomal trisomies represent the largest (about 50%) single class of chromosomal complements in cytogenetically early pregnancy failure. That is, 25% of all miscarriages are trisomic, given half of all abortuses have a chromosomal abnormality. Frequencies of various trisomies are listed in Table 33.1.

TABLE 33.1 Chromosomal Completion in Spontaneous Abortions Recognized Clinically in the First Trimester.

Chromosomal Complement	Frequency	Percent
Normal 46,XX or 46,XY	–	54.1
Triploidy	–	7.7
69,XXX	2.7	–
69,XYX	0.2	–
69,XXY	4.0	–
Other	0.8	–
Tetraploidy	–	2.6
92,XXX	1.5	–
92,XXYY	0.55	–
Not stated	0.55	–
Monosomy X	–	18.6
Structural abnormalities	–	1.5
Sex chromosomal polysomy	–	0.2
47,XXX	0.05	–
47,XXY	0.15	–
Autosomal monosomy (G)	–	0.1
Autosomal trisomy for chromosomes	–	22.3
1	0	–
2	1.11	–
3	0.25	–
4	0.64	–
5	0.04	–
6	0.14	–
7	0.89	–
8	0.79	–
9	0.72	–
10	0.36	–
11	0.04	–
12	0.18	–
13	1.07	–
14	0.82	–
15	1.68	–
16	7.27	–
17	0.18	–
18	1.15	–
19	0.01	–
20	0.61	–
21	2.11	–
22	2.26	–
Double trisomy	–	0.7
Mosaic trisomy	–	1.3
Other abnormalities or not specified	–	0.9
	–	100.0

Data from Simpson JL, Bombard AT. Chromosomal abnormalities in spontaneous abortion: frequency, pathology and genetic counseling. In: Edmonds K, ed. Spontaneous Abortion. London: Blackwell; 1987.

3. **Answer: b**

(see *Gabbe's Obstetrics* 8e: ch33)

Embryos implant 6 days after conception. Even immediately after implantation, determined chemically by the presence of β-human chorionic gonadotropin (β-hCG) in maternal serum, about 30% of pregnancies are lost. Physical signs are not generally appreciated until 5–6 weeks after the last menstrual period.[1] After clinical recognition, 10%–12% are lost. Most clinical pregnancy losses occur before 8 weeks.

4. **Answer: d**

(see *Gabbe's Obstetrics* 8e: ch33)

Certain maternal laboratory tests are recommended by ACOG in the setting of a stillbirth (Box 33.1).[2] Even if the cause of the stillbirth may seem obvious (e.g., diabetes mellitus), it is prudent to order recommended laboratory tests because the ostensible diagnosis may prove erroneous. Of note, ACOG does not recommend testing for antinuclear antibodies, for certain serologies (toxoplasmosis, rubella, cytomegalovirus, herpes simplex virus), or for genetic tests other than a karyotype.

BOX 33.1 Maternal Laboratory Tests Recommended by ACOG Following Stillbirth

All Mothers Having Stillbirths
- Complete blood count
- Kleihauer-Betke or other test for fetal cells in maternal circulation
- Human parvovirus-B19 immunoglobulin G; immunoglobulin M antibody
- Syphilis
- Lupus anticoagulant
- Anticardiolipin antibody
- Thyroid-stimulating hormone

Selected Mothers Having Stillbirths
- Thrombophilia
  - Factor V Leiden
  - Prothrombin gene mutation
  - Antithrombin III
  - Homocysteine (fasting)
- Protein S and protein C activity
- Parental karyotypes
- Indirect Coombs test
- Glucose screening (oral glucose tolerance test, hemoglobin A1c)
- Toxicology screen

Data from ACOG Practice Bulletin No. 102: management of stillbirth. 2009.

---

5. **Answer: c**

(see *Gabbe's Obstetrics* 8e: ch33)

Approximately 25% of stillbirths have been attributed to genetic etiologies.[3,4] The most common cytogenetic abnormalities are similar to those seen in liveborn infants and include 45X, trisomy 21, trisomy 18, and trisomy 13.

6. **Answer: e**

(see *Gabbe's Obstetrics* 8e: ch33)

After three miscarriages, evaluation is usually indicated. Chromosomal rearrangements exist in 2%–3% of recurrent early pregnancy loss (REPL) L couples. Ideally all parents should have their karyotype evaluated for chromosomal rearrangements, but this is not considered cost effective by RCOG. There is not a routine recommendation for universal diabetes or thyroid screening among women with sporadic or REPL. Luteal phase defects are no longer considered a likely explanation and thus progesterone level measurements are of no use in the management of REPL.

7. **Answer: d**

(see *Gabbe's Obstetrics* 8e: ch33)

Alcohol consumption may increase pregnancy loss slightly, but the evidence is limited. Considerable controversy exists regarding the relation between maternal caffeine intake during pregnancy and the risks of miscarriage. Any active smoking is associated with increased risk of miscarriage (relative risk (RR) ratio 1.23; 95% confidence interval (CI) 1.16–1.30) and that risk increases with the amount smoked (1% increase in relative risk per cigarette smoked per day).[5] The use of antidepressants in early pregnancy has been associated in some studies with a slightly increased risk of miscarriage.[6] However, this link has not been shown to be causal.

8. **Answer: d**

(see *Gabbe's Obstetrics* 8e: ch33)

The most common acquired thrombophilia in pregnancy is the antiphospholipid syndrome (APS), an autoimmune disease characterized by the presence of antiphospholipid antibodies (aPLs), such as LAC antibodies, aCL, or anti-β2–glycoprotein antibodies (aβ2GPI). Values for the latter two should be greater than the 99th percentile, of moderate or higher titers, and at least 12 weeks apart, in order to make a diagnosis that the syndrome is present. A systematic review and metaanalysis have shown that for women with APS and at least two prior pregnancy losses, the combination of heparin and aspirin confers a significant benefit in live births against first-trimester losses (OR 0.39; 95% CI 0.24–0.65).[7]

9. Answer: c

(see *Gabbe's Obstetrics* 8e: ch33)

Müllerian fusion defects are in fact an accepted cause of second-trimester losses and pregnancy complications. In a study published in 2001, women with a subseptate uterus were found to have a significantly higher proportion of first-trimester loss compared with women with a normal uterus, whereas women with an arcuate uterus had a significantly greater proportion of second-trimester loss.[8] None of the unification defects reduce fertility, but some are associated with miscarriage and preterm delivery, leading the authors to conclude that arcuate uteri are specifically associated with second-trimester miscarriage. There is no increase in risk of early pregnancy loss among those with leiomyomas compared to those without.

10. Answer: d

(see *Gabbe's Obstetrics* 8e: ch33)

See Table 33.2.

TABLE 33.2   Approximate Recurrence Risk Figures Useful for Counseling Women with Repeated Spontaneous Abortions.

	Prior Abortions	Risk (%)
Women with live-born infant	0	5–10
	1	20–25
	2	25
	3	30
	4	30
Women without live-born infant	3	30–40

Recurrence risks are slightly higher for older women.
Data from Regan L: A prospective study on spontaneous abortion. In: Beard RW, Sharp F, eds. Early Pregnancy Loss: Mechanisms and Treatment. London: Springer-Verlag; 1988: 22. Warburton D, Fraser FC. Spontaneous abortion risks in man: data from reproductive histories collected in a medical genetic unit. Am J Hum Genet. 1964;16:1-25. and Poland BJ, Miller JR, Jones DC, Trimble BK. Reproductive counseling in patients who have had a spontaneous abortion. *Am J Obstet Gynecol.* 1977;127:685-691.

REFERENCES

1. Jauniaux E, Poston L, Burton GJ. Placental-related diseases of pregnancy: involvement of oxidative stress and implications in human evolution. *Hum Reprod Update.* 2006;12:747-755.
2. Stillbirth Collaborative Research Network Writing Group. Association between stillbirth and risk factors known at pregnancy confirmation. *JAMA.* 2011;306:2469-2479.
3. Wapner RJ. Genetics of stillbirth. *Clin Obstet Gynecol.* 2010;53: 628-634.
4. Stillbirth Collaborative Research Network Writing Group. Causes of death among stillbirths. *JAMA.* 2011;306:2459-2468.
5. Pineles BL, Park E, Samet JM. Systematic review and meta-analysis of miscarriage and maternal exposure to tobacco smoke during pregnancy. *Am J Epidemiol.* 2014;179:807-823.
6. Kjaersgaard MI, Parner ET, Vestergaard M, et al. Prenatal antidepressant exposure and risk of spontaneous abortion - a population-based study. *PLoS One.* 2013;8:e72095.
7. Ziakas PD, Pavlou M, Voulgarelis M. Heparin treatment in antiphospholipid syndrome with recurrent pregnancy loss: a systematic review and meta-analysis. *Obstet Gynecol.* 2010;115: 1256-1262.
8. Woelfer B, Salim R, Banerjee S, Elson J, Regan L, Jurkovic D. Reproductive outcomes in women with congenital uterine anomalies detected by three-dimensional ultrasound screening. *Obstet Gynecol.* 2001;98:1099-1103.

34

Stillbirth

Alyssa Stephenson-Famy

(see *Gabbe's Obstetrics: Normal and Problem Pregnancies*, 8e: ch34)

QUESTIONS

1. At which maternal age is the risk of stillbirth the lowest?

   a. <15 years old

   b. 15–19 years old

   c. 20–29 years old

   d. 30–34 years old

   e. >35 years old

2. A 24-year-old G1P0 presents at 22 weeks gestation with preterm labor, fever, and uterine tenderness, and rapidly delivers a fetus without cardiac activity at birth. What is the most likely cause of the intrapartum demise?

   a. *Escherichia coli* infection

   b. Listeria infection

   c. Syphilis infection

   d. Malaria infection

   e. Rubella infection

3. A 23-year-old G1P0 presents at 36 weeks gestation for routine prenatal care and is found to have a fetal demise. Ultrasound findings are consistent with hydrops fetalis. Her pregnancy has been complicated by subclinical hypothyroidism and an early diagnosis of gestational diabetes that is diet-controlled. She works in a preschool and had a low-grade fever and rash a few weeks ago. What is the most likely cause of this outcome?

   a. Aneuploidy

   b. Placental abnormalities

   c. Viral illness

   d. Hyperglycemia

   e. Hypothyroidism

4. A 32-year-old G1P0 at 35 weeks gestation presents with diffuse, severe itching. Her liver function enzymes are mildly elevated and fasting bile acids are ordered. At which bile acid level does the risk of adverse fetal outcome increase significantly?

   a. <10 mol/L

   b. 10–19 mol/L

   c. 20–29 mol/L

   d. 30–39 mol/L

   e. >40 mol/L

5. A 25-year-old woman is diagnosed with a deep venous thrombosis in the first trimester and undergoes thrombophilia testing. Which thrombophilia has the highest risk of stillbirth?

   a. Factor V Leiden mutation

   b. Prothrombin G20210A mutation

   c. Protein C deficiency

   d. Protein S deficiency

   e. Anti-β2-glycoprotein-I antibodies

6. A 39-year-old woman who is late to prenatal care presents for ultrasound at 21 weeks and is found to have a fetal demise. Ultrasound suggests multiple fetal abnormalities including absent nasal bone, cardiac defect and double-bubble sign. What is the most likely karyotypic abnormality associated with this finding?

   a. Trisomy 13

   b. Trisomy 18

   c. Trisomy 21

   d. 45,X

   e. 69,XXX

7. A 29-year-old woman delivers a stillborn fetus at 37 weeks. Her pregnancy was uncomplicated until the day of delivery, when she had a large-volume hemorrhage. What is the most likely finding on placental pathology?

   a. Single umbilical artery

   b. Velamentous cord insertion

   c. Chorioamnionitis

   d. Villous immaturity

   e. Retroplacental hematoma

8. A woman delivers a 42-week stillborn fetus. On gross evaluation there is a tight nuchal cord, but no other abnormal findings. Pathologic evaluation of the cord fails to show grooving of the cord, constriction of the umbilical vessels, edema, congestion, or thrombosis. What is the most appropriate conclusion from this finding?

   a. The nuchal cord was the etiology of the stillbirth.

   b. The nuchal cord was not the etiology of the stillbirth.

   c. The isolated finding of a nuchal cord is insufficient evidence that cord accident is the cause of the stillbirth.

   d. Further pathologic evaluation of the cord is needed before making a conclusion.

9. What study is the single most useful test to order for evaluation after a stillbirth?

   a. Pathology of the placenta, cord, and membranes

   b. Autopsy

   c. Microarray

   d. TORCH titers

   e. Antiphospholipid infection antibodies

   f. Oral glucose tolerance test

10. A 30-year-old woman undergoes a fetal microarray following a term stillbirth in a pregnancy that was previously uncomplicated. She should be counseled that microarray will not detect which genetic abnormality?

    a. Chromosomal aneuploidy

    b. Single gene mutations

    c. Duplications>50 kilobases

    d. Deletions>50 kilobases

    e. Balanced translocation

11. A 37-year-old G3P2 is diagnosed with an intrauterine fetal demise at 32 weeks. She has had one vaginal delivery and one previous cesarean section. What is the safest plan for delivery in this situation?

    a. Await spontaneous labor

    b. Dilation and evacuation

    c. Induction of labor with misoprostol

    d. Induction of labor with Foley balloon and oxytocin

    e. Repeat cesarean section

12. A 33-year-old G2P1 is at 36 weeks gestation. She has a history of a previous term stillbirth 10 years ago in the setting of limited prenatal care. What is the most appropriate recommendation for timing of delivery in this pregnancy?

    a. 37 weeks

    b. 39 weeks

    c. 41 weeks

    d. Expectant management

    e. Timing of delivery determined only by antepartum testing

ANSWERS

1. **Answer: d**

   (See *Gabbe's Obstetrics* 8e: ch34)

   Maternal age has a U-shaped relationship with stillbirth. Stillbirth rates are highest for women younger than 15 years and women aged 45 years and older. Women aged 30–34 years are the lowest-risk group.

2. **Answer: a**

   (See *Gabbe's Obstetrics* 8e: ch34)

   Maternal infections with group B *Streptococcus* and *E. coli* are the most common causes of chorioamnionitis which can cause preterm stillbirth or periviable neonatal demise. Listeria is less common in the United States. Syphilis and malaria are more common causes of infection-related stillbirth in endemic areas and low-resource settings.

3. **Answer: c**

   (See *Gabbe's Obstetrics* 8e: ch34)

   Infection is associated with approximately 10%–20% of stillbirths in developed countries and a much higher percentage in developing countries. In developed countries, infection accounts for a greater percentage of preterm stillbirths than term stillbirths. Pathogens may result in stillbirth by producing direct fetal infection, placental dysfunction, severe maternal illness, or by stimulating spontaneous preterm birth at a periviable gestational age.

4. Answer: e

(See *Gabbe's Obstetrics* 8e: ch34)

Intrahepatic cholestasis of pregnancy (ICP) has been associated with an increased stillbirth rate of 12 to 30/1000 affected pregnancies. Women with bile acid levels greater than 40 mol/L have significantly higher rates of fetal complications, such as asphyxia, spontaneous preterm delivery, and meconium staining of amniotic fluid, placenta, and membranes, compared with women with normal bile acid levels and women with mild ICP (bile acid levels of 40 mol/L or less).

5. Answer: e

(See *Gabbe's Obstetrics* 8e: ch34)

Current data suggest a weak association, if any, between heritable thrombophilias and stillbirth, while elevated levels of anticardiolipin and anti-β2-glycoprotein-I antibodies in maternal serum are associated with a three- to five-fold increased odds of stillbirth.

6. Answer: c

(See *Gabbe's Obstetrics* 8e: ch34)

The distribution of chromosomal abnormalities associated with stillbirth in descending order is: trisomy 21, 31%; monosomy X, 22%; trisomy 18, 22%; other chromosomal abnormalities 19%, and trisomy 13, 6%.

7. Answer: e

(See *Gabbe's Obstetrics* 8e: ch34)

Histologic evaluation of the placenta can be helpful in documenting abruption. Placental abruption may be considered the cause of death when there are clinical signs of a large abruption, or when histopathologic examination of the placenta shows extensive signs of abruption (≥75%). In cases of chronic abruption, there may be hemosiderin deposits in the placenta. In other cases, there may be evidence of abnormal placental vasculature, thrombosis, and reduced placental perfusion (e.g., infarction).

8. Answer: c

(See *Gabbe's Obstetrics* 8e: ch34)

Examination of a tight knot or nuchal cord at the time of stillbirth may show grooving of the cord and constriction of the umbilical vessels in long-standing cases, and edema, congestion, or thrombosis in more acute ones. Thus, the isolated finding of a nuchal cord or a true knot at the time of birth is insufficient evidence that cord accident is the cause of the stillbirth in the absence of such changes.

9. Answer: a

(See *Gabbe's Obstetrics* 8e: ch34)

Gross and histologic evaluation of the placenta, umbilical cord, and fetal membranes by a trained pathologist is the single most useful aspect of the evaluation of stillbirth and is considered an essential component of the evaluation. Placental weight should be documented and noted in relation to the norms for gestational age. Gross evaluation may reveal conditions such as abruption, umbilical cord thrombosis, velamentous cord insertion, and vasa previa.

10. Answer: e

(See *Gabbe's Obstetrics* 8e: ch34)

Chromosomal microarray is considered the first-line genetic test for stillbirth, if cost is not problematic. Microarray technology does not detect balanced translocations or low-level mosaicism. A microarray detects deletions and duplications as small as 50 kilobases.

11. Answer: d

(See *Gabbe's Obstetrics* 8e: ch34)

For women with a previous low transverse incision, and a uterus greater than 28 weeks size, oxytocin protocols may be used, and cervical ripening with Foley catheter balloon may be considered. Patients may choose a repeat cesarean delivery in the setting of a stillbirth, but the risks and benefits must be carefully considered and discussed with the patient. Ideally, cesarean delivery is avoided.

12. Answer: b

(See *Gabbe's Obstetrics* 8e: ch34)

Following a history of stillbirth, management of a subsequent pregnancy includes serial ultrasounds for fetal growth, antepartum surveillance, and, if the pregnancy is uncomplicated, elective induction at 39 weeks gestation.

35

Cervical Insufficiency

Eva K. Pressman

(see *Gabbe's Obstetrics: Normal and Problem Pregnancies*, 8e: ch35)

QUESTIONS

1. A 26-year-old G3P0111 comes to the office to establish prenatal care at 10 weeks gestation. Her past obstetric history includes a 19-week loss following painless cervical dilation and a 28-week preterm delivery after preterm premature rupture of membranes (PPROM) and preterm labor. She also has a history of systemic lupus erythematosus which is well controlled on hydroxychloroquine. Which of the following etiologies is least likely to be associated with this obstetric history?

    a. Autoimmune disease

    b. Genetics

    c. Infection

    d. Local hormone effects

    e. Weakened internal os

2. A 32-year-old G2P0010 comes to the office at 8 weeks gestation for her first prenatal visit. Her first pregnancy was a 16-week fetal demise treated by dilation and evacuation. Ultrasound shows this pregnancy is a dichorionic, diamniotic twin gestation. She is concerned about losing another pregnancy and wants to know if there are tests or treatments that might improve her chances of a successful pregnancy outcome. Which of the following is the most appropriate statement?

    a. Transabdominal cervical length screening would be recommended if she develops symptoms of preterm labor.

    b. Transvaginal cervical length screening is recommended since she had a prior 16-week loss.

    c. Transvaginal cervical length screening is standard practice in twin gestations.

    d. Vaginal progesterone may be beneficial if she is found to have a shortened cervix on transvaginal cervical length measurement.

    e. Vaginal progesterone is known to be beneficial in twin pregnancies regardless of cervical length.

3. A 29-year-old G3P2002 comes to the office at 18 weeks gestation for a routine prenatal visit. Her medical history includes well-controlled type 2 diabetes mellitus (DM), a cervical biopsy for an abnormal Pap smear, and dilatation and curettage for a retained placenta after her second delivery. Ultrasound shows no evidence of fetal anomalies, but her cervical length on transvaginal imaging is 1.8 cm. Which risk factors may be contributing to her clinical situation?

    a. Abnormal Pap smear

    b. Cervical biopsy

    c. Diabetes mellitus

    d. Dilation and curettage

    e. Pregnancy history

4. Which of the following tests can reliably predict the diagnosis of cervical insufficiency?

    a. #8 Hegar dilator passes into the cervical canal without resistance

    b. There is no validated test for cervical insufficiency

    c. Transvaginal ultrasound prior to the first trimester of pregnancy

    d. Transvaginal ultrasound prior to pregnancy

    e. Q-tip passes easily through the external os prior to pregnancy

5. A 27-year-old G4P0121 at 18 weeks gestation comes to the office for a prenatal visit. Her first pregnancy was complicated by a loss at 19 weeks after presenting with increased vaginal discharge and finding "hour glassing" membranes through the cervix. Her second pregnancy was complicated by preterm labor and delivery at 31 weeks but that child is doing well. In her third pregnancy she was treated with 17-hydroxyprogesterone injections weekly, starting at 17 weeks. At 20 weeks she was noted to have a cervical length of 2.1 cm and a McDonald cerclage was placed. She experienced rupture of membranes 1 week later, developed a fever, and underwent a pregnancy termination due to chorioamnionitis. On today's ultrasound, the cervix is noted to be 0.9 cm in length on transvaginal ultrasound. What is the most appropriate treatment for this patient in the current pregnancy?

a. A single McDonald cerclage

b. Amniocentesis prior to cerclage placement

c. An abdominal cerclage

d. McDonald cerclage with two sutures

e. Repeat transvaginal ultrasound in 1 week

6. A 37-year-old G2P0101 comes to the office at 14 weeks for a routine prenatal visit. Her prior pregnancy was complicated by preterm labor starting at 30 weeks, with subsequent delivery at 32 weeks. She would like to avoid a recurrent preterm delivery and asks if cerclage would be beneficial in her situation. Which is the most appropriate response?

a. Cerclage has been shown to be beneficial in all patients with prior preterm birth.

b. Cerclage has been shown to be beneficial only in women with cervical dilation after 24 weeks.

c. Cervical length screening is not indicated since she delivered her prior pregnancy after 24 weeks.

d. Cerclage may be beneficial if her cervix appears <25 mm on transvaginal ultrasound prior to 24 weeks.

e. No therapies have been found to decrease the risk of recurrent preterm birth.

7. A 36-year-old G1P0 comes to labor and delivery at 17 weeks reporting increased vaginal discharge. Her pregnancy has been uncomplicated. Examination shows the cervix to be 1-cm dilated, with membranes visible at the external os. Ultrasound is performed showing normal amniotic fluid volume, appropriate fetal growth, and no fetal anomalies. The patient is offered an examination-indicated cerclage and asks what the risks would be. Which of the following is not a risk of cerclage placement in this clinical situation?

a. Cervical laceration

b. Chorioamnionitis

c. Failure to dilate in labor

d. Fetal laceration

e. Premature rupture of membranes

8. A 27-year-old G2P0101 comes to the office at 20 weeks for ultrasound evaluation. Her prior pregnancy was complicated by preterm labor and delivery at 33 weeks. She is currently receiving 17-hydroxyprogesterone injections weekly. Ultrasound reveals normal fetal anatomy, growth, and amniotic fluid volume. The transvaginal cervical length shown below. What is the most appropriate treatment for this patient?

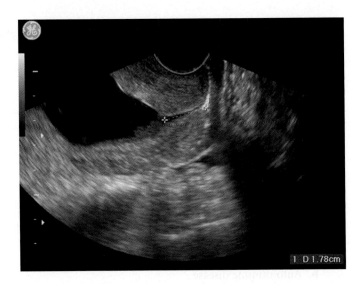

a. Abdominal cerclage placement

b. Vaginal progesterone daily

c. Cervical pessary insertion

d. McDonald cerclage placement

e. Strict activity restriction with bedrest

9. A 33-year-old G3P1102 comes to the office at 19 weeks gestation for a prenatal visit. Her first pregnancy delivered at term but her second pregnancy was complicated by preterm labor and delivery at 33 weeks. She was started on intramuscular (IM) progesterone 2 weeks ago and is not having any cramping or change in vaginal discharge. What is the best way to predict and prevent another preterm birth in this patient?

a. Digital cervical examination

b. Speculum examination

c. Transabdominal ultrasound

d. Translabial ultrasound

e. Transvaginal ultrasound

10. A 29-year-old G2P0101 comes to the office at 16 weeks gestation for a prenatal visit. Her prior pregnancy was complicated by PPROM at 28 weeks and induction of labor at 34 weeks due to risk of chorioamnionitis. An ultrasound shows normal fetal anatomy, normal growth and amniotic fluid, and the cervical length shown below. Which of the following treatments is most appropriate?

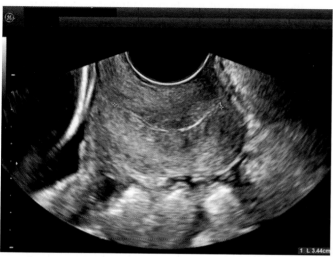

Fig. 35.2 Normal cervical length as measured by transvaginal ultrasound.

   a. Abdominal cerclage
   b. Bed rest
   c. IM progesterone
   d. McDonald cerclage
   e. Vaginal progesterone

11. A 37-year-old G2P0101 comes to the office at 20 weeks gestation for an ultrasound examination. Her prior pregnancy was complicated by PPROM at 28 weeks, with preterm labor and delivery at 32 weeks. She has been receiving IM progesterone since 17 weeks. On ultrasound, her cervix appears closed and 1.5 cm in length. Which of the following statements is most accurate regarding next steps in her management?

   a. Adding tocolytics and antibiotics would not decrease risk of preterm birth.
   b. Adding vaginal progesterone would decrease the risk of preterm birth.
   c. No additional treatment is needed at this time.
   d. Placing a cerclage would decrease the risk of preterm birth.
   e. The IM progesterone should be changed to vaginal progesterone.

ANSWERS

1. Answer: a

(see *Gabbe's Obstetrics* 8e: ch35)

In a proposed model of cervical competence as a continuum, a poor obstetric history attributed to cervical insufficiency likely results from a process of premature cervical ripening induced by myriad underlying processes that include a weakened internal os, infection, inflammation, local or systemic hormonal effects, or even genetic predisposition. This new description defines cervical insufficiency by the presence of both (1) transvaginal ultrasound cervical length less than 25 mm and/or cervical changes detected on physical examination before 24 weeks of gestation, and (2) prior spontaneous preterm birth at less than 37 weeks.

2. Answer: d

(see *Gabbe's Obstetrics* 8e: ch35)

Currently, the most appropriate groups to be considered for transvaginal ultrasound cervical length screening are asymptomatic singleton pregnancies without prior spontaneous preterm birth, asymptomatic singleton pregnancies with prior spontaneous preterm birth, and symptomatic singleton pregnancies. A recent individual patient-level metaanalysis demonstrated that vaginal progesterone in women carrying twins with a cervical length <25 mm decreased the risk of preterm birth, as well as neonatal morbidity and mortality. This finding has prompted some centers to adopt cervical length screening in asymptomatic twin pregnancies, but it is not currently standard practice.

3. Answer: **c**

(see *Gabbe's Obstetrics* 8e: ch35)

Risk Factors for cervical insufficiency include prior cervical destructive surgery (i.e., loop electrosurgical excision procedure, laser conization, and cold-knife cone biopsy), prior induced or spontaneous first- and second-trimester abortions, other procedures requiring mechanical cervical dilation (e.g. hysteroscopy), uterine anomalies, multiple gestations, or even prior spontaneous preterm births that did not meet typical clinical criteria for cervical insufficiency.

4. Answer: **b**

(see *Gabbe's Obstetrics* 8e: ch35)

There is no universally applicable standard for the diagnosis of cervical insufficiency, and because the results of such tests were never evaluated and linked to a proven effective treatment, their clinical utility was at best theoretic. Because no test for cervical insufficiency in the nonpregnant patient has been validated, none of these tests can be recommended.

5. Answer: **c**

(see *Gabbe's Obstetrics* 8e: ch35)

A McDonald technique is recommended as the first-line procedure for cerclages for all indications. Currently, no strong evidence suggests that placing two sutures results in better outcomes than placing one. It appears that for a history-indicated cerclage, the rate of subclinical intraamniotic infection (IAI) is very low, and amniocentesis does not seem justifiable. In patients with a prior failed vaginal cerclage, an abdominal cerclage is recommended.

6. Answer: **d**

(see *Gabbe's Obstetrics* 8e: ch35)

Because of its unproven efficacy in randomized controlled trials (RCTs) and the attendant surgical risks, the recommendation for history-indicated cerclage should be limited to women with multiple midtrimester spontaneous preterm births when a careful history and physical examination suggest a dominant cervical component. Most women with prior spontaneous preterm birth(s) can be instead followed with transvaginal ultrasound cervical length screening, with ultrasound-indicated cerclage if the cervical length is found to be <25 mm before 24 weeks. Shortened cervical length (<25 mm) before 24 weeks is diagnostic of cervical insufficiency if it occurs in a singleton gestation and in a patient with a prior spontaneous preterm birth.

7. Answer: **d**

(see *Gabbe's Obstetrics* 8e: ch35)

Cervical lacerations at the time of delivery are one of the most common complications from a cerclage and occur in 1%–13% of patients. Three percent of patients require cesarean delivery because of the inability of the cervix to dilate secondary to cervical scarring and dystocia. Although the risk of infection is minimal with a history-indicated cerclage, the risk increases significantly in cases of advanced dilation with exposure of membranes to the birth canal. However, this infectious morbidity may be the result of the final expression of subclinical chorioamnionitis. Even though cerclage placement is considered a benign procedure, a maternal death from sepsis in a patient with PPROM and retained cerclage has been reported.

8. Answer: **d**

(see *Gabbe's Obstetrics* 8e: ch35)

The validity of bed rest for treatment has not been scientifically proven, and some data suggest worse outcomes in patients with a short cervical length placed on bed rest. We must await the results of these ongoing RCTs before pessary use can be recommended in women with a short transvaginal ultrasound cervical length, but results overall are encouraging. RCTs are also needed to assess the efficacy of pessary compared with other interventions, such as cerclage, progesterone, and others. Two RCTs have compared the effectiveness of vaginal progesterone to cerclage in preventing preterm birth in women with singleton gestations, prior spontaneous preterm birth, and short transvaginal ultrasound cervical length <25 mm before 24 weeks. Both show null findings, but trends towards a longer latency to delivery of about 1–2 weeks for cerclage compared with progesterone.

9. Answer: **e**

(see *Gabbe's Obstetrics* 8e: ch35)

Transvaginal ultrasound cervical length screening has been shown to have superior cost-effectiveness compared with transabdominal ultrasound because transvaginal ultrasound is associated with better prevention of preterm birth. The transabdominal ultrasound cervical length measurement is less sensitive in detecting a short cervical length and is noted to overestimate cervical length and underdiagnose short cervical length. Translabial ultrasound is also less sensitive and less predictive than transvaginal ultrasound. Given this evidence, neither transabdominal ultrasound nor translabial ultrasound should be used for cervical length screening. Moreover, transvaginal ultrasound has been shown to be more predictive of spontaneous preterm birth compared with digital manual examination of the cervix.

10. Answer: **c**

(see *Gabbe's Obstetrics* 8e: ch35)

All women with a prior spontaneous preterm birth should be recommended IM progesterone prophylaxis starting at 16 weeks and continuing until 36 weeks. The validity of bed rest for treatment has not been scientifically proven, and some data suggest worse outcomes in patients with a short cervical length placed on bed rest. Shortened cervical length <25 mm before 24 weeks is diagnostic of cervical insufficiency if it occurs in a singleton gestation and in a patient with a prior spontaneous preterm birth. Two RCTs have compared the effectiveness of vaginal progesterone to cerclage in preventing preterm birth in women with singleton gestations, prior spontaneous preterm birth, and short transvaginal ultrasound cervical length <25 mm before 24 weeks. Both show null findings, but trends for a longer latency to delivery of about 1–2 weeks for cerclage compared to progesterone.

11. Answer: **e**

(see *Gabbe's Obstetrics* 8e: ch35)

Progesterone and cerclage seem to be associated with better prevention of preterm birth than either intervention used alone in women with singleton gestations, prior spontaneous preterm birth (an indication for the progesterone), and with a short cervical length before 24 weeks despite the progesterone (an indication for cerclage). In an RCT, indomethacin and antibiotics have been shown to be associated with a further decrease in preterm birth in women with singleton gestations and physical exam indicated cerclage, compared to placebos.

Pregnancy and Coexisting Disease

Preterm Labor and Birth

Eva K. Pressman

(see *Gabbe's Obstetrics: Normal and Problem Pregnancies*, 8e: ch36)

QUESTIONS

1. Which of the following factors contribute to a decrease in the rate of preterm birth (PTB) since 2006?

a. Improvements in ultrasound dating

b. Decreases in multifetal gestations

c. Increases in indicated preterm delivery

d. Improvements in tocolytic therapy

e. Decreased use of cerclage

2. Which of the following risk factors are present in most women with PTB?

a. A history of previous preterm delivery

b. Multifetal gestation

c. Bleeding after the first trimester

d. No apparent risk factors

e. Short cervical length (CL)

3. Which of the following interventions has not been shown to reduce perinatal morbidity and mortality?

a. Transfer of the mother to an appropriate hospital before PTB

b. Administration of maternal antibiotics to prevent neonatal group B *Streptococcus* infection

c. Administration of maternal corticosteroids to reduce neonatal respiratory distress syndrome (RDS), intraventricular hemorrhage (IVH), and neonatal mortality

d. Administration of maternal magnesium sulfate to reduce the incidence of cerebral palsy.

e. Administration of tocolytic agents to reduce the rate of PTB

4. A 27-year-old G2P0101 comes to the office for prenatal care at 12 weeks gestation. Her previous pregnancy was complicated by preterm premature rupture of membranes (PPROM) at 28 weeks and preterm labor resulting in vaginal delivery at 30 weeks. She is concerned about her risk of recurrent PTB. Which of the following approaches is most appropriate to decrease her risk of recurrent PTB?

a. Bed rest for the duration of the pregnancy

b. Avoidance of sexual activity

c. Supplementation of vitamins C and E

d. Antibiotic treatment for bacterial vaginosis

e. Weekly injections of 17-α-hydroxyprogesterone

5. A 26-year-old G1P0 comes to the office for her first prenatal visit at 10 weeks gestation. She has no medical problems but reports that her husband was born prematurely at 32 weeks and she is concerned that this will put her at risk for PTB. Which of the following statements is most accurate about her risk for preterm delivery?

a. Heritability of PTB appears to be the result of maternal, rather than paternal, lineage.

b. The pattern of PTBs that occur in family pedigrees suggests that the most likely form of inheritance is Mendelian.

c. Insights into the genetics of PTB have led to influences in clinical care.

d. The magnitude of her increased risk is inversely related to the gestational age of her husband's birth.

e. There is no data supporting a genetic contribution to PTB.

6. A 29-year-old G1P0 comes to the labor and delivery unit at 29 weeks gestation with pelvic pressure and vaginal spotting. Her pregnancy is notable for dichorionic twins conceived with in vitro fertilization, due to anovulation secondary to polycystic ovarian syndrome. She reports having an upper respiratory infection last week that resolved after 3 days but has otherwise been well. On cervical examination, she is noted to be 2 cm dilated and 75% effaced, and the vertex of twin A is at 0 station. What is the most likely pathologic process responsible for her clinical presentation?

   a. Intrauterine infection

   b. Vascular disorder

   c. Uterine overdistension

   d. Cervical insufficiency

   e. Endocrine disorder

7. A 37-year-old G3P1011 at 33 weeks gestation comes to the labor and delivery unit with regular uterine contractions every 3 minutes. Her pregnancy was conceived through in vitro fertilization but has otherwise been uncomplicated. Her previous pregnancies were conceived spontaneously, with the first delivering at term and the second ending in an 8-week miscarriage. She works as an intensive care unit as an attending physician and typically works three 12-hour shifts per week. A cervical examination reveals her cervix to be 3 cm dilated, 80% effaced and the fetal vertex is at +1 station. Which of the following patient characteristics are most likely to have contributed to her clinical situation?

   a. Her prior term delivery

   b. Her prior miscarriage

   c. Her use of in vitro fertilization

   d. Her high level of education

   e. Her long work hours

8. A 25-year-old G1P0 at 33 weeks gestation comes to the labor and delivery unit with leakage of clear fluid from her vagina for the past hour. Her pregnancy has been uncomplicated until this point, with a normal anatomic ultrasound at 19 weeks. She has not had any vaginal bleeding or contractions and reports normal fetal movement. Testing of the vaginal fluid shows a positive nitrazine and ferning. What is the most likely mechanism for her presentation?

   a. Decreased levels of matrix metalloproteinases

   b. Increased expression of antiapoptosis genes

   c. Decreased amounts of collagen I, III and V

   d. Decreased expression of tenascin

   e. Increased release of fetal fibronectin

9. A 29-year-old G1P0 at 33 weeks gestation comes to the labor and delivery unit with leakage of clear fluid from her vagina for 4 hours. Her pregnancy has been uncomplicated and she has no medical history. She denies vaginal bleeding or contractions, but shortly after arrival, she begins having contractions every 2 minutes and is noted to have a temperature of 38.7°C (101.7 F). She is treated with antibiotics and betamethasone but progresses to a vaginal delivery of a 1900-g male infant with Apgar scores of 7 and 9 after 4 hours of labor. Placental pathology reveals acute chorioamnionitis and funisitis. Which of the following clinical findings is most predictive of long-term morbidity for the infant?

   a. Gestational age greater than 32 weeks

   b. Maternal administration of antibiotics

   c. Maternal administration of betamethasone

   d. One minute Apgar of 7

   e. Funisitis on placental pathology

10. A 24-year-old G2P0010 18 weeks gestation comes to the office at with red vaginal bleeding for the last hour that filled less than half of a small sanitary pad. Speculum examination shows no active bleeding. Ultrasound reveals a 2-cm subchorionic collection. The bleeding resolves, although she reports occasional dark brown spotting for the next 2 weeks. She does well for the next several weeks, although she is diagnosed with gestational diabetes at 28 weeks. At 29 weeks gestation, she comes to the labor and delivery unit with cramping and is noted to be contracting every 3 minutes. Cervical examination shows her cervix to be 3 cm dilated and 80% effaced and the fetal vertex is at 0 station. What is the most likely cause of her current pregnancy complications?

   a. Thrombin stimulating myometrial contractility

   b. Intrauterine infection due to multiple cervical examinations

   c. Uterine overdistension due to the subchorionic collection

   d. Uteroplacental insufficiency due to placental separation

   e. Endocrine imbalance due to gestational diabetes

11. A 27-year-old G2P1001 at 30 weeks gestation comes to the labor and delivery unit with contractions every 10 minutes and vaginal spotting. Cervical examination shows her cervix to be 1 cm dilated and 50% effaced and the presenting part to be at −3 station. There is a small amount of blood in the vagina and no pooling of fluid. Of her symptoms and examination characteristics, which is most strongly associated with preterm delivery?

   a. Cervical dilation

   b. Contraction frequency

   c. Effacement

   d. Prior pregnancy history

   e. Vaginal bleeding

12. A 22-year-old G2P1001 at 31 weeks gestation comes to the labor and delivery unit with contractions every 5 minutes. Cervical examination shows her cervix to be 1 cm dilated and 50% effaced and the presenting part to be at −3 station. There is no pooling of fluid or blood in the vagina. Which of the following findings on diagnostic testing increases her chances of delivering preterm to the greatest degree?

    a. Transvaginal ultrasound (TVU) CL measurement of 20 mm

    b. Negative fetal fibronectin test of the cervicovaginal fluid

    c. Transabdominal ultrasound (TAU) CL measurement of 35 mm

    d. Amniotic fluid glucose of 45 mg/dL

    e. No change in cervical examination after 2 hours

13. A 28-year-old G2P0101 at 35 weeks gestation comes to the labor and delivery unit in active preterm labor. Her prior pregnancy was complicated by labor and delivery at 31 weeks. She has not had any other complications this pregnancy and has been receiving weekly 17-hydroxyprogesterone injections. On arrival, her cervix is 3 cm dilated and 90% effaced and the vertex is at +1 station. She reports that she received betamethasone and tocolytics prior to her prior preterm delivery and asks if she will be receiving these treatments this time as well. Which is the most appropriate answer?

    a. Betamethasone is recommended but tocolytics are not.

    b. Both betamethasone and tocolytics are recommended.

    c. Neither tocolytics nor betamethasone is recommended.

    d. Tocolytics are recommended but betamethasone is not.

    e. 17-hydroxyprogesterone injections should be stopped.

14. A 24-year-old G1P0 at 32 weeks gestation comes to the labor and delivery unit with contractions. She has not had any pregnancy complications to date. On examination, she is 3 cm dilated, 100% effaced and 0 station. She is started on nifedipine for tocolysis, betamethasone for fetal lung maturation, and penicillin for group B *Streptococcus* prophylaxis. Which of the following maternal effects are expected from these treatments?

    a. Decrease in blood glucose

    b. Decrease in heart rate

    c. Elevation in blood pressure

    d. Elevation in platelet count

    e. Elevation in white blood cell (WBC) count

15. A 32-year-old G1P0 at 33 weeks gestation comes to the labor and delivery unit with leakage of clear fluid and regular uterine contractions every 3 minutes. She is noted to have a temperature of 38.4°C (101.12 F), pulse of 106, blood pressure of 140/90, and fetal heart rate of 170 beats per minute with minimal variability and no decelerations. On examination, she has mild uterine tenderness, her cervix is 2 cm dilated and 50% effaced and the fetal vertex is at −1 station. A small amount of bleeding is noted from the external surface of the cervix. Why would tocolysis be contraindicated in this patient?

    a. Abnormal fetal heart rate tracing

    b. Chorioamnionitis

    c. Gestational hypertension

    d. Gestational age >32 weeks

    e. Hemorrhage

16. A 30-year-old G2P0101 at 25 weeks gestation comes to the labor and delivery unit with regular uterine contractions every 4 minutes. Her pregnancy has been uncomplicated, but her prior delivery occurred at 30 weeks due preterm labor after PPROM. She is given betamethasone for fetal lung maturation, magnesium sulfate for fetal neuroprotection, indomethacin for tocolysis, and penicillin for group B *Streptococcus* prophylaxis. Which of the following are possible side effects of these medications?

    a. Development of oligohydramnios

    b. Neonatal hyperglycemia

    c. Neonatal pulmonary hypotension

    d. Neonatal intraventricular hemorrhage (IVH)

    e. Persistent patency of the ductus arteriosus

ANSWERS

1. Answer: **b**

(see *Gabbe's Obstetrics* 8e: ch36)

Contributors to the decline in PTBs that have occurred since 2006 include the decline in multifetal gestations related to fertility care and increased use of progesterone and cervical cerclage. The rise in PTBs between 1990 and 2006 in singletons was almost entirely explained by an increased rate of indicated PTBs between 34 and 36 weeks gestation. The principal driver of this increase was an increased willingness to consider scheduled birth as a safer option than continuing the pregnancy in women with various pregnancy complications.

2. Answer: **d**

(see *Gabbe's Obstetrics* 8e: ch36)

Approximately half of women who deliver preterm have no obvious risk factors. CL as measured by TVU is inversely related to the risk of PTB, with a relative risk of up to 7. The strongest historic risk factor is a previous birth between 16 and 36 weeks gestation. This history is often reported to confer a 1.5- to 2-fold increased risk but varies widely according to the number, sequence, and gestational age of prior PTBs. Women who experience unexplained vaginal bleeding after the first trimester have an increased risk of subsequent PTB that increases with the number of bleeding episodes. Multifetal gestation is one of the strongest risk factors for PTB, with 50% of women with twins delivering prior to 37 weeks. The risk of early birth rises with the number of fetuses, which suggests uterine overdistension and fetal signaling as potential pathways to the early initiation of labor.

3. Answer: **e**

(see *Gabbe's Obstetrics* 8e: ch36)

No studies have shown that any tocolytic can reduce the rate of PTB. Meta-analyses of studies of individual tocolytic drugs typically report limited prolongation of pregnancy but no decrease in PTB, and they rarely offer information about whether prolongation of pregnancy was accompanied by improved infant outcomes. Delayed delivery for 48 hours to allow antenatal transport and corticosteroids to reduce neonatal morbidity and mortality are thus the main rationale for use of these drugs.

4. Answer: **e**

(see *Gabbe's Obstetrics* 8e: ch36)

Randomized trials have demonstrated an approximately 40% decrease in the rate of PTB in women with a prior PTB who were treated with intramuscular 17-α-hydroxy-progesterone caproate 250 mg weekly between 16 and 36 weeks gestation. Grobman and coworkers reported no relation between reduced activity and frequency of PTB. Yost and colleagues found no relationship between coitus and risk of recurrent PTB. Trials of supplemental vitamins C and E and calcium have not demonstrated a reduction in PTB risk. Screening and antibiotic treatment of women with abnormal genital flora have been largely ineffective to prevent PTB. Maternal activity restriction has not shown a benefit in obstetrical outcomes regardless of the indication.

5. Answer: **a**

(see *Gabbe's Obstetrics* 8e: ch36)

The notion of some genetic contribution to PTB is based on several observations. First, a woman's family history of PTB influences her own risk. Porter and colleagues found that a mother who was herself born preterm had an increased risk for delivering a child preterm; the magnitude of that increased risk was inversely related to the gestational age of her own birth. This heritability appears to be the result of maternal, rather than paternal, lineage. The pattern of PTBs that occur in family pedigrees suggests that the most likely form of inheritance is nonmendelian; rather, the observed pedigrees are more consistent with the influence of many genes. Insights into the complex genetics of PTB hold promise for giving insight into pathophysiology and, potentially, to risk identification; at present, neither of these potential benefits influences clinical care.

6. Answer: c

(see *Gabbe's Obstetrics* 8e: ch36)

Multifetal gestation is one of the strongest risk factors for PTB. Slightly more than 50% of women with twins deliver before 37 weeks gestation. The risk of early birth rises with the number of fetuses, which suggests uterine overdistension as a potential pathway to the early initiation of labor. The mechanisms responsible for the increased frequency of PTB in multiple gestations and other disorders associated with uterine overdistension are unknown. Central questions are how the uterus senses stretch and how these mechanical forces induce biochemical changes that lead to parturition. Increased expressions of oxytocin receptor, connexin 43, and the *c-fos* messenger RNA (mRNA) have been consistently demonstrated in the rat myometrium near term. Progesterone blocks stretch-induced gene expression in the myometrium. Mitogen-activated protein kinases have been proposed to mediate stretch-induced *c-fos* mRNA expression in myometrial cells.

7. Answer: c

(see *Gabbe's Obstetrics* 8e: ch36)

The strongest historic risk factor is a previous birth between 16 and 36 weeks gestation. A nearly twofold increased risk of PTB is observed in singleton pregnancies conceived with all methods of fertility care, including ovulation promotion and in vitro fertilization. Similarly, a nearly twofold difference is seen in the rate of PTB between women with the highest and lowest levels of education. The risk of PTB is increased among women who work more than 42 hours per week (odds ratio [OR], 1.33; confidence interval [CI], 1.1 to 1.6) and who were required to stand for more than 6 hours per day (OR, 1.26; CI, 1.1 to 1.5). Kudela M1, Větr M, Fingerová H. [The EUROPOP Project. European Programme of Occupational Risks and Pregnancy Outcomes]. Ceska Gynekol. 1998 Jun;63(3):167-9.

8. Answer: c

(see *Gabbe's Obstetrics* 8e: ch36)

Although rupture of the membranes normally occurs during the first stage of labor, histologic studies of prematurely ruptured membranes show decreased amounts of collagen types I, III, and V; increased expression of tenascin, expressed during tissue remodeling and wound healing; and disruption of the normal wavy collagen pattern, which suggests that preterm rupture is a process that precedes the onset of labor. Degradation of the extracellular matrix, assessed by the detection of fetal fibronectin (FFN), is part of the common pathway of parturition. The presence of FFN or pathogen-associated molecular patterns in cervicovaginal secretions between 22 and 37 weeks gestation is evidence of disruption of the decidual-chorionic interface and is associated with an increased risk of PTB. The precise mechanism of membrane/decidua activation is uncertain, but matrix-degrading enzymes and apoptosis—programmed cell death—have been proposed. Increased levels of matrix metalloproteinases (MMPs) and their regulators (tissue inhibitors of MMPs) have been documented in the amniotic fluid of women with PPROM.

9. Answer: e

(see *Gabbe's Obstetrics* 8e: ch36)

Microorganisms that gain access to the fetus may elicit a systemic inflammatory response, the fetal inflammatory response syndrome (FIRS), characterized by increased concentrations of interleukin-6 and other cytokines, as well as cellular evidence of neutrophil and monocyte activation. FIRS is a subclinical condition originally described in fetuses of mothers with preterm labor and intact membranes and PPROM. Fetuses with FIRS have a higher rate of neonatal complications and are frequently born to mothers with subclinical microbial invasion of the amniotic cavity. Evidence of multisystemic involvement in cases of FIRS includes increased concentrations of fetal plasma MMP-9, neutrophilia, a higher number of circulating nucleated red blood cells, and higher plasma concentrations of granulocyte-colony stimulating factor. The histologic hallmark of FIRS is inflammation in the umbilical cord (funisitis) or chorionic vasculitis. The systemic fetal inflammatory response may result in multiple organ dysfunction, septic shock, and death in the absence of timely delivery. Newborns with funisitis are at increased risk for neonatal sepsis and long-term handicaps that include bronchopulmonary dysplasia (BPD) and cerebral palsy.

10. **Answer: a**

(see *Gabbe's Obstetrics* 8e: ch36)

After inflammation, the most common abnormalities seen in placental pathology specimens from spontaneous preterm births (sPTBs) are vascular lesions of the maternal and fetal circulations. Decidual necrosis and hemorrhage can activate parturition through production of thrombin, which stimulates myometrial contractility in a dose-dependent manner. Thrombin also stimulates production of MMP-1, urokinase-type plasminogen activator, and tissue-type plasminogen activator by endometrial stromal cells in culture. Directly or indirectly, these factors can digest important components of the extracellular matrix (ECM) in the chorioamniotic membranes. Thrombin/antithrombin complexes, a marker of in vivo generation of thrombin, are increased in the plasma and amniotic fluid of women with preterm labor and PPROM. The decidua is a rich source of tissue factor, the primary initiator of coagulation and of thrombin activation. These observations are consistent with clinical associations among vaginal bleeding, retroplacental hematomas, and preterm delivery.

11. **Answer: e**

(see *Gabbe's Obstetrics* 8c: ch36)

The inability to accurately distinguish women with an episode of preterm labor who will deliver preterm from those who deliver at term has greatly hampered the assessment of therapeutic interventions because as many as 50% of untreated (or placebo-treated) subjects do not actually deliver preterm. Optimal criteria for initiation of treatment are unclear. A contraction frequency of six or more per hour, cervical dilation of 3 cm, effacement of 80%, ruptured membranes, and bleeding are symptoms of preterm labor most often associated with preterm delivery.

12. **Answer: a**

(see *Gabbe's Obstetrics* 8e: ch36)

Symptomatic women whose cervical dilation is less than 2 cm and whose effacement is less than 80% present a diagnostic challenge. Diagnostic accuracy may be improved in these patients by testing other features of parturition such as cervical ripening; measurement of CL by TVU; and decidual activation, tested by an assay for FFN in cervicovaginal fluid. Both tests aid diagnosis primarily by reducing false-positive results. TAU has poor reproducibility for cervical measurement and should not be used clinically without confirmation by a TVU. If the examination is properly performed, a CL of 30 mm or more by endovaginal sonography indicates that preterm labor is unlikely in symptomatic women. Similarly, a negative FFN test in women with symptoms before 34 weeks' gestation with cervical dilation less than 3 cm can also reduce the rate of false-positive diagnosis. Amniotic fluid glucose (levels <20 mg/dL suggest intraamniotic infection) and Gram stain for bacteria, cell count, and culture may be used.

13. **Answer: a**

(see *Gabbe's Obstetrics* 8e: ch36)

Recent data also suggest that betamethasone can be beneficial in pregnant women at high risk of late PTB, between 34 0/7 weeks and 36 6/7 weeks of gestation, who have not received a prior course of antenatal corticosteroids. Tocolysis was not given, and delivery was not delayed for obstetric indications. The administration of steroids led to a decrease in the need for neonatal respiratory support. A larger decrease was demonstrated for severe respiratory complications, from 12.1% in the placebo group to 8.1% in the betamethasone group (relative risk, 0.67; 95% CI, 0.53–0.84; p < 0.001). There were also improvements in transient tachypnea of the newborn; bronchopulmonary dysplasia; a composite of RDS, transient tachypnea of the newborn and RDS; and the need for postnatal surfactant. There was no increase in proven neonatal sepsis, chorioamnionitis, or endometritis, with late preterm betamethasone. Hypoglycemia was more common in the infants exposed to betamethasone.

14. Answer: e

(see *Gabbe's Obstetrics* 8e: ch36)

Antenatal glucocorticoids produce a transient rise in maternal platelet and WBC counts that lasts 72 hours; a WBC count in excess of 20,000 is rarely due to steroids. Maternal glucose tolerance is also challenged, and treatment often requires insulin therapy to maintain euglycemia in those with previously well-controlled gestational or pregestational diabetes. Maternal blood pressure is unaffected by antenatal steroid treatment; neither betamethasone nor dexamethasone has a significant mineralor corticoid effect.

15. Answer: a

(see *Gabbe's Obstetrics* 8e: ch36)

Common maternal contraindications to tocolysis include preeclampsia or gestational hypertension with severe features, hemorrhage, and significant maternal cardiac disease. Although vaginal spotting may occur in women with preterm labor because of cervical effacement or dilation, any bleeding beyond light spotting is rarely due to labor alone. Fetal contraindications to tocolysis include gestational age of greater than 37 weeks, fetal demise or lethal anomaly, chorioamnionitis, and evidence of acute or chronic fetal compromise.

16. Answer: a

(see *Gabbe's Obstetrics* 8e: ch36)

Three principal side effects of indomethacin raise concern: (1) in utero constriction of the ductus arteriosus, (2) oligohydramnios, and (3) neonatal pulmonary hypertension. Other potential complications—including necrotizing enterocolitis, small bowel perforation, patent ductus arteriosus (PDA), jaundice, and IVH—have been observed when indomethacin administration was outside of standardized protocols that did not limit the duration of treatment or that used the drug after 32 weeks gestation. No association with IVH was noted in studies in which standard protocols were used.

37

Premature Rupture of the Membranes

Rini Banerjee Ratan

(see *Gabbe's Obstetrics: Normal and Problem Pregnancies*, 8e: ch37)

QUESTIONS

1. In all women with premature rupture of the membrane (PROM) before 34 weeks, over 90% will deliver spontaneously within which period of time?

a. 24 hours

b. 48 hours

c. 3 days

d. 7 days

e. 14 days

2. Which of the following is the most common maternal complication after preterm PROM?

a. Chorioamnionitis

b. Abruptio placentae

c. Hemorrhage from retained placenta

d. Maternal sepsis

e. Maternal death

3. A 32-year-old G1P0 at 35 weeks gestation presents to the labor and delivery unit in spontaneous preterm labor. She appears uncomfortable with contractions, which occur every 2–3 minutes. She reports leakage of clear fluid for the past 8 hours. Her cervix is 8 cm dilated and 90% effaced, with the vertex at 0/+5 station. Maternal temperature is 100.4F/38°C. Fetal heart rate is category II with intermittent variable decelerations lasting 30 seconds. She receives epidural anesthesia for pain relief and undergoes spontaneous vaginal delivery of a 2700-g male infant with Apgar scores of 6 at 1 minute and 7 at 5 minutes. Which of the following complications is this newborn most likely to encounter?

a. Sepsis

b. Umbilical cord prolapse

c. Respiratory distress syndrome

d. Necrotizing enterocolitis

e. Intellectual disabilities

4. A 27-year-old G1P0 at 40 weeks gestation presents to the labor and delivery unit with leakage of clear fluid for the past 3 hours. On speculum examination, amniotic fluid can be seen passing out of the cervical canal, and the pH of the posterior fornix is >6.5. The cervix is visualized and appears closed. She is afebrile with a nontender abdomen. Fetal heart rate tracing is category I. Only occasional contractions are present. Which of the following is the most appropriate next step in management?

a. Expectant management

b. Early delivery with continuous oxytocin infusion

c. Transcervical amnioinfusion of warm normal saline solution

d. Prostaglandin therapy for cervical ripening

e. Immediate cesarean delivery

5. A 29-year-old G2P1 at 33 weeks gestation presents to the labor and delivery unit after noticing a big gush of clear fluid 5 hours ago. On speculum examination, amniotic fluid is seen pooling in the posterior fornix. She is afebrile. Her abdomen is nontender. Bedside ultrasound shows oligohydramnios. The cervix appears 1 cm dilated on visualization. Fetal heart rate tracing is category I. Which of the following is the most appropriate next step in management?

a. Vaginal pool specimen collection to test for fetal lung maturity

b. Administration of antenatal corticosteroid therapy

c. Amniocentesis to test specimen for presence of pulmonary phospholipids

d. Oxytocin induction of labor

e. Immediate cesarean delivery

6. A 29-year-old G2P1 at 33 weeks gestation presents to the labor and delivery unit after noticing a big gush of clear fluid 2 hours ago. Her past obstetrical history is notable for one prior vaginal delivery at 32 weeks gestation in the setting of preterm labor. In the current pregnancy, she had an examination-indicated McDonald cerclage placed at 18 weeks when a shortened cervix was noted on ultrasound. On speculum examination, amniotic fluid is seen pooling in the posterior fornix. The cervix appears 1 cm dilated on visualization. The cerclage is visible and does not appear to be under tension. She is afebrile. Her abdomen is non-tender. Bedside ultrasound shows oligohydramnios. Fetal heart rate tracing is category I. Only occasional uterine contractions are noted on tocometer. Which of the following is the most appropriate next step in management?

   a. Cerclage removal

   b. Cerclage retention unless evidence of chorioamnion-itis develops

   c. Cerclage retention unless preterm labor ensues

   d. Amnioinfusion of warm normal saline solution with cerclage in place

   e. Immediate cesarean delivery

7. Which of the following outcomes is associated with oxytocin induction after PROM?

   a. Increased cesarean delivery

   b. Increased postpartum fever

   c. Decreased chorioamnionitis

   d. Decreased patient satisfaction

   e. No change in latency from membrane rupture to delivery

8. A 19-year-old G1P0 at 28 weeks gestation presents to the labor and delivery unit with leakage of clear fluid for the past 12 hours. On speculum examination, amniotic fluid is seen pooling in the posterior fornix. The cervix appears closed. Ferning of the pooled fluid specimen is seen on microscopic examination. She is afebrile. Her abdomen is nontender. Admission and antenatal corticosteroid admin-istration are advised. Fetal heart rate tracing is category I. Which of the following is the most appropriate next step in management?

   a. 1 day of intravenous azithromycin

   b. 2 days of intravenous ampicillin and erythromycin

   c. 5 days of oral amoxicillin and erythromycin

   d. 7 days of oral erythromycin

   e. 10 days of oral amoxicillin-clavulanic acid

9. A 24-year-old G2P1 at 30 weeks gestation presents to the labor and delivery unit with loss of clear fluid for the past 6 hours. On speculum examination, the cervix appears closed. pH of the vaginal sidewall is >6.0. Bedside ultra-sound shows oligohydramnios. She is afebrile and appears comfortable. Her abdomen is nontender. Fetal heart rate is 155, with moderate variability and spontaneous accel-erations present. Intermittent variable decelerations last-ing 30 seconds are noted. Mild contractions occur every 4–5 minutes. Which of the following is the most appropri-ate next step in management?

   a. Magnesium sulfate for neuroprotection

   b. Therapeutic tocolysis

   c. 17-hydroxyprogesterone therapy to prolong latency

   d. Oxytocin infusion

   e. Transcervical amnioinfusion of warm normal saline solution

10. Preterm PROM occurs after elective cerclage placement in what percentage of patients?

    a. 1%

    b. 5%

    c. 10%

    d. 25%

    e. 50%

11. A 42-year-old G1P0 at 24 weeks gestation presents to the antenatal testing center for surveillance ultrasound. She was diagnosed with preterm PROM at 18 weeks and now is complaining of vaginal bleeding. She strongly desired conservative management and has been undergoing serial ultrasounds every 2 weeks. All have shown persistent severe oligohydramnios. This fetus is at greatest risk for developing which of the following outcomes?

    a. Intraventricular hemorrhage (IVH)

    b. Retinopathy of prematurity

    c. Limb contractures

    d. Necrotizing enterocolitis

    e. Lethal pulmonary hypoplasia

12. In what percentage of all pregnancies does membrane rupture occur spontaneously before the onset of labor?

    a. 1%–2%

    b. 5%–7%

    c. 8%–10%

    d. 20%–25%

    e. 45%–50%

13. A 40-year-old G1P0 Hispanic woman at 33 weeks gestation presents to the labor and delivery unit with leakage of clear fluid, and preterm PROM is diagnosed. The cervix is visualized and appears closed. Maternal temperature is 38°C. Her abdomen is nontender. She was recently diagnosed with gestational diabetes, thus far controlled with diet. Pre-pregnancy body mass index (BMI) was 38. She smokes one half-pack of cigarettes daily. Fetal heart rate tracing is category I. Only occasional contractions are present. Fingerstick blood glucose level was 98 mg/dL on admission. Which of the following risk factors is most strongly associated with preterm PROM?

a. Maternal age

b. Hispanic race

c. Gestational diabetes

d. Maternal obesity

e. Maternal cigarette smoking

ANSWERS

1. Answer: d

(see *Gabbe's Obstetrics* 8e: ch37)

Brief latency from membrane rupture to delivery is one of the hallmarks of PROM. On average, latency increases with decreasing gestational age at membrane rupture. At term, half of expectantly managed gravidas deliver within 33 hours, and 95% deliver within 94 to 107 hours of membrane rupture.[29] Of all women with PROM before 34 weeks, 93% deliver in less than 1 week.

2. Answer: a

(see *Gabbe's Obstetrics* 8e: ch37)

Chorioamnionitis is the most common maternal complication after preterm PROM. Abruptio placentae can cause PROM or can occur subsequent to membrane rupture, and it affects 4% to 12% of these pregnancies.[1] Uncommon but serious complications of PROM managed conservatively near the limit of viability include retained placenta and hemorrhage requiring dilation and curettage (12%), maternal sepsis (0.8%), and maternal death (0.14%).[2]

3. Answer: c

(see *Gabbe's Obstetrics* 8e: ch37)

The frequency and severity of newborn complications after PROM vary inversely with gestational age at membrane rupture and at delivery. Respiratory distress syndrome (RDS) is the most common serious newborn complication after PROM at any gestational age. Necrotizing enterocolitis (NEC), IVH, and sepsis are common with early preterm birth but are relatively uncommon when PROM and delivery occur near term.

4. Answer: b

(see *Gabbe's Obstetrics* 8e: ch37)

Women with PROM at term should be offered early delivery, generally with a continuous oxytocin infusion, to reduce the risk for maternal and newborn complications. Adequate time for latent phase of labor should be allowed. During labor, transcervical amnioinfusion of warm normal saline solution may prove useful if significant umbilical cord compression is suspected based on the fetal heart rate tracing, and immediate delivery is not required.[3,4]

5. Answer: a

(see *Gabbe's Obstetrics* 8e: ch37)

At 32 to 33 weeks gestation, it can be helpful to assess fetal pulmonary maturity and to treat with antenatal corticosteroids those pregnancies without documented fetal maturity. Either vaginal pool or amniocentesis specimens can be used for testing. Vaginal pool specimen collection is preferable if an adequate specimen can be obtained. Because of the increased risk for infectious morbidity and potential for occult umbilical cord compression with conservative management, delivery should be pursued before complications ensue if there is documented fetal pulmonary maturity after PROM at 32 to 33 weeks.

6. **Answer: a**

(see *Gabbe's Obstetrics* 8e: ch37)

Preterm PROM is a common complication after cervical cerclage placement, and it affects about one in four elective cerclages and half of emergent procedures.[5] Retrospective studies reveal that perinatal complications are similar to PROM without a cerclage if the stitch is removed on admission.[6] Retrospective studies that compared stitch removal and retention after preterm PROM have been small but have yielded consistent patterns.[7,8] Each has found insignificant trends toward increased maternal infections and only brief pregnancy prolongation; one study noted increased infant mortality and death due to sepsis when the cerclage was retained after PROM.[7] Because no well-controlled study has found cerclage retention to improve newborn outcomes after PROM, early cerclage removal is recommended when PROM occurs. The risks and benefits of short-term cerclage retention during antenatal corticosteroid are unknown.

7. **Answer: c**

(see *Gabbe's Obstetrics* 8e: ch37)

The largest prospective study to date has found that oxytocin induction after PROM at term reduces the duration of membrane rupture after PROM (median, 17 vs. 33 hours), and the frequencies of chorioamnionitis (4% vs. 8.6%) and postpartum fever (1.9% vs. 3.6%) (p ≤0.008) for each, without increasing cesarean deliveries (14% each) or neonatal infections (2% vs. 2.8%).[9]

8. **Answer: b**

(see *Gabbe's Obstetrics* 8e: ch37)

Antibiotic treatment significantly prolongs latency after membrane rupture and reduces chorioamnionitis. Treatment also reduces the frequencies of newborn complications including neonatal infection, the need for oxygen or surfactant therapy, and IVH. There is a role for a 7-day course of parenteral followed by oral antibiotic therapy with erythromycin and amoxicillin-ampicillin during conservative management of PROM remote from term, to prolong latency and to reduce infectious and gestational age–dependent neonatal complications. Extended-spectrum ampicillin-clavulanic acid treatment is not recommended because it may be harmful.

9. **Answer: a**

(see *Gabbe's Obstetrics* 8e: ch37)

Infants born at 23 to 31 weeks gestation are at increased risk for perinatal death, and survivors commonly suffer acute and long-term complications. Inpatient conservative management is generally attempted unless intrauterine infection, significant vaginal bleeding, or advanced labor is evident or if fetal testing becomes nonreassuring. Administration of magnesium sulfate before early preterm birth will improve long-term infant outcomes and is recommended for anticipated deliveries before 32 weeks gestation after PROM regardless of attempts at conservative management.[10,11] Pending further study, tocolysis and progesterone therapy are not recommended during conservative management of preterm PROM.

10. **Answer: d**

(see *Gabbe's Obstetrics* 8e: ch37)

Preterm PROM is a common complication after cervical cerclage placement, and it affects about one in four elective cerclages and half of emergent procedures.[12]

11. **Answer: e**

(see *Gabbe's Obstetrics* 8e: ch37)

Overall, infant survival after conservatively managed periviable PROM occurs in 44% of cases, but this varies with gestational age at membrane rupture (14.4% before 22 weeks vs. 57.7% at 22 to 24 weeks). Newborn complications include pulmonary hypoplasia (19%), RDS (66%), grade III or IV IVH (5%), sepsis (19%), and NEC (4%), as well as long-term complications such as bronchopulmonary dysplasia (29%), stage III retinopathy of prematurity (5%), and contractures (3%). Persistent severe oligohydramnios is a strong marker for subsequent development of lethal pulmonary hypoplasia.

12. **Answer: c**

(see *Gabbe's Obstetrics* 8e: ch37)

Membrane rupture that occurs spontaneously before the onset of labor is described as PROM regardless of the gestational age at which it occurs. PROM complicates about 8% to 10% of pregnancies overall.

13. Answer: e

(see *Gabbe's Obstetrics* 8e: ch37)

A number of risk factors have been associated with the occurrence of preterm PROM. Among these are low socioeconomic status, uterine overdistension, second- and third-trimester bleeding, low BMI, nutritional deficiencies of copper and ascorbic acid, maternal cigarette smoking, cervical conization or cerclage, pulmonary disease in pregnancy, connective tissue disorders (e.g., Ehlers-Danlos syndrome), and preterm labor or symptomatic contractions in the current gestation.

REFERENCES

1. Gonen R, Hannah ME, Milligan JE. Does prolonged preterm premature rupture of the membranes predispose to abruptio placentae? *Obstet Gynecol.* 1989;74:347.
2. Waters TP, Mercer BM. The management of preterm premature rupture of the membranes near the limit of fetal viability. *Am J Obstet Gynecol.* 2009;201:230.
3. Strong TH Jr, Hetzler G, Sarno AP, Paul RH. Prophylactic intrapartum amnioinfusion: a randomized clinical trial. *Am J Obstet Gynecol.* 1990;162:1370.
4. Schrimmer DB, Macri CJ, Paul RH. Prophylactic amnioinfusion as a treatment for oligohydramnios in laboring patients: a prospective randomized trial. *Am J Obstet Gynecol.* 1991;165:972.
5. Treadwell MC, Bronsteen RA, Bottoms SF. Prognostic factors and complication rates for cervical cerclage: a review of 482 cases. *Am J Obstet Gynecol.* 1991;165:555.
6. Yeast JD, Garite TR. The role of cervical cerclage in the management of preterm premature rupture of the membranes. *Am J Obstet Gynecol.* 1988;158:106.
7. Ludmir J, Bader T, Chen L, et al. Poor perinatal outcome associated with retained cerclage in patients with premature rupture of membranes. *Obstet Gynecol.* 1994;84:823.
8. McElrath TF, Norwitz ER, Lieberman ES, Heffner LJ. Perinatal outcome after preterm premature rupture of membranes with in situ cervical cerclage. *Am J Obstet Gynecol.* 2002;187:1147.
9. Hannah ME, Ohlsson A, Farine D, et al. Induction of labor compared with expectant management for prelabor rupture of membranes at term. *N Engl J Med.* 1996;334:1005.
10. Doyle LW, Crowther CA, Middleton P, Marret S, Rouse D. Magnesium sulphate for women at risk of preterm birth for neuroprotection of the fetus. *Cochrane Database Syst Rev.* 2009;(1):CD004661.
11. Rouse DJ, Hirtz DG, Thom E, et al; Eunice Kennedy Shriver NICHD Maternal-Fetal Medicine Units Network. A randomized, controlled trial of magnesium sulfate for the prevention of cerebral palsy. *N Engl J Med.* 2008;359:895-905.
12. Shen TT, DeFranco EA, Stamilio DM, Chang JJ, Muglia LJ. A population-based study of race-specific risk for preterm premature rupture of membranes. *Am J Obstet Gynecol.* 2008;199:373.

38

Preeclampsia and Hypertensive Disorders

Thaddeus P. Waters

(see *Gabbe's Obstetrics: Normal and Problem Pregnancies*, 8e: ch38)

QUESTIONS

1. A 22-year-old G1P0 presents at 35 weeks gestation to the labor and delivery unit for evaluation of contractions. Her prenatal care and past medical history are unremarkable. The patient has a blood pressure (BP) of 165/105 and reports no symptoms of headache, blurry vision, or other concerns beyond her contractions. The patient received 5 mg of IV hydralazine and now has a BP of 130/87. Laboratory assessment noted a protein/creatinine (P/C) ratio of 0.15, with a normal-for-the-gestational-age complete metabolic profile and complete blood count. Which of the following is the most accurate statement?

   a. The patient has preeclampsia with severe features.

   b. The patient does not have a diagnosis at this time and requires admission for evaluation.

   c. The patient may have preeclampsia with severe features but only if a 24-hour urine collection suggests greater than 300 mg of protein.

   d. The patient has gestational hypertension and can be started on an antihypertensive medication and be discharged with close follow-up.

2. A 31-year-old G3P1011 presents for prenatal care at 10 weeks gestation. She has a past medical history of chronic hypertension. Prior to pregnancy, the patient had a preconception consult with a maternal-fetal medicine provider, who recommended baseline assessments of her urinary protein and renal function. Which of the following is most accurate regarding assessment of clinically significant proteinuria?

   a. Proteinuria can only be determined by a 24-hour urine collection greater than 300 mg.

   b. Proteinuria is established with a P/C ratio greater than 0.3.

   c. Proteinuria is established with a single dipstick measurement of at least 1+.

   d. All patients with chronic hypertension require serial assessment of their renal function in each trimester as protein excretion increases during pregnancy.

3. All of the following are accurate regarding proteinuria excretion in pregnancy except:

   a. Protein excretion in the urine increases in normal pregnancy from approximately 5 mg/dL in the first and second trimesters to 15 mg/dL in the third trimester.

   b. Normal third-trimester urinary protein excretion is identified on a urine dipstick as trace or +1.

   c. The concentration of urinary protein is influenced by contamination with vaginal secretions, blood, or bacteria.

   d. Urinary protein excretion varies by maternal exercise and posture.

4. A 42-year-old G5P2113 presents for a routine evaluation at 34 weeks gestation. Her BP is 153/92 and she reports no complaints. Her medical history is significant for chronic hypertension, managed with labetalol 300 mg BID. Her prior BP was always approximately 130/80 throughout her prenatal care. A urine dipstick notes 2+ protein. In reviewing her chart, you note the patient had a baseline P/C ratio of 0.26 and a serum creatinine of 0.6. Which of the following is most accurate?

   a. The patient has superimposed preeclampsia at this time.

   b. Superimposed preeclampsia can be confirmed with a repeat 24-hour urine collection of >500 mg or a P/C ratio of >0.5.

   c. Superimposed preeclampsia can be confirmed with a repeat 24-hour urine collection >300 mg or a P/C ratio of >0.3.

   d. Preeclampsia can only be confirmed by evidence of laboratory changes or persistent severe hypertension >160/110.

5. A healthy 25-year-old G2P0010 presents for a routine prenatal visit at 35 weeks. Her pregnancy has been uncomplicated to date, she has no significant past medical history, and she reports feeling well, with active fetal movements. Her BP is 110/72 and a urine dipstick notes 1+ protein. Prior urine dips have been negative except for a positive 1+ result 2 weeks ago at her last visit. A clean catch urinalysis confirms 1+ protein and is otherwise normal. All of the following are acceptable for this patient except:

   a. The patient should complete either a P/C ratio or 24-hour urine collection to confirm new-onset proteinuria.

   b. The patient has gestational proteinuria and should be treated as having possible preeclampsia.

   c. No change to routine obstetric care is needed unless the patient develops other evidence of preeclampsia.

   d. The patient requires twice weekly assessments for BP and laboratory assessment for Hemolysis Elevated Liver Enzymes Low Platelet count (HELLP) syndrome.

6. Which of the following is part of the criteria for atypical preeclampsia?

   a. Gestational proteinuria without hypertension

   b. Fetal growth restriction with hypertension

   c. Gestational proteinuria with fetal growth restriction

   d. Fetal growth restriction with evidence of maternal hemolysis

7. A 38-year-old G2P1102 presents to the emergency department for evaluation of a severe headache. Her recent delivery was complicated by chronic hypertension, with superimposed preeclampsia with severe features. Her BP on arrival is 195/131. Which of the following is most accurate for this patient?

   a. The optimal drug in this setting is labetalol.

   b. Lowering the BP too rapidly may produce cerebral ischemia, stroke, or coma.

   c. The aim of therapy is to lower the BP to <160/110 as quickly as possible.

   d. The diagnosis will only be confirmed with CT imaging.

8. A 26-year-old G1P0 with a history of chronic hypertension presents at 12 weeks for prenatal care. She was previously taking a thiazide diuretic but discontinued her medication when she discovered a positive home pregnancy test. Her BP is 145/92. Baseline assessments note no evidence of proteinuria and a serum creatinine of 0.4. What is the best course of action?

   a. The patient should be started on an antihypertensive medication to keep systolic BP between 130 and 140 mm Hg and diastolic BP between 80 and 90 mm Hg.

   b. No medication is needed at this time.

   c. The recommended drug of choice for hypertensive control in pregnancy is labetalol.

   d. For women with uncontrolled hypertension on a maximum dose of labetalol, a thiazide can be added.

9. A 38-year-old G2P1001 presents for evaluation of a missed period. A urine pregnancy test is positive. Her medical history is significant for chronic hypertension managed on a low dose of lisinopril and nifedipine. A bedside ultrasound confirms an intrauterine gestation measuring 8 weeks with normal fetal heart tones. Which of the following is the most appropriate management at this time?

   a. The patient can be counseled that randomized trials have clearly demonstrated which antihypertensive therapies are the best.

   b. The medications taken by the patient should be altered, with discontinuation of her lisinopril, but are not associated with any fetal risk at this time.

   c. The patient should be counseled on the risks of fetal anomalies at this time related to her first-trimester nifedipine exposure.

   d. The patient should be counseled on the risks of fetal hydramnios related to her first-trimester angiotensin-converting enzyme (ACE) exposure.

10. A 39-year-old G2P1001 presents for preconception counseling. The patient reports a history of chronic hypertension managed with labetalol, with no associated cardiac or renal disease. Her baseline electrocardiogram (EKG) is normal sinus rhythm (NSR) with a P/C ratio of 0.1 and a serum creatinine of 0.7. Her current BP is 127/75. Which of the following is most accurate regarding benefits of BP control during pregnancy?

   a. In a large multicenter study of women with chronic hypertension, women with less-tight control of their chronic hypertension had a higher rate of small for gestational age (SGA) infants.

   b. In a large multicenter study of women with chronic hypertension, women with tighter control of their chronic hypertension had higher rate of progression to severe hypertension.

   c. In a large multicenter study of women with chronic hypertension, women with less-tight control of their chronic hypertension had a higher rate of progression to severe hypertension.

   d. In a large multicenter study of women with chronic hypertension, all women with some control of their chronic hypertension had clear maternal and fetal benefit, including pregnancy loss, neonatal intensive care unit admissions, and serious maternal complications

11. All of the following are accurate statements regarding maternal and fetal risks for women with chronic hypertension except:

    a. They are at risk for the development of preeclampsia.

    b. They are at risk for placental abruption.

    c. They are at risk for fetal growth restriction.

    d. The overall risk of complications including superimposed preeclampsia, is strongly correlated to maternal demographic factors.

12. A 19 year old G1P0 presents to the emergency department for evaluation after a family member witnessed seizure-like activity. The patient is currently post-ictal and has started to receive her magnesium loading dose. Her BP is 152/104. A laboratory evaluation for preeclampsia is pending. A bedside ultrasound noted an active fetus with a single deepest pocket of 4 cm and fetal heart tones in the 150 beats per minute range. During your ultrasound evaluation, the patient experiences a tonic-clonic seizure lasting 20 seconds, with fetal heart rate of 70 beats per minute by ultrasound. Which of the following is incorrect regarding this situation?

a. 10% of eclamptic women have a second convulsion after receiving magnesium sulfate.

b. Fetal heart rate changes, including a transient bradycardia, are common, but late decelerations are not and warrant emergent delivery.

c. Maternal hypoxemia and hypercarbia can be observed during the seizure.

d. Maternal and fetal changes related to the seizure usually resolve by 10 minutes after the end of the seizure activity.

13. The patient from above presents for a 6-week postpartum visit. During the delivery hospitalization, the patient was treated with magnesium for 24-hours postdelivery for seizure prophylaxis, and she had persistent hypertension of 140/90 managed without antihypertensive therapy. Her current BP is 110/70, and she is recovering well from her delivery and eclampsia. Which of the following is incorrect regarding her subsequent pregnancy counseling at this time?

a. The rate of preeclampsia in subsequent pregnancies is about 25%.

b. The rate of eclampsia in a subsequent pregnancy is about 2%.

c. Baby aspirin may reduce her risk of eclampsia in a subsequent pregnancy.

d. At present, no preventative therapies can be offered that will reduce her risk of eclampsia in a subsequent pregnancy.

14. A 27-year-old G3P0020 presents at 26 weeks gestation with a headache. The patient's prenatal care has been complicated by early fetal growth restriction, identified at her routine anatomic ultrasound survey. The patient reports a headache that has been persistent for 3 days, with no relief after using Tylenol. Her BP is 148/95 and the patient has a P/C ratio of 1.2. Which of the following statements is correct?

a. Her risk of an eclamptic seizure is reduced by the absence of severe hypertension.

b. The patient has an increased risk for lifelong morbidities, including renal disease and cardiovascular disease, but not diseases related to insulin resistance, such as diabetes.

c. Outpatient management can be considered if the patient has no evidence of HELLP syndrome and normal fetal surveillance.

d. A renal biopsy in this patient has a higher likelihood of identifying underlying renal disease.

15. A 25-year-old G1P0 presents at 37 weeks for a routine prenatal care visit. Her BP is 142/90. A review of her records is significant for a BP of 145/90 1 week ago. The patient reports no symptoms and feels well, with active fetal movements. Based upon the findings, you recommended an evaluation for preeclampsia and induction of labor at this time. The patient is concerned about delivery prior to her due date. With regard to expectant management versus delivery for gestational hypertension or preeclampsia, all of the following are correct except:

a. Data regarding the risks or benefits of induction versus expectant care are largely based upon observational studies.

b. Women who undergo induction of labor at 37 weeks have a lower risk of cesarean delivery.

c. Women managed expectantly have a high risk of morbidity, including severe preeclampsia.

d. The incidence of eclampsia is similar for expectantly managed patients versus those who are induced

16. All of the following are correct statements regarding eclampsia except:

a. The risk of an eclamptic seizure is equal antepartum and postpartum through 96 hours postdelivery.

b. Eclampsia that occurs before the 20th week of gestation is generally associated with molar pregnancy.

c. Cerebral imaging findings in eclampsia are similar to those found in patients with hypertensive encephalopathy.

d. Two competing theories may explain ecliptic seizures: forced dilation of cerebral vessels and vasospasm of intracranial vessels.

17. A 28-year-old G0P0 presents for a routine annual examination. The patient is currently using birth control and is considering becoming pregnant. She is concerned as her older sister had a pregnancy complicated by preeclampsia and is curious about screening tests to identify women at risk for preeclampsia prior to pregnancy. All of the following are correct regarding tools for the prediction of preeclampsia except:

a. Several prospective and nested case-control studies have found that certain maternal risk factors, biophysical clinical factors, and serum biomarkers obtained in the first trimester are associated with subsequent development of hypertensive disorders of pregnancy.

b. Evaluation of maternal clinical factors and other biophysical and biomarkers measured in the first trimester is useful to predict any hypertensive disorder of pregnancy prior to 39 weeks.

c. A major concern of screening for preeclampsia is the unintended consequences of those identified as at risk, particularly for a test with a very high false-positive rate.

d. A major concern of screening for preeclampsia is the very low positive predictive value.

18. A 24-year-old G2P0101 presents at 17 weeks gestation for prenatal care. She reports that her last pregnancy was complicated by preeclampsia with severe features, at 35 weeks gestation. In counseling the patient about the benefits of a daily low-dose aspirin (LDA), which of the following is correct?

a. The patient can start LDA, but the benefits are reduced compared to women who start at 12 weeks gestation.

b. The rationale for LDA is the vasospasm and coagulation abnormalities in preeclampsia are caused by an imbalance in the TXA2/prostacyclin ratio.

c. LDA reduces the risk of preeclampsia by up to 10%.

d. The benefit of LDA is related to the dose (81 mg vs. 150 mg).

19. While seeing patients during your routine obstetric clinic, you are asked to speak with a family medicine colleague, who asks for your assistance regarding an obstetric patient at 13 weeks. The provider is unclear regarding which patients are recommended to receive LDA for the prevention of preeclampsia. All of the following are appropriate candidates for LDA except:

a. Women with a history of hypertension, renal disease, or diabetes

b. Women with autoimmune diseases

c. Multifetal gestation pregnancies

d. A 15 year-old-nulliparous patient

20. A 21-year-old G3P0020 presents at 28 weeks to the labor and delivery unit for evaluation of new-onset epigastric pain. Her initial evaluation is notable for new onset severe hypertension (170/95) and proteinuria (3+ on dipstick). An evaluation including assessment for HELLP syndrome is recommended with treatment of her hypertension and initiation of betamethasone therapy with magnesium for seizure prophylaxis. All of the following are correct regarding the laboratory changes seen with preeclampsia with severe features except:

a. Elevated liver studies are the most common hematologic abnormality identified.

b. A mild elevation of serum transaminases is most common liver abnormality identified.

c. Hemolysis is defined as the presence of microangiopathic hemolytic anemia with an elevated total Lactate dehydrogenase (LDH) >600 U/L.

d. Plasma D-dimer levels are higher in women with preeclampsia than in normotensive pregnant women.

ANSWERS

1. Answer: a

(see *Gabbe's Obstetrics* 8e: ch38)

Severe gestational hypertension (GH) is defined as systolic BP of at least 160 or diastolic BP of at least 110 mm Hg on at least two occasions at least 4 hours apart or only once if acute antihypertensive medications are given prior to 4 hours. In addition, there should be absent proteinuria, absent maternal symptoms, and normal platelet count, serum creatinine, and liver enzymes. In the most recent American College of Obstetrics and Gynecology (ACOG) Task Force, women who have severe gestational hypertension are considered to have preeclampsia with severe features.

2. Answer: b

(see *Gabbe's Obstetrics* 8e: ch38)

Proteinuria may be present before pregnancy, or it may be newly diagnosed during pregnancy. The definition of proteinuria is the same no matter when it occurs: greater than 0.3 g in a 24-hour urine collection or P/C ratio greater than 0.3. If it is not possible to measure 24-hour protein or P/C ratio, proteinuria can be defined as a dipstick measurement of at least 1+ on two occasions.

3. Answer: b

(see *Gabbe's Obstetrics* 8e: ch38)

Protein excretion in the urine increases in normal pregnancy from approximately 5 mg/dL in the first and second trimesters to 15 mg/dL in the third trimester. These low levels are not detected by dipstick. The concentration of urinary protein is influenced by contamination with vaginal secretions, blood, bacteria, or amniotic fluid. It also varies with urine-specific gravity and pH, exercise, and posture. In addition, it is influenced by accuracy of the collection method, and total volume of urine collected.

4. Answer: c

(see *Gabbe's Obstetrics* 8e: ch38)

Women with chronic hypertension may develop superimposed preeclampsia, which increases morbidity for both the mother and fetus. The diagnosis of superimposed preeclampsia is based on one or both of the following findings: development of new-onset proteinuria, defined as the urinary excretion of 0.3 g or more of protein in a 24-hour specimen or a P/C ratio greater than 0.3 in women with hypertension and no proteinuria before 20 weeks' gestation; or, in women with hypertension and proteinuria before 20 weeks, severe exacerbation in hypertension plus development of new onset of symptoms or thrombocytopenia, or abnormal liver enzymes.

5. Answer: c

(see *Gabbe's Obstetrics* 8e: ch38)

Gestational proteinuria is defined as new-onset urinary protein excretion of at least 300 mg per 24-hour timed collection, P/C ratio greater than 0.3, or persistent proteinuria (≥1+ on dipstick on at least two occasions at least 4 hours apart). In the absence of other pathology, the patient should be treated as having possible preeclampsia. Ongoing evaluation can include blood tests and frequent monitoring of BP (at least twice per week or, alternatively, ambulatory home BP measurements).

6. Answer: d

(see *Gabbe's Obstetrics* 8e: ch38)

The criteria for atypical preeclampsia include gestational proteinuria plus one or more of the following symptoms of preeclampsia: hemolysis, thrombocytopenia, elevated liver enzymes, signs and symptoms of preeclampsia-eclampsia earlier than 20 weeks, and late postpartum preeclampsia-eclampsia (>48 hours postpartum).

7. Answer: b

(see *Gabbe's Obstetrics* 8e: ch38)

Hypertensive encephalopathy is usually seen in patients with a systolic BP above 220 mm Hg or a diastolic BP above 130 mm Hg. The only reliable clinical criterion to confirm the diagnosis of hypertensive encephalopathy is prompt response of the patient to antihypertensive therapy. The headache and sensorium often clear dramatically, sometimes within 1 to 2 hours after the treatment. The aim of therapy is to lower mean BP by no more than 15% to 25%. Small reductions in BP in the first 60 minutes, working toward a diastolic level of 100 to 110 mm Hg, have been recommended. In chronically hypertensive women who have a rightward shift of the cerebral autoregulation curve secondary to medial hypertrophy of the cerebral vasculature, lowering BP too rapidly may produce cerebral ischemia, stroke, or coma. The drug of choice in a hypertensive crisis is sodium nitroprusside.

8. Answer: b

(see *Gabbe's Obstetrics* 8e: ch38)

In women without target-organ damage, the aim of antihypertensive therapy is to keep systolic BP between 140 and 150 mm Hg and diastolic BP between 90 and 100 mm Hg. The recommended drug of choice for control of hypertension in pregnancy is labetalol. If maternal BP is not controlled with maximal doses of labetalol, a second drug such as a thiazide diuretic or nifedipine may be added.

9. Answer: b

(see *Gabbe's Obstetrics* 8e: ch38)

Evidence for the long-term effects on children exposed to antihypertensive drugs during pregnancy are lacking except for limited information concerning the use of methyldopa and nifedipine. The potential adverse effects of most commonly prescribed antihypertensive agents are either poorly established or unclearly quantified. Most of the evidence on harm associated with antihypertensives in pregnancy is limited to case reports. The available evidence suggests that the use of calcium channel blockers, particularly nifedipine, in the first trimester was not associated with increased rates of major birth defects. Limited data in the literature suggest potential adverse fetal effects, such as oligohydramnios and fetal-neonatal renal failure, when ACE inhibitors are used in the second or third trimester.

10. Answer: c

(see *Gabbe's Obstetrics* 8e: ch38)

No available data suggest that short-term antihypertensive therapy is beneficial for the mother or the fetus in the setting of low-risk hypertension except for a reduction in the rate of exacerbation of hypertension. The benefits of tight BP control versus less BP control in women with chronic hypertension in pregnancy were studied in a large multicenter study, the Control of Hypertension in Pregnancy Study. The investigators found no difference between groups in primary outcome (pregnancy loss or high-level neonatal care) or in serious maternal complications. However, women in the less-tight control group had a higher rate of progression to severe hypertension. In contrast, the tight control group had a significantly higher rate of SGA infants.

11. Answer: d

(see *Gabbe's Obstetrics* 8e: ch38)

Pregnancies complicated by chronic hypertension are at increased risk for the development of superimposed PE, placental abruption, and fetal growth restriction. The reported rates of PE in mild hypertension range from 14% to 28%. The overall rate of superimposed preeclampsia can be 25% and is greater in women who had hypertension for at least 4 years, in those who had preeclampsia during a previous pregnancy, and in those whose diastolic BP was 100 mm Hg or higher.

12. Answer: b

(see *Gabbe's Obstetrics* 8e: ch38)

About 10% of eclamptic women have a second convulsion after receiving magnesium sulfate. Maternal hypoxemia and hypercarbia cause FHR and uterine activity changes during and immediately after a convulsion. The FHR tracing may reveal bradycardia, transient late decelerations, decreased beat-to-beat variability, and compensatory tachycardia. Uterine contractions can increase in frequency and tone. These changes usually resolve spontaneously within 3 to 10 minutes after the termination of convulsions. The patient should not be rushed to emergency cesarean delivery based on these findings.

13. Answer: c

(see *Gabbe's Obstetrics* 8e: ch38)

Women with a history of eclampsia are at increased risk for all forms of PE in subsequent pregnancies (Table 38.1). In general, the rate of PE in subsequent pregnancies is about 25%, with substantially higher rates if the onset of eclampsia was in the second trimester. The rate of recurrent eclampsia is about 2%. Because of these risks, these women should be informed that they are at increased risk for adverse pregnancy outcome in subsequent pregnancies. At present, no preventive therapy exists for recurrent antepartum eclampsia.

TABLE 38.1   Recurrent Preeclampsia-Eclampsia in Women With Eclampsia.

	Chesley[1]	Lopez-Ilera and Horta[2]	Adelusi and Ojengbede[3]	Sibai et al.[4]
No. of women	171	110	64	182
No. of pregnancies	398	110	64	366
Eclampsia (%)	1.0	—	15.6	1.9
Preeclampsia (%)	23	35	27	22

From Sibai BM. Diagnosis, differential diagnosis and management of eclampsia. *Obstet Gynecol.* 2005;105:402.

14. Answer: d

(see *Gabbe's Obstetrics* 8e: ch38)

Evidence suggests that women with preeclampsia remote from term are at particular increased risk for cardiovascular disease, including chronic hypertension later in life. Microvascular dysfunction, which is associated with insulin resistance, may be a predisposing vascular mechanism for both coronary heart disease and preeclampsia. In addition, these patients—particularly those with recurrent PE—are more likely to have underlying renal disease. In a recent report, 86 Japanese women who had severe hypertension, severe proteinuria, or both, during pregnancy had a postpartum renal biopsy. The authors found that women who had gestational proteinuria or PE before 30 weeks gestation were more likely to have had underlying renal disease.

15. Answer: a

(see *Gabbe's Obstetrics* 8e: ch38)

The Hypertension and Preeclampmsia Intervention Trial At Term (HYPITAT) was a multicenter, open-label randomized controlled trial conducted at 6 academic and 32 nonacademic hospitals in the Netherlands of women with mild gestational hypertension randomized to induction or expectant care. No cases of maternal, fetal, or neonatal death and no cases of eclampsia or abruption were reported in either group. However, women randomized to the induction group had a significant reduction in the primary outcome of a composite morbidity, primarily due to a decrease in the rates of severe hypertension. Moreover, in the induction group, the rate of cesarean delivery was lower.

16. Answer: a

(see *Gabbe's Obstetrics* 8e: ch38)

The onset of eclamptic convulsions can be during the antepartum, intrapartum, or postpartum period. The reported frequency of antepartum convulsions among recent series has ranged from 38% to 53%, whereas the frequency of postpartum eclampsia has ranged from 11% to 44%. Although most cases of postpartum eclampsia occur within the first 48 hours, some cases can develop beyond 48 hours postpartum.

17. Answer: b

(see *Gabbe's Obstetrics* 8e: ch38)

Based on the available data, evaluation of maternal clinical factors and other biophysical and biomarkers measured in the first trimester is useful only for the prediction of those who will ultimately progress to PE that will require delivery prior to 34 weeks of gestation.

18. Answer: b

(see *Gabbe's Obstetrics* 8e: ch38)

The rationale for recommending LDA prophylaxis is the theory that the vasospasm and coagulation abnormalities in preeclampsia are caused partly by an imbalance in the TXA2/prostacyclin ratio. In women considered at increased risk for preeclampsia, the U.S. preventative services task force (USPSTF) members found that LDA administered after 12 weeks gestation reduced the risk of PE by an average of 24% and beneficial effects of LDA were not dependent on the dose of LDA, and they were evident when LDA was used between 12 and 28 weeks gestation. In an updated individual patient data metaanalysis, they found no difference in benefit between an aspirin dose of <75 mg or >75 mg/d, and no difference whether LDA was started at <16 weeks or ≥16 weeks gestation.

19. Answer: d

(see *Gabbe's Obstetrics* 8e: ch38)

USPSTF recommended that those with a history of preeclampsia, preexisting chronic hypertension or renal disease, pregestational diabetes, autoimmune disease, and multifetal gestation or those with more than moderate risk factors such as nulliparity and obesity should receive LDA (81 mg/day) starting at 12 to 28 weeks until delivery to reduce the likelihood of developing subsequent PE, preterm birth, or FGR. This recommendation has also been adopted by ACOG.

20. Answer: a

(see *Gabbe's Obstetrics* 8e: ch38)

Thrombocytopenia is the most common hematologic abnormality in women with severe PE. It is correlated with the severity of the disease process and the presence or absence of placental abruption. When liver dysfunction does occur in PE, mild elevation of serum transaminases is most common. Many authors have used elevated total LDH (usually >600 U/L) as diagnostic criteria for hemolysis. Several studies have evaluated the hematologic abnormalities in women with preeclampsia. Plasma fibrinopeptide A, D-dimer levels, and circulating thrombin-antithrombin complexes are higher in women with PE than in normotensive gravidas.

REFERENCES

1. Black MH, Zhou H, Sacks DA, et al. Prehypertension prior to or during early pregnancy is associated with increased risk for hypertensive disorders in pregnancy and gestational diabetes. *J Hypertens.* 2015;33:1860-1867.

2. Ankumah NE, Sibai BM. Chronic hypertension in pregnancy: diagnosis, management, and outcomes. *Clin Obstet Gynecol.* 2017 Mar;60(1):206-214.

3. Magee LA, von Dadelszen P, Rey E, et al. Less-tight versus tight control of hypertension in pregnancy. *N Engl J Med.* 2015;372:407-417.

4. Mayama M, Uno K, Tano S, et al. Incidence of posterior reversible encephalopathy syndrome in eclamptic and patients with preeclampsia with neurologic symptoms. *Am J Obstet Gynecol.* 2016;215:239.e1-e5.

39

Multiple Gestations

Rini Banerjee Ratan

(see *Gabbe's Obstetrics: Normal and Problem Pregnancies*, 8e: ch39)

QUESTIONS

1. Among natural conceptions, what is the rate of monozygotic twinning?

   a. 0.05%

   b. 0.4%

   c. 1.0%

   d. The rate is affected by family history and race

   e. The rate increases with maternal age

2. A 37-year-old G3P2 at 8 weeks gestation presents to her obstetrician's office to establish prenatal care. An ultrasound shows one intrauterine gestational sac with a thin dividing membrane and two fetuses.
   Which of the following is the most likely diagnosis?

   a. Monochorionic monoamniotic twin pregnancy

   b. Monochorionic diamniotic twin pregnancy

   c. Dichorionic diamniotic (DCDA) twin pregnancy

   d. Twin pregnancy, chorionicity cannot be determined until second trimester

3. Which of the following maternal physiologic adaptations to pregnancy is thought to be associated with the increased risk for gestational diabetes in multifetal gestations?

   a. Increased production of human chorionic gonadotropin by the placenta

   b. Higher levels of maternal cortisol

   c. Expansion of plasma volume and total body water

   d. Increased human placental lactogen (hPL)

   e. Higher renal protein excretion

4. A 26-year-old G1P0 at 8 weeks gestation presents to her obstetrician's office to establish prenatal care. An ultrasound shows an intrauterine gestational sac with a thin dividing membrane and two fetuses. A follow-up ultrasound is performed 4 weeks later, at which time only one fetus is seen. The fetus appears active, with normal cardiac motion. The patient is concerned about further risks in pregnancy following spontaneous loss of one twin. Which of the following is the most likely outcome for this patient's pregnancy?

   a. Healthy term or near-term baby

   b. Higher likelihood of preterm delivery

   c. Higher likelihood of intrauterine fetal demise of surviving twin

   d. Possible ischemic-hypoxic injury to surviving twin

   e. Increased risk of placental abruption

5. A 31-year-old G2P1 at 35 weeks gestation with a monochorionic diamniotic twin pregnancy presents to the antenatal testing unit for routine ultrasound. An intrauterine fetal demise (IUFD) of one twin is noted. Etiology of the demise is not apparent. The surviving twin has a biophysical profile (BPP) of 10/10. In addition to providing emotional support to the patient, which of the following is the most appropriate next step in management?

   a. Advise weekly ultrasound with Doppler studies of surviving twin.

   b. Offer MRI for evaluation of surviving twin's central nervous system in 2–3 weeks.

   c. Perform serial growth scan in 4 weeks.

   d. Counsel the patient that neurologic injury to the survivor has likely already occurred.

   e. Recommend delivery at this time.

6. At what gestational age is delivery recommended for uncomplicated DCDA twin pregnancies?

    a. 34 weeks

    b. 36 weeks

    c. 37 weeks

    d. 38 weeks

    e. 39 weeks

7. A 41-year-old G3P2 at 36 weeks gestation with a DCDA twin pregnancy presents to the labor and delivery unit in spontaneous active labor. A bedside ultrasound confirms that the twins are concordantly grown, in vertex/vertex presentation. Her cervix is 4 cm dilated, 80% effaced, and −1/5 station. Both fetal heart rate (FHR) tracings are category I. Her past obstetric history is notable for two prior normal spontaneous vaginal deliveries at term. She desires a trial of labor and is willing to undergo breech extraction of the second twin if required. She did not have epidural anesthesia with her previous deliveries and does not wish to have an epidural now. She requests intermittent monitoring so that she may have as natural a birth as possible. Which of the following is the most appropriate recommendation for this patient?

    a. Epidural anesthesia is not advocated by the American College of Obstetrics and Gynecology (ACOG) for a trial of labor.

    b. Fetal and maternal outcomes are improved with cesarean delivery of twins.

    c. If a trial of labor is elected, both fetuses must be continuously monitored.

    d. Cesarean delivery would be advised if the second twin does not deliver within 15 minutes after the first twin is born.

    e. The likelihood of combined vaginal-caesarean delivery is 20%.

8. A 38-year-old G1P0 at 20 weeks gestation with a triplet pregnancy presents to her obstetrician's office for a routine prenatal visit. Genetic testing was normal in all triplets, and ultrasound showed normal anatomy in all three. The triplets appear to be concordantly grown at this time. She feels fetal movements and denies contractions, bleeding, or leakage of fluid. Which of the following is the most appropriate antenatal surveillance to recommend?

    a. Weekly BPPs beginning at 34 weeks

    b. Serial ultrasounds for growth every 3 weeks beginning at 24 weeks

    c. Weekly non-stress test (NST)s beginning at 32 weeks

    d. Twice-weekly BPPs beginning at 32 weeks

    e. Weekly BPPs beginning at 28 weeks

9. Which of the following calculations demonstrates the correct way to determine discordance in growth between twins?

    a. $\dfrac{\text{Weight of larger twin} - \text{Weight of smaller twin}}{\text{Weight of larger twin}}$

    b. $\dfrac{\text{Weight of both twins} - \text{Weight of larger twin}}{\text{Weight of smaller twin}}$

    c. $\dfrac{\text{Weight of larger twin} - \text{Weight of smaller twin}}{\text{Weight of smaller twin}}$

    d. $\dfrac{\text{Weight of larger twin} - \text{Weight of smaller twin}}{\text{Weight of both twins}}$

10. A 38-year-old G4P0030 at 12 weeks gestation with a DCDA pregnancy presents to her obstetrician's office for her first prenatal visit. Her cervical length on ultrasound is 3 cm. Her pregnancy was conceived using in vitro fertilization. Her past obstetric history is notable for three prior first-trimester pregnancy losses. Which of the following is the most appropriate recommendation to reduce the risk of spontaneous preterm birth for this patient?

    a. Insertion of a vaginal pessary at 16–20 weeks

    b. Weekly 17-hydroxyprogesterone caproate injections from 16 to 37 weeks

    c. Vaginal progesterone in the midtrimester

    d. Placement of a prophylactic cerclage

    e. Serial transvaginal cervical length (TVCL) measurements from 18 to 24 weeks

11. A 25-year-old G2P1 at 10 weeks gestation presents to her obstetrician's office to establish prenatal care. Ultrasound shows a DCDA twin pregnancy. Her body mass index (BMI) is 38 kg/m². What is the total weight gain recommended by the Institute of Medicine for her current pregnancy?

    a. 11–20 lb

    b. 15–25 lb

    c. 25–42 lb

    d. 31–50 lb

    e. 37–54 lb

12. A 28-year-old G2P1 with a monochorionic diamniotic twin pregnancy at 18 weeks gestation presents to the antenatal testing unit for routine ultrasound. Oligohydramnios in one amniotic sac and polyhydramnios in the other amniotic sac is noted. The bladder is not visible in the twin with oligohydramnios. Doppler studies of both twins are normal. Which of the following is the most appropriate next step in management?

a. Follow-up ultrasound surveillance in 2 weeks

b. Serial amnioreduction

c. Laser photocoagulation

d. Selective termination via cord occlusion

13. A 33-year-old G1P0 at 10 weeks gestation presents to her obstetrician's office to establish prenatal care. An ultrasound shows one intrauterine gestational sac with two fetuses. No dividing membrane is visible. Which of the following is the most likely cause of perinatal mortality for this twin gestation?

a. Premature delivery

b. Fetal growth restriction

c. Congenital anomalies

d. Umbilical cord entanglement

14. A 22-year-old G1P0 at 20 weeks gestation with a DCDA twin pregnancy presents to her obstetrician's office for a routine prenatal visit. Both twins appear to be concordantly grown with normal fetal anatomy. She feels fetal movements and denies contractions, bleeding, or leakage of fluid. Which of the following is the most appropriate surveillance regimen to evaluate fetal growth?

a. Ultrasound evaluation every 2 weeks beginning now

b. Ultrasound evaluation every 4 weeks beginning now

c. Ultrasound evaluation at 28 and 36 weeks

d. Ultrasound evaluation every 2 weeks beginning at 24 weeks

e. Ultrasound evaluation every 2 weeks beginning at 28 weeks

ANSWERS

1. Answer: b

(see *Gabbe's Obstetrics* 8e: ch39)

Among natural conceptions, dizygotic (DZ) twins arise in about 1% to 1.5% of pregnancies, and monozygotic (MZ) twins occur in 0.4% of pregnancies. Rates of spontaneous DZ twinning are affected by maternal age, family history, and race. MZ twinning rates are constant across all population and demographic variables, with the exception of assisted reproduction. Against a spontaneous rate of 0.4% in the general population, studies of MZ twinning report rates more than 10-fold higher in pregnancies conceived by assisted fertility.

2. Answer: b

(see *Gabbe's Obstetrics* 8e: ch39)

Between 6 and 10 weeks, counting the number of gestational sacs and evaluating the thickness of the dividing membrane is the most reliable method of determining chorionicity (Table 39.1). Two separate gestational sacs, each containing a fetus, and a thick dividing membrane represent a DCDA pregnancy, whereas one gestational sac with a thin dividing membrane and two fetuses suggests a monochorionic diamniotic pregnancy.

TABLE 39.1 Determination of Chorionicity and Amnionicity in First-Trimester Pregnancies.

Placentation	Gestational Sacs	Amniotic Cavities	Yolk Sacs
Dichorionic diamniotic	2	2 (thick dividing membrane)	2
Monochorionic diamniotic	1	2 (thin dividing membrane)	2
Monochorionic monoamniotic	1	1	1[a]

[a]Although this is nearly always true, there have been case reports of two yolk sacs in early pregnancy in twins later confirmed to be monoamniotic.

3. Answer: d

(see *Gabbe's Obstetrics* 8e: ch39)

Levels of maternal progesterone, estriol, cortisol, and human chorionic somatomammotropin (placental lactogen) are higher in multiple gestations than in singletons. Increased hPL modifies maternal metabolism and is thought to be associated with the increased risk for gestational diabetes seen in multifetal pregnancies.

4. Answer: a

(see *Gabbe's Obstetrics* 8e: ch39)

The so-called vanishing twin refers to the loss of one fetus in a multiple gestation early in pregnancy. It is a fairly common occurrence and is typically either asymptomatic or associated with spotting or mild bleeding. A reasonable approach to counseling and managing a pregnancy complicated by a first-trimester vanishing twin is to reassure the parents that the most likely outcome will be a healthy term or near term baby. Because of the reports of smaller birthweights and increased risk of SGA, a third trimester growth scan is reasonable.

5. Answer: e

(see *Gabbe's Obstetrics* 8e: ch39)

In the authors' practices, a single IUFD in a monochorionic diamniotic pregnancy at or after 34 weeks would be an indication for delivery. If IUFD of one twin occurs in the second or early third trimester of an otherwise uncomplicated monochorionic diamniotic gestation, a typical recommendation is delivery at 37 weeks if growth and antenatal testing are reassuring, but with a low threshold to deliver after 34 weeks.

6. Answer: d

(see *Gabbe's Obstetrics* 8e: ch39)

Numerous population-based studies suggest that the nadir of perinatal complications occurs at earlier gestational ages in multiple gestations compared with singletons. The 2011 Eunice Kennedy Shriver National Institute of Child Health and Human Development (NICHD) and Society for Maternal-Fetal Medicine (SMFM) publication on timing of indicated late-preterm and early-term birth recommends delivery of uncomplicated DC twins at 38 weeks.[1] The 2016 Practice Bulletin on Multifetal Gestations offers a similar recommendation for delivery at 38 weeks for uncomplicated DC gestations.[2]

7. Answer: c

(see *Gabbe's Obstetrics* 8e: ch39)

Retrospective and prospective data on mode of delivery in diamniotic twin gestations with a cephalic-presenting first twin show that in selected women, under appropriate conditions and with experienced obstetricians and supporting staff, no benefit to routine cesarean delivery is evident. If a trial of labor is elected, both fetuses must be continuously monitored. Epidural anesthesia for labor and delivery is also advisable and is advocated by ACOG.[2] Although some second twins may require rapid delivery, most can be safely followed with fetal heart rate surveillance and can remain undelivered for substantial periods of time.

8. Answer: e

(see *Gabbe's Obstetrics* 8e: ch39)

The 2009 NICHD document lists initiation of antenatal testing at 28 weeks as a reasonable strategy for triplets.[3] The authors' preferentially perform BPPs instead of NSTs in triplets or higher plurality because of the difficulty in consistently and efficiently obtaining and interpreting NSTs with more than two fetuses.

9. Answer: a

(see *Gabbe's Obstetrics* 8e: ch39)

Significant discordance in weight between twins is most commonly defined as a greater than 20% difference in actual or estimated twin weights (the difference between the weights divided by the weight of the larger twin).

10. Answer: e

(see *Gabbe's Obstetrics* 8e: ch39)

The use of ultrasound TVCL measurements can help stratify preterm birth (PTB) risk in multiple gestations. A TVCL of 20 mm or less between 20 and 24 weeks gestation was the best predictor of PTB before 32 and before 34 weeks. The degree of change in the cervical length over time may also be an important predictor of PTB in twins. No studies have shown any benefit associated with the use of 17-OH-P in multiple gestation.[4–8] The authors' interpretation of the available literature on progesterone to prevent PTB in twins is that there is no evidence to support the use of intramuscular 17-OH-P in any multifetal gestation, nor should any form of progesterone be used in unselected multiples. There is no role for "prophylactic" cerclage solely for the indication of multifetal gestation. At the present time, there is no conclusive evidence upon which to base a strong recommendation for ultrasound- or examination-indicated cerclage in twins. The 2016 ACOG Practice Bulletin on Multifetal Gestation states that "use of prophylactic cervical pessary is not recommended in multifetal pregnancies."

11. Answer: c

(see *Gabbe's Obstetrics* 8e: ch39)

See Table 39.2.

TABLE 39.2 2009 Institute of Medicine Recommendations for Weight Gain in Pregnancy.

Prepregnancy BMI	BMI (kg/m²) WHO Criteria	Total Weight Gain: Singleton (lb)	Total Weight Gain: Twins (lb)
Underweight	<18.5	28–40	No recommendations made
Normal weight	18.5–24.9	25–35	37–54
Overweight	25.0–29.9	15–25	31–50
Obese	≥30.0	11–20	25–42

BMI, Body mass index; *WHO*, World Health Organization.
From Rasmussen KM, Yaktine AL, editors. *Institute of Medicine (Committee to Reexamine IOM Pregnancy Weight Guidelines, Food and Nutrition Board and Board on Children, Youth, and Families). Weight Gain During Pregnancy: Reexamining the Guidelines.* Washington, DC: National Academies Press; 2009.

12. Answer: c. Laser photocoagulation

(see *Gabbe's Obstetrics* 8e: ch39)

For twin-twin transfusion syndrome (TTTS) stage II or greater, laser photocoagulation is the preferred treatment for pregnancies <26 weeks gestation and is considered standard of care when technically feasible. Serial amnioreduction is considered in cases in which laser cannot be done, either because of advanced gestational age or due to technical limitations. In rare cases, selective termination via cord occlusion can be considered. This would generally be reserved for previable twins with an extremely high risk of donor twin loss.

13. Answer: d

(see *Gabbe's Obstetrics* 8e: ch39)

Historically, perinatal mortality rates for monoamniotic (MA) twins have been reported to approach 50%, attributed to premature delivery, growth restriction, and congenital anomalies (seen in up to 25% of MA twin pregnancies) but mostly to umbilical cord entanglement.

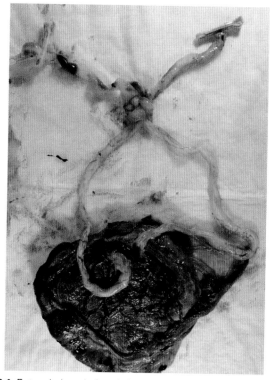

Fig. 39.1 Entangled cords found during emergent cesarean delivery in a case of monochorionic monoamniotic twins at 32 weeks. Both babies did well.

14. Answer: b

(see *Gabbe's Obstetrics* 8e: ch39)

All patients with twins should undergo ultrasound evaluation of fetal growth at least every 4 weeks after 20 weeks gestation. Additionally, ultrasounds should be performed every 2 weeks in monochorionic twins beginning at 16 weeks to screen for TTTS.

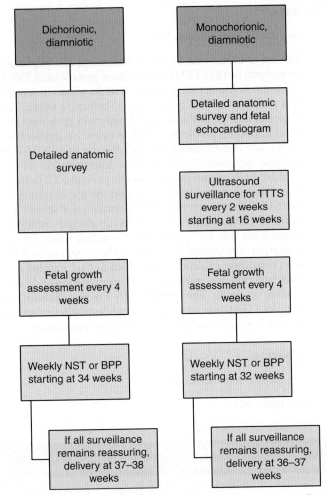

Fig. 39.2 Antenatal surveillance and delivery timing for uncomplicated diamniotic twins. biophysical profile (BPP), ●●●. Figure adapted from Unal ER. Fetal surveillance and timing of delivery for multiples. *Clin Obstet Gynecol.* 2015 Sep;58(3):676-689. Used with permission.

REFERENCES

1. Spong CY, Mercer BM, D'Alton M, et al. Timing of indicated late-preterm and early-term birth. *Obstet Gynecol.* 2011;118:323-333.
2. Multifetal gestations: twin, triplet, and higher-order multifetal pregnancies. Practice Bulletin No. 169. American College of Obstetricians and Gynecologists. *Obstet Gynecol.* 2016;128:e131-e146.
3. Signore C, Freeman RK, Spong CY. Antenatal testing—a reevaluation. *Obstet Gynecol.* 2009;113:687-701.
4. Senat MV, Porcher R, Winer N, et al. Prevention of preterm delivery by 17 alpha-hydroxyprogesterone caproate in asymptomatic twin pregnancies with a short cervix: a randomized controlled trial. *Am J Obstet Gynecol.* 2013;208:194.e1-e8.
5. Lim AC, Schuit E, Bloemenkamp K, et al. 17-Hydroxyprogesterone caproate for the prevention of adverse neonatal outcome in multiple pregnancies: a randomized controlled trial. *Obstet Gynecol.* 2011;118:513-520.
6. Combs CA, Garite T, Maurel K, et al. 17-hydroxyprogesterone caproate for twin pregnancy: a double-blind, randomized clinical trial. *Am J Obstet Gynecol.* 2011;204:221.e1-e8.
7. Caritis SN, Rouse DJ, Peaceman AM, et al. Prevention of preterm birth in triplets using 17 alpha-hydroxyprogesterone caproate: a randomized controlled trial. *Obstet Gynecol.* 2009;113:285-292
8. Rouse DJ, Caritis SN, Peaceman AM, et al. A trial of 17 alpha-hydroxyprogesterone caproate to prevent prematurity in twins. *N Engl J Med.* 2007;357:454-461.

40

Red Cell Alloimmunization

Vanita D. Jain

(see *Gabbe's Obstetrics: Normal and Problem Pregnancies*, 8e: ch40)

QUESTIONS

1. The Centers for Disease Control and Prevention (CDC) reports decreased incidence of RhD alloimmunization due to the advent of:

    a. Routine administration of antenatal and postpartum rhesus immune globulin (RhIG)

    b. Increased intrauterine transfusion

    c. Improved management of neonatal jaundice

    d. Increased rate of cesarean sections with decreased immunization occurring with delivery

2. What percentage of deliveries of RhD-positive fetuses result in RhD alloimmunization in RhD-negative women who did not receive RhIG?

    a. 1%

    b. 13%

    c. 27%

    d. 93%

3. A 22-year-old G1P0 Hispanic female presents for routine obstetric care at 9 weeks. She has completed her first trimester new prenatal laboratory work. Her type and screen return as A+; however, there is a note from the blood bank that the patient is "weak D positive." Her antibody screen is negative. The next best step is:

    a. Nothing, routine prenatal care

    b. Administer RhIG and repeat administration at delivery if the neonate is RhD positive.

    c. Do NOT given RhIG now but test neonate at delivery and give RhIG if the neonate is RhD positive.

    d. Counsel the patient that her neonate is at risk for hydrops, start serial middle cerebral artery (MCA) Doppler ultrasound studies.

4. A 23-year-old G1P0 presents at 30 weeks. Her laboratory work is reviewed and noted to have a 1-hour glucose tolerance test of 102, hemoglobin of 12 mg/dL, and a normal ferritin value. She is blood type A−, antibody screen negative. You discuss the need for RhIG prophylaxis. The patient asks what is the chance that her fetus is RhD positive. Dad's blood type is unknown. You discuss that approximately what percentage of Rh-negative pregnant women carry an Rh-negative fetus:

    a. 10%

    b. 20%

    c. 30%

    d. 40%

5. All of the following are cited as an indication by the American College of Obstetrics and Gynecology (ACOG) to administer RhIG (if the mother is RhD negative) except:

    a. Spontaneous miscarriage

    b. Elective termination of pregnancy

    c. Ectopic pregnancy

    d. Prior to amniocentesis

    e. Placenta previa, with no vaginal bleeding

6. A 32-year-old G3P2002 presents at 28 weeks gestation after a motor vehicle accident with a placental abruption seen on sonogram. She is B−, and antibody screen is negative. She is a candidate for RhIG administration. However, to calculate the dosing, you obtain a rosette test, which is positive. A Kleihauer -Betke test (KB) is then obtained and the KB stain is calculated at 5%. How many vials of 300 μg Rh Immune Globulin (RhIG) are needed?

    a. 9 vials = 2700 μg

    b. 6 vials = 1800 μg

    c. 4 vials = 1200 μg

    d. 1 vial = 300 μg

7. A 32-year-old G1P0 presents for counseling after her prenatal laboratories at 12 weeks reveal a blood type of A−, antibody screen positive to the D antigen with a titer of 32. She notes a history of a blood transfusion after a skiing accident and a broken femur about 2 years ago. Her partner, and identified father of the current pregnancy, is B+. The most appropriate next step is:

a. Cell free fetal DNA to determine RhD status

b. chorionic villus sampling (CVS)

c. Amniocentesis

d. Intrauterine transfusion therapy

8. A 29-year-old G1P0 is 24 weeks gestational age. She is A−, antibody screen positive at a titer of 4, from her first trimester laboratory work. Today, at 24 weeks, her titer returns at 32. The father is unavailable for testing. A cell free fetal DNA test is ordered and returns that the fetus is RhD negative and female. The most appropriate next step is:

a. Repeat cell free fetal DNA to confirm

b. Admit the patient and plan for umbilical cord blood sampling

c. Amniocentesis to determine blood type

d. Refer to Maternal Fetal Medicine for serial MCA-PSV Dopplers

9. A 29-year-old G2P1001 is planning to have a periumbilical blood sample and intrauterine transfusion after discussion with Maternal Fetal Medicine, due to her antibody status of 32 to RhD, and MCA Dopplers peak systolic velocity (PSV) at 1.65 Multiples of Median (MoM). She is very nervous at her routine obstetric visit today with you, but you reassure her that the total perinatal loss rate is:

a. 1%–3%

b. 10%–15%

c. 15%–20%

d. 90% and she should cancel the procedure

10. The difference between the RhD algorithm for management and the Kell algorithm for management is that with Kell the critical titer is considered:

a. 8

b. 16

c. 32

d. 64

ANSWERS

1. Answer: **a**

(see *Gabbe's Obstetrics* 8e: ch40)

The advent of the routine administration of antenatal and postpartum RhIG has resulted in a marked reduction in cases of red-cell alloimmunization in industrialized countries. The CDC last required the reporting of rhesus alloimmunization as a medical complication of pregnancy on U.S. birth certificates in the year 2002.[1] In that year, the most recent for which epidemiologic data are available, the incidence was reported to be 6.7 cases of rhesus alloimmunization per 1000 live births. Rh hemolytic disease of the fetus and newborn (HDFN) continues to contribute to worldwide perinatal morbidity and mortality due to the unavailability of RhIG in countries like India and China.[2] One estimate of its effect includes 41,000 stillbirths, 90,000 neonatal deaths, and 48,000 cases of kernicterus annually.

2. Answer: **b**

(see *Gabbe's Obstetrics* 8e: ch40)

In most cases of red cell alloimmunization, a fetomaternal hemorrhage (FMH) occurs in the antenatal period or, more commonly, at the time of delivery. If a maternal ABO blood type incompatibility exists between the mother and her fetus, anti-A and/or anti-B antibodies lyse the fetal cells in the maternal circulation and destroy the RhD antigen. Even if this protective effect is not present, only 13% of deliveries of RhD-positive fetuses result in RhD alloimmunization in RhD-negative women who do not receive RhIG.

3. Answer: b

(see *Gabbe's Obstetrics* 8e: ch40)

All pregnant patients should undergo determination of blood type and an antibody screen at the first prenatal visit. In the past, all Rh-negative patients underwent additional testing to see if they were *Du positive*. This terminology was later changed to classify these patients as *weak Rh-positive* individuals. In one series of 500 pregnant patients, this occurred in 1% of whites, 2.6% of blacks, and 2.7% of Hispanics. The recommendation in the past was that these individuals should be considered Rh positive, and RhIG was not indicated. Subsequent research found that the *weak D* individuals can belong to one of two groups:

(a) Some of these patients have intact D antigens that are expressed in reduced numbers on the surface of the red cells (Fig. 40.1). These individuals are *not* at risk for rhesus alloimmunization.

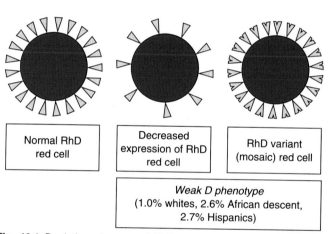

▷ = Normal RhD antigen   ▷ = RhD antigen with missing epitope

Normal RhD red cell

Decreased expression of RhD red cell

RhD variant (mosaic) red cell

Weak D phenotype
(1.0% whites, 2.6% African descent, 2.7% Hispanics)

Fig. 40.1 Depiction of a normal RhD-positive red cell as well as red cells noted in individuals with weak D variants.

(b) In others with a weak D phenotype, the individual has inherited a gene that results in a variant expression of the D antigen. In these cases, one or more of the D antigen epitopes are missing, and the patient can become alloimmunized to these missing portions of the D antigen. Severe HDFN has been reported in these cases when a maternal antibody develops to the missing epitope.

Although clinical trials have not been undertaken, the current recommendation is that these patients should all receive RhIG as it would be unknown if they fall into group a or b.

4. Answer: d

(see *Gabbe's Obstetrics* 8e: ch40)

Approximately 40% of Rh-negative pregnant women will carry an Rh-negative fetus; thus RhIG would not be indicated in the antepartum period if this can be accurately determined.

5. Answer: e

(see *Gabbe's Obstetrics* 8e: ch40)

Although not well studied, level A scientific evidence has been cited by ACOG to address additional indications for the antepartum administration of RhIG. These include spontaneous miscarriage, elective abortion, ectopic pregnancy, genetic amniocentesis, chorionic villus sampling, and cordocentesis (Table 40.1).

TABLE 40.1 Indications for Rhesus Immune Globulin.

Indication	Level of Evidence[a]
Spontaneous miscarriage	A
Elective abortion	A
Threatened miscarriage	C
Ectopic pregnancy	A
Hydatidiform mole	B
Genetic amniocentesis	A
Chorion villus biopsy	A
Cordocentesis	A
Placenta previa with bleeding	C
Suspected abruption	C
Intrauterine fetal demise	C
Blunt trauma to the abdomen	C
At 28 weeks gestation unless father of fetus is RhD negative	A
Amniocentesis for fetal lung maturity	A
External cephalic version	C
Within 72 hours of delivery of an RhD-positive infant	A
After administration of RhD-positive blood component	C

[a]A = high, B = moderate, C = low.
Modified from Prevention of Rh D alloimmunization. *Am Coll Obstet Gynecol Pract Bull.* 2017;181:1-14.

6. Answer: a

(see *Gabbe's Obstetrics* 8e: ch40)

A qualitative yet sensitive test for FMH, the *rosette test*, is first performed. Results return as positive or negative; a negative result warrants administration of a standard 300 μg dose of RhIG. If the rosette is positive, a KB stain or fetal cell stain using flow cytometry is undertaken to quantitate the amount of the fetal maternal hemorrhage (FMH). The American Association of Blood Banks then recommends that the percentage of fetal blood cells be multiplied by a factor of 50 (to account for an estimated maternal blood volume of 5000 mL) to calculate the volume of the FMH. This volume is divided by 30 to determine the number of vials of RhIG to be administered. A decimal point is rounded up or down for values greater than 0.5 or less than 0.5, respectively. Because this calculation includes an inaccurate estimation of the maternal blood volume, one additional vial of RhIG is added to the calculation. In this example, the KB returns at 5%, and we assume maternal blood volume (MBV) at 5 L. Thus, 5% multiplied by 50 means 250 mL of FMH has occurred. 250/30 = 8.3, round down to 8, and then add one additional vial = 9 vials.

7. Answer: a

(see *Gabbe's Obstetrics* 8e: ch40)

Once a maternal antibody screen reveals the presence of an anti-D antibody, a titer is the first step in the evaluation of the RhD-sensitized patient during the first affected pregnancy. A *critical titer* is defined as the anti-red cell titer associated with a significant risk for hydrops fetalis. When this is present, further fetal surveillance is warranted. This value will vary with institution and methodology; however, in most centers, a critical titer for anti-D between 8 and 32 is usually used. Several techniques have been used to determine the fetal blood type if the patient's partner is determined to be heterozygous for the involved red cell antigen. In 50% of cases in which the fetus is found to be antigen negative, further maternal and fetal testing is unnecessary. The initial step in determining the fetal RhD type involves an assessment of paternity and paternal zygosity. Once undertaken using serologic testing and population statistics, molecular techniques can now be used to accurately determine the paternal genotype at the *RHD* locus.[3] However, some authorities have argued that issues with paternity can be averted by omitting this step and testing every pregnancy with cell free DNA testing for fetal *RHD* determination. Thus, cell free fetal DNA is considered the next best step given reliable results and minimal risk to the fetus.

8. Answer: d

(see *Gabbe's Obstetrics* 8e: ch40)

An *RHD*-positive cell free DNA result can be considered reliable since there should not be any *RHD* DNA in the maternal circulation. In the case of a *RHD*-negative cell free DNA result, the detection of the *SRY* gene from a male fetus confirms the presence of fetal DNA (Fig. 40.2). An *RHD*-negative, female result is more problematic since this could be due to amplification of the maternal DNA in the absence of fetal DNA. Many cell free DNA assays used in Europe use single nucleotide polymorphisms (SNPs) to determine if this is a valid result. A difference between maternal SNPs and fetal SNPs (paternal in origin) in the sample confirms the presence of fetal DNA. SNPs are not employed in the current U.S. assay. Thus, an *RHD*-negative female result is reported with a qualifying statement. If a critical maternal anti-D titer of 32 or more is present and the cell free DNA result returns *RHD* negative, female, or *indeterminate*, the fetal *RHD* status should be determined by amniocentesis or, alternatively, surveillance with serial MCA-PSV Dopplers can be undertaken. In general, as most patients wish to avoid invasive testing, starting with MCA-PSV would be the next best step.

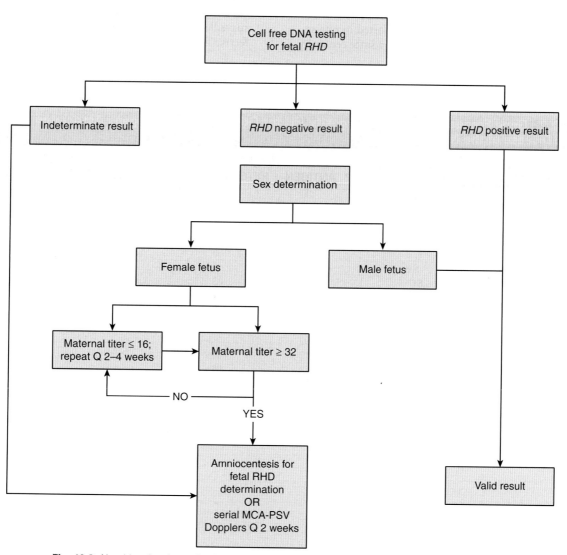

Fig. 40.2 Algorithm for determination of the fetal RHD status using circulating cell free fetal DNA.

9. Answer: a

(see *Gabbe's Obstetrics* 8e: ch40)

Cordocentesis allows direct access to the fetal circulation to obtain important laboratory values such as fetal blood type, hematocrit, direct Coombs test, reticulocyte count, and total bilirubin. Although serial cordocentesis was once proposed as a primary method of fetal surveillance after a maternal critical titer is reached, it has been associated with a 1% to 2% rate of fetal loss and up to a 50% risk for FMH with subsequent worsening of the alloimmunization.[4] For these reasons, cordocentesis is reserved for patients with elevated peak systolic MCA Doppler velocities. Complications from intrauterine transfusion (IUT) are uncommon. Survival after IUT varies with the center, its experience, and the presence of hydrops fetalis. An overall survival rate of 97% has been reported in one series of over 900 procedures performed at a since center in the Netherlands.

10. Answer: a

(see *Gabbe's Obstetrics* 8e: ch40)

The majority of cases of K1 sensitization are secondary to previous maternal blood transfusion, usually as a result of postpartum hemorrhage in a previous pregnancy. Because 92% of individuals are Kell negative, the initial management of the K1-sensitized pregnancy should entail paternal red-cell typing and genotype testing. If the paternal typing returns K1-negative (kk) and paternity is assured, no further maternal testing is undertaken. The majority of Kell-positive individuals will be heterozygous (Table 40.2). Amniocentesis can be used to determine the fetal genotype in these cases because ccffDNA for fetal Kell typing is currently only available in Europe. A lower maternal critical antibody value of 8 has been proposed to begin fetal surveillance. Serial MCA Doppler studies have proven effective in detecting fetal anemia.

TABLE 40.2 Gene Frequencies (%) and Zygosity (%) for Other Red Cell Antigens Associated With Hemolytic Disease of the Neonate.

	WHITE		BLACK		HISPANIC	
	ANTIGEN +	HETEROZYGOUS	ANTIGEN +	HETEROZYGOUS	ANTIGEN +	HETEROZYGOUS
C	70	50	30	32	81	51
c	80	50	96	32	76	51
E	32	29	23	21	41	36
e	97	29	98	21	95	36
K (K1)	9	97.8	2	100		
k (K2)	99.8	8.8	100	2		
M	78	64	70	63		
N	77	65	74	60		
S	55	80	31	90		
s	89	50	97	29		
U	100	—	99	—		
Fy^a	66	26	10	90		
Fy^b	83	41	23	96		
Jk^a	77	36	91	63		
Jk^b	72	32	43	21		

Modified from Moise KJ. Hemolytic disease of the fetus and newborn. In Creasy RK, Resnik R, Iams J, eds. *Maternal-Fetal Medicine: Principles and Practice.* 5th ed. Philadelphia: Elsevier; 2004.

CHAPTER 40

REFERENCES

1. Martin JA, Hamilton BE, Sutton PD, Ventura SJ, Menacker F, Munson ML. Births: final data for 2002. National vital statistics reports: from the Centers for Disease Control and Prevention, National Center for Health Statistics, National Vital Statistics System. *Natl Vital Stat Rep.* 2003;52(10):1-113.

2. Zipursky A, Paul VK. The global burden of Rh disease. *Arch Dis Child Fetal Neonatal Ed.* 2011;96(2):F84-F85.

3. Pirelli KJ, Pietz BC, Johnson ST, Pinder HL, Bellissimo DB. Molecular determination of RHD zygosity: predicting risk of hemolytic disease of the fetus and newborn related to anti-D. *Prenat Diagn.* 2010;30(12–13):1207–1212.

4. Weiner CP, Williamson RA, Wenstrom KD, et al. Management of fetal hemolytic disease by cordocentesis. II. Outcome of treatment. *Am J Obstet Gynecol.* 1991;165(5 Pt 1):1302-1307.

41

Maternal Mortality: A Global Perspective

Audrey Merriam

(See *Gabbe's Obstetrics: Normal and Problem Pregnancies*, 8e: ch41)

QUESTIONS

1. What is the leading cause of death among adolescent girls in developing countries?

a. Accidents

b. Suicide

c. Infections

d. Pregnancy complications

e. Diarrheal illnesses

2. A 22-year-old comes in for a routine visit at 15 weeks gestation. She has just finished college and has plans to start a physics PhD program in August. She says she cannot have a child right now and she and the father are not together currently. She is asking about pregnancy termination, but she is concerned about her risk of death from the procedure because a person on the way in told her that she has a 1 in 100 chance of death from the procedure. What do you tell her?

a. There are fewer than 60 deaths annually in Europe and North America combined, so the risk of mortality is exceedingly low.

b. The risk of mortality is actually closer to 1 in 1000, so it is still very safe.

c. About one-third of all abortion-related maternal mortality occurs in the US.

d. The information she heard on the way in is correct and the risk of mortality from abortion in the US is approximately 1 in 100.

e. Because only 40% of women have access to safe abortion, the risk of death from abortion is actually closer to 1 in 60.

3. You are preparing for a medical mission trip to a rural area of Tanzania. You remember from your last trip that postpartum hemorrhage (PPH) is a major risk to women undergoing childbirth there. What medication do you chose to bring as a primary means to control PPH?

a. Tranexamic acid

b. Carboprost

c. Misoprostol

d. Methylergonivine

e. Pitocin

4. You are traveling to Uganda to a medical center that cares for a large population of women who typically deliver at home unless there are complications. Your supervising physician has told you that many women present after having a seizure at home in the peripartum period. She wants you to develop a protocol to help decrease the number of women presenting with eclampsia. What is the most important part of your algorithm?

a. Getting drug companies to donate magnesium sulfate to be administered as seizure prophylaxis

b. Education materials for home birth attendants about the signs and symptoms of preeclampsia

c. Ask your hospital to donate oral immediate-release nifedipine that you can distribute to the home birth attendants

d. Ask a medical supply company to donate home blood pressure (BP) cuffs so women can monitor their BP themselves since home birth attendants cannot monitor BP

e. Go to the local drug store and buy as much aspirin as you can to decrease the risk of preeclampsia in this population

5. The rising maternal mortality in the US has been a keen interest of yours, and you are planning to organize a lobby day at your state capital to ask your state legislature to fund a maternal mortality review committee and resources to institute the committee's recommendations. Which of the following facts *does not* support your argument?

   a. The US is one of the few developed countries where maternal mortality has been increasing in recent years.

   b. Indicators of severe maternal morbidity are increasing.

   c. There are indications that most deaths are preventable, and evaluation of these deaths would provide valuable information.

   d. Emphasis on patient safety and quality improvement improves maternal outcomes.

   e. Many of the errors leading to maternal deaths are individual physician mistakes, and studying them would help to identify bad physicians.

6. A 22-year-old female presents to you for her annual gynecological examination. Her body mass index is 53 kg/m^2 and her BP in your office is 142/86. She tells you that she is healthy and is just here for her Pap smear because her primary care doctor would not do it. She is engaged and getting married in the next 6 months. Upon review of her medical record, you see that her primary care physician has recently diagnosed her with type 2 diabetes and she has a history of asthma requiring hospitalization and intravenous (IV) steroid administration. Her only medication listed is albuterol. You enquire about this history and she says she does not believe it and is not taking medication or changing her diet or exercising. You then ask her about her childbearing plans and she states she does want children soon. What do you tell her?

   a. Over a quarter of maternal deaths are due to causes not directly related to obstetric conditions, and optimizing her health prior to conception could save her life.

   b. You are trying to help her primary care doctor by also counseling her on her medical issues.

   c. It is difficult to do examinations on morbidly obese women and you prefer she lose weight.

   d. You are just trying to figure out why she lied to you and said she was healthy.

   e. You are trying to determine when you will have to do her cesarean section because you will need the bariatric equipment.

7. While you are working in a clinic in Uganda, a 14-year-old G1P0 presents in labor. She is accompanied by a birth attendant. They have walked from home because she has been 9–10 cm dilated at 0 station for the past 10 hours. As per the birth attendant, there is no fetal heart rate. You confirm the lack of fetal heart rate by an ultrasound. You perform your own examination and see that she also has a type III female genital mutilation (FGM) and you agree with the labor examination performed by the birth attendant. You initiate misoprostol and are able to deliver the fetus vaginally and the young woman returns home the following day. Long-term, what risk are you most worried about to the mother?

   a. Pelvic organ prolapse

   b. Infertility

   c. Fistula formation

   d. Fecal incontinence

   e. Preterm birth in a subsequent pregnancy

8. You are in a remote prenatal clinic in India. An 18-year-old G1P1001 who is postpartum day 1 presents after delivering at home. Through a translator, you learn that her mother delivered her child because the closest hospital is 5 hours away and she was in labor for 48 hours. She looks very unwell and can barely answer your questions. She has not been able to eat or drink since delivery and she tells you her abdomen is very sore. You are able to obtain vital signs and her temperature is 103°F (39.5C), pulse is 120 bpm, respiration rate is 20, and BP is 88/50. What two interventions were most likely to avoid this outcome?

   a. Delivery in a hospital and delivery by a physician

   b. Delivery in a hospital and delivery by a midwife

   c. Hot water and a safe birth kit

   d. Safe birth kit and delivery by a skilled birth attendant

   e. Safe birth kit and oral antibiotics

9. You are on a medical mission in an obstetrics clinic in Kenya. Your next patient is a 21-year-old G1P0 at 38 weeks gestation. She presents with fevers, abdominal pain, nausea, and vomiting and is feeling generally unwell. She tells you that this feels like when she had malaria 5 years ago. You detect fetal heart tones at 155 on auscultation. Which of the following *is not* a risk to the current pregnancy with an active malarial infection?

   a. Fetal ventriculomegaly

   b. Stillbirth

   c. Low birth weight

   d. Maternal anemia

   e. Preterm delivery

10. You are on a medical mission trip in India and are rounding on the postpartum ward. You are seeing a 23-year-old woman who has just had her third cesarean delivery in 4 years. She is uncertain about starting on contraception because she has never used it before. You have combined oral contraceptive pills, levonorgestrel-releasing intrauterine devices (IUDs), and etonogestrel implants with you and discuss their risks and benefits. In addition to discussing health benefits of contraception and pregnancy spacing, what else do you tell her about the benefits of contraception?

    a. Mirena IUD insertion is painless and you can do it before she goes home.

    b. Combined oral contraceptive pills can be started immediately postpartum.

    c. The Nexplanon will stop her periods and she will feel better without them.

    d. She should just have her tubes tied while she is at the hospital.

    e. Access to contraception reduces maternal, newborn, and child morbidity and mortality and results in improvements in women's earnings and children's education.

11. You have been asked to give a presentation on the high cesarean delivery rate in your state, with strategies to decrease the rate. Your state's cesarean delivery rate is 33%, down from a max of 38% 5 years prior. After the presentation, one of the state public health administrators that attended the presentation says, "I am glad our state's cesarean delivery rate is decreasing, but we should aim to make it 5% to decrease maternal morbidity related to cesarean deliveries!" What is your response?

    a. "That is a great idea! We will work on it!"

    b. "That will take years to do! There is no way to do it!"

    c. "While I appreciate your enthusiasm and agree the cesarean delivery rate still has room for improvement, a World Health Organization (WHO) study has shown a cesarean delivery rate of 10% is the minimum standard for safe motherhood services."

    d. "We probably can't get to 5%, but maybe we can get to 8%."

    e. "You must be joking?!"

12. You are asked to be a part of your hospital team tasked with designing and building a birth health center in Guatemala. Your health-care system has a long-standing relationship with physicians and midwives in that country through an education program they started years ago. The team is excited about the level of fundraising they accomplished to help build a labor and delivery area to hopefully decrease maternal mortality in the country. The team would like to build the hospital in Guatemala City because it will be easiest and cheapest to build there. What is one concern you have about this endeavor, based on the plans you have heard?

    a. There will not be any trained staff to deliver babies.

    b. Many women in Guatemala City already deliver in health-care facilities and you are afraid this facility will not be situated in a rural area of the country where maternal morbidity and mortality is highest.

    c. You think that the infection rates are higher when delivering in hospitals, so more women should be delivering at home to decrease morbidity and mortality from infection.

    d. You are worried about narcotics being stolen from the facility and sold on the street.

    e. You are worried your residents will want to go train there and you won't be able to cover services at your current hospital.

13. You are asking for supplies and medications to take with you on a mission trip to Bangladesh. You have asked drug companies for medications, and they offer IV antibiotics and some old dressings. You know that on the trip, you will be primarily working in clinics caring for reproductive-aged women and you are interested in making a long-term impact on the region. What class of medication could be useful to improve the physical and social well-being of women and children overtime?

    a. Contraceptives

    b. PPH medications

    c. Highly active antiretroviral therapy (HAART)

    d. Chemotherapeutics

    e. Prenatal vitamins

14. The "three delays" model refers to what?

    a. Power, passenger, and pelvis

    b. Patient, health-care provider, and health-care systems

    c. Physicians, nurses, and midwives

    d. Transportation, medical records, and patients

    e. Maternal age, maternal comorbidities, and maternal medications

ANSWERS

1. Answer: d

(see *Gabbe's Obstetrics* 8e: ch41)

Maternal death is now the leading cause of mortality for young girls in developing countries. Compared with mothers aged 20 to 24 years, girls between 10 and 19 years have higher risks of obstructed labor, eclampsia, puerperal sepsis, systemic infection, and preterm delivery and their babies also fare worse.

2. Answer: a

(see *Gabbe's Obstetrics* 8e: ch41)

About two-thirds of abortion-related deaths occur in sub-Saharan Africa and one-third in Asia. In high-resource regions of the world offering safe and legal services, deaths are extremely rare, with fewer than 60 deaths in total in Europe and North America combined.

3. Answer: c

(see *Gabbe's Obstetrics* 8e: ch41)

Misoprostol, a synthetic prostaglandin E1 analogue, has been listed by the WHO as an essential medicine for its key role in the management of miscarriage and prevention of PPH. Unlike oxytocin, it is low cost, stable at high temperatures, not degraded by ultraviolet light, and can be used orally or rectally, which makes it particularly useful in areas where skilled health-care providers and resources are less available. Although tranexamic acid shows promise for treatment of hemorrhage, its cost and method of administration are somewhat prohibitive to its use in developing countries.

4. Answer: b

(see *Gabbe's Obstetrics* 8e: ch41)

Training health-care and community workers about the signs and symptoms of preeclampsia has shown a reasonable ability to identify women at increased risk of adverse maternal outcomes associated with hypertensive disorders and has been shown to be effective in reducing the associated case fatality rate.

5. Answer: e

(see *Gabbe's Obstetrics* 8e: ch41)

The US is one of the few countries whose maternal mortality rate has increased in recent years. Indicators of severe pregnancy complications that place women at risk are increasing. There is a critical need for better data to provide a more accurate accounting and a more nuanced explanation for causes and trends. Patient safety research demonstrates that placing an emphasis on continuous quality improvement, and implementing consistent protocols for diagnosis and management is critical to improving patient outcomes. Effective maternal mortality committees are not punitive toward individual physicians.

6. Answer: a

(see *Gabbe's Obstetrics* 8e: ch41)

An estimated 73% of maternal deaths are due to direct obstetric causes (i.e., due only to the mother being pregnant). The remaining 27% are due to preexisting medical or psychiatric conditions aggravated or exacerbated by the pregnant state and are defined as indirect deaths. These causes are now being bolstered by conditions adversely affected by poorer lifestyles, such as acquired cardiac disease, hypertension, type 2 diabetes, liver disease, alcohol and drug dependency, and other disorders associated with obesity.

7. Answer: c

(see *Gabbe's Obstetrics* 8e: ch41)

In low-resourced countries, over 95% of fistulas are associated with childbirth. They are most common in young girls with poorly developed pelvises and are a direct result of prolonged obstructed labor where the pressure of the impacted fetus leads to destruction of the vesicovaginal/rectovaginal septum. Type III FGM involves narrowing the vaginal orifice, creating a covering seal by incising and appositioning the labia minora and/or the labia majora, which increases the risk of obstructed labor and fistula formation.

8. Answer: d

(see *Gabbe's Obstetrics* 8e: ch41)

The WHO guidelines on "the five cleans" needed during delivery (clean delivery surface + clean hands + clean cord cut + clean cord tie + clean cord stump) have led to the introduction of clean birth kits that contain soap, plastic sheeting, gloves, sterile gauze, a razor, and cord ties for use at home births, and these kits have reduced infectious morbidity and mortality in mothers and infants. The best practices to decrease infectious complications at delivery in developing countries are safe birth kits and delivery by skilled birth attendants.

9. Answer: a

(see *Gabbe's Obstetrics* 8e: ch41)

Women with malarial infection during pregnancy are at risk for severe maternal anemia, infants with low birth weight, stillbirth, and preterm delivery. These risks also appear to be more common in primigravidas. Malarial infection does not cause fetal neurologic sequelae.

10. Answer: e

(see *Gabbe's Obstetrics* 8e: ch41)

Access to contraception improves health outcomes (reduced maternal and neonatal/childhood morbidity and mortality) and has positive economic effects, including improved earnings for women, improved childhood education, and enhanced economic growth nationally.

11. Answer: c

(see *Gabbe's Obstetrics* 8e: ch41)

A recent WHO study cited that cesarean delivery rates lower than 10%–15% lead to increased maternal morbidity and mortality. Conversely, elevated cesarean delivery rates also lead to increased maternal morbidity and mortality with, about 6.2 million unnecessary operations performed in higher income countries worldwide.

12. Answer: b

(see *Gabbe's Obstetrics* 8e: ch41)

Most maternal deaths occur in rural areas, as these women lack transport to and access to skilled health care providers and facilities, so building a new hospital in an area where transportation is more readily available may not improve outcomes, as access will still be an issue for many women in the country.

13. Answer: a

(see *Gabbe's Obstetrics* 8e: ch41)

If women's contraceptive needs were met, the number of maternal deaths would fall by two-thirds and newborn deaths by more than three-quarters. The transmission of HIV from mothers to newborns would also be virtually eliminated. Meeting the unmet need for contraception could prevent an additional 104,000 deaths per year, thus preventing a further 29% of maternal mortality.

14. Answer: b

(see *Gabbe's Obstetrics* 8e: ch41)

The "three delay" model refers to problems that can arise at the client, health-care provider, and health systems level that can impact the quality and timeliness of care a patient receives. This model is ideal for examining systems errors, maternal morbidity/mortality, near misses, and sentinel safety events.

42

Heart Disease in Pregnancy

Thaddeus P. Waters

(See *Gabbe's Obstetrics: Normal and Problem Pregnancies*, 8e: ch42)

QUESTIONS

1. Which of the following is most accurate regarding maternal mean arterial pressure (MAP)?
   a. MAP falls sharply in the first trimester, reaching a nadir by midpregnancy.
   b. MAP is constant through all trimesters of pregnancy.
   c. MAP is stable throughout pregnancy, with a routine increase in the third trimester.
   d. MAP in pregnancy is significantly lower in all trimesters when compared to the nonpregnant state.

2. All of the following are normal maternal hemodynamic responses during labor except:
   a. Maternal tachycardia
   b. Redistribution of 400–500 mL of blood from the uterus to the central circulation with each contraction
   c. Increase in cardiac output
   d. Decrease in blood pressure (BP)

3. Which of the following maternal cardiac conditions does not benefit from a reduction in vascular resistance?
   a. Cardiomyopathy
   b. Aortic regurgitation
   c. Intracardiac shunt
   d. Mitral regurgitation

4. A 20-year-old G1P0 presents for initial prenatal care at 8 weeks of gestation. She is concerned, as a family member recently had a myocardial infarction (MI). All of the following are indications for a screening echocardiogram in pregnancy except:
   a. Patient has a personal history of cardiac disease
   b. Cardiopulmonary symptoms in excess of what is anticipated as part of normal pregnancy
   c. Clinical evidence of cardiopulmonary failure
   d. A midsystolic grade 2 cardiac murmur

5. A 24-year-old woman with a history of a repaired tetralogy of Fallot presents for preconception counseling. All of the following are appropriate in this situation except:
   a. A fetal echocardiogram in the second trimester
   b. Discouraging pregnancy if the patient reports ordinary physical activity results in shortness of breath.
   c. A screening echocardiogram
   d. A baseline B-type natriuretic peptide (BNP)

6. A 31-year-old G2P1001 is at 34 weeks, with a history of unrepaired aortic stenosis. She is asymptomatic at this time. Which of the following is most appropriate with regard to her intrapartum/postpartum plan of care?
   a. Postpartum hemodynamic monitoring for 24–48 hours
   b. Cesarean delivery
   c. Antibiotic prophylaxis for endocarditis intrapartum
   d. No regional anesthesia

7. A 25-year-old nulligravida presents for preconception counseling. She has a history of a corrected ventriculoseptal defect in childhood. She reports that she did not need follow-up with cardiology. She is New York Heart Associate (NYHA) class 1 on your review of symptoms. Which of the following is incorrect regarding her future pregnancy?
   a. She is considered to have a major risk in pregnancy, due to suspected severe left outflow obstruction from her surgical correction.
   b. Men and women with congenital heart disease are at increased risk for having children with congenital heart disease.
   c. The risk of congenital heart disease with a future pregnancy is estimated at 3%.
   d. Specific parental congenital heart defects are not generally associated with the same defect in the child.

8. A 21-year-old G2P0010 at 5 weeks gestation presents for her initial obstetric visit. Her medical history is significant for an elective termination and Marfan syndrome. She is NYHA class 1. Which of the following situations is most correct for this patient?

 a. An aortic root diameter of 45 mm would require prophylactic aortic graft and valve replacement in the first trimester.

 b. Her fetus is not at risk for Marfan syndrome because it is an autosomal recessive genetic disorder.

 c. Vaginal delivery is considered safe if the aortic root diameter is 45 mm.

 d. Pregnancy is contraindicated if the aortic root diameter is greater than 45 mm.

9. You are called to the emergency room to evaluate a 41-year-old G3P0020 who has had no prenatal care. She has a fundal height of 32 cm. She is complaining of shortness of breath, chest pain, and hemoptysis. She reports a history of a heart problem, with a hole in her heart, asthma, and hypertension. Her BP is 165/105, heart rate (HR) is 105, respiratory rate is 28, and oxygen saturation is 82%. Fetal heart rate is category II. She is receiving O_2 supplementation, with minimal improvement in her O_2 saturation. She received labetalol 20 mg IV, with improvement in her BP to 145/85. STAT laboratory tests are pending. An electrocardiogram (EKG) demonstrates frequent premature atrial contractions. A bedside maternal echocardiogram being performed by the cardiology fellow demonstrates a large Ventricular Septal Defect (VSD) and increased pulmonary artery pressure. Which of the following is the most appropriate next step in management?

 a. Magnesium sulfate for seizure prophylaxis due to preeclampsia with severe features

 b. Immediate anticoagulation due to high likelihood of a pulmonary embolism

 c. Immediate transfer to intensive care unit (ICU) for stabilization of the mother prior to determining delivery timing

 d. Immediate cesarean delivery to improve maternal outcomes

10. A patient presents to the emergency room 5 weeks postpartum complaining of new-onset dyspnea and orthopnea. She had an uncomplicated vaginal delivery 5 weeks ago and developed these symptoms within the last week. Her vital signs are significant for tachypnea and an O_2 saturation of 92% on room air. Her chest X-ray demonstrates vascular congestion bilaterally and an enlarged cardiac silhouette. Her labs demonstrated an Hgb of 9.5 g/dL, platelets 155 k/uL, normal comprehensive metabolic panel, negative troponins, blood and protein on her urinalysis, and an elevated BNP. Which of the following is incorrect?

 a. She has pulmonary edema from atypical preeclampsia.

 b. Her medical management can include an angiotensin-converting enzyme (ACE) inhibitor, digoxin, β-blocker, and a diuretic.

 c. She needs an immediate echocardiogram and EKG with transfer to a cardiac ICU.

 d. Her mortality rate can be 50%.

11. A 45-year-old nulligravida presents to you for in vitro fertilization (IVF) clearance. She has a history of diabetes, hypertension, and previous MI. Her diabetes is currently well controlled on insulin. Her hypertension has been well controlled with labetalol. Her MI was 4 years ago and required an angioplasty and stenting of the left coronary artery. She is taking aspirin daily. Which of the following is the *most* correct statement?

 a. Coronary angioplasty and stenting during pregnancy should not be withheld when appropriate for the mother's condition.

 b. If she experiences another MI during a viable point in her pregnancy, delivery would be recommended within 2 weeks of the event to improve maternal outcomes.

 c. She should stop her aspirin while undergoing IVF and then restart at 12–14 weeks to decrease her risk of preeclampsia.

 d. A maternal echocardiogram would be recommended to diagnose a cardiac event in pregnancy because elevated creatine kinase myocardial band (CK-MB) and EKG abnormalities (such as ST-segment elevations) can be seen during the third trimester of pregnancy.

12. A 32-year-old G3P2002 at 10 weeks gestation presents to your hospital with complaints of nausea/vomiting and occasionally feeling short of breath with regular activity. She recently immigrated to this country and has not yet established prenatal care. She is normotensive and slightly tachycardic. Her physical examination is unremarkable except for auscultation of a cardiac murmur. An EKG demonstrates normal sinus rhythm. A maternal echocardiogram demonstrates normal ejection fraction, a small patent ductus arteriosus, and otherwise normal cardiac measurements and pressure readings. After further evaluation, you determine that she has a NYHA class I–II functional status. Which of the following correctly classifies her World Health Organization (WHO) maternal cardiovascular risk?

a. WHO I

b. WHO II

c. WHO III

d. WHO IV

ANSWERS

1. **Answer: a**

(see *Gabbe's Obstetrics* 8e: ch42)

Mean arterial pressure (MAP) falls sharply in the first trimester, reaching a nadir by midpregnancy. Thereafter, BP increases slowly, reaching near nonpregnant levels by term. Cardiac output (CO) rises throughout the first and second trimesters, reaching a maximum by the middle of the third trimester. In the supine position, a pregnant woman in the third trimester may experience significant hypotension due to venocaval occlusion by the gravid uterus. In normal pregnancy, venocaval occlusion may produce symptoms such as diaphoresis, tachycardia, or nausea, but will rarely result in significant complications.

2. **Answer: d**

(see *Gabbe's Obstetrics* 8e: ch42)

Labor, delivery, and the postpartum period are times of acute hemodynamic changes. Tachycardia is a normal response. Significant catecholamine release increases afterload. Each uterine contraction acutely redistributes 400 to 500 mL of blood from the uterus to the central circulation. Robson and colleagues describe the hemodynamic changes associated with unmedicated labor. HR, BP, and CO all increase with uterine contractions, with the magnitude of the change increasing as labor advances.

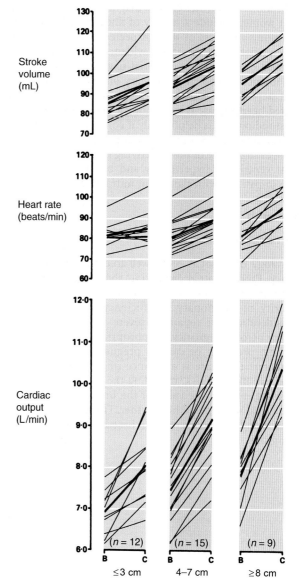

Fig. 42.1 Changes in hemodynamic parameters at three different points during labor (≤3 cm, 4–7 cm, and ≥8 cm). Each line represents the change in an individual subject. *B*, Before contraction; *C*, during contraction. (From Robson S, Dunlop W, Boys R, Hunter S. Cardiac output during labour. *BMJ.* 1987;295:1169.)

3. Answer: c

(see *Gabbe's Obstetrics* 8e: ch42)

Reduction in vascular resistance may be beneficial to some patients; afterload reduction reduces cardiac work. Cardiomyopathy, aortic regurgitation, and mitral regurgitation all benefit from reduced afterload. Alternatively, patients with intracardiac shunts, in which right and left ventricular pressures are nearly equal when not pregnant, may reverse their shunt during pregnancy and desaturate because of right to left shunting from a decrease in vascular resistance.

4. Answer: d

(see *Gabbe's Obstetrics* 8e: ch42)

Indications for further cardiac diagnostic testing in pregnant women include a history of known cardiac disease, symptoms in excess of those expected in a normal pregnancy, a pathologic murmur, evidence of heart failure on physical examination, or arterial oxygen desaturation in the absence of known pulmonary disease. The preferred next step in the evaluation of pregnant women with suspected heart disease is transthoracic echocardiography. A chest radiograph is helpful only if congestive heart failure is suspected. An EKG may be nonspecific but could have changes suggestive of the underlying heart disease, such as right ventricular hypertrophy and biatrial enlargement, seen in patients with significant mitral stenosis.

5. Answer: b

(see *Gabbe's Obstetrics* 8e: ch42)

Tetralogy of Fallot is often well tolerated during pregnancy. Preconceptual evaluation should include assessment of right and left ventricular size and function, severity of pulmonary insufficiency or stenosis, with consideration for repair of severe pulmonary insufficiency before pregnancy, if appropriate. The decision to become pregnant or carry a pregnancy in the context of maternal disease is a balance of two forces: (1) the objective medical risk, including the uncertainty of that estimate, and (2) the value of the birth of a child to an individual woman and her partner. This patient is NYHA class II and of low overall risk based upon her reported symptoms.

6. Answer: a

(see *Gabbe's Obstetrics* 8e: ch42)

Given that most cases of aortic stenosis in young women are congenital in origin, fetal echocardiography is indicated. Although some controversy persists, cesarean delivery is generally reserved for obstetrical indications. Pain during labor and delivery can be safely managed with regional analgesia, using a low-dose bupivacaine and narcotic technique. Postpartum, patients should be monitored hemodynamically for 24 to 48 hours.

7. Answer: a

(see *Gabbe's Obstetrics* 8e: ch42)

Major cardiac risks in pregnancy include (1) cyanosis, (2) left (or systemic) ventricular dysfunction and poor functional status, (3) pulmonary hypertension and Eisenmenger syndrome, particularly with right ventricular dysfunction, and (4) severe left (or systemic) outflow tract obstruction. Her NYHA class I status is also of low risk for pregnancy complications.

8. Answer: d

(see *Gabbe's Obstetrics* 8e: ch42)

Marfan syndrome is an autosomal dominant genetic disorder caused by an abnormal gene for fibrillin on chromosome 15. Given the data available, a precise risk for death from aortic dissection or rupture cannot be quantified, although patients with a prior aortic dissection or an AD greater than 4.5 cm likely are at highest risk. Patients with aortic roots less than 4.0 cm can be delivered vaginally, reserving cesarean delivery for obstetrical indications.

9. Answer: c

(see *Gabbe's Obstetrics* 8e: ch42)

Acute treatment of cardiomyopathy is directed at improving cardiac function and, when present, treating the inciting event. Patients usually present with signs and symptoms of pulmonary edema: dyspnea, cough, orthopnea, tachycardia, and occasionally, hemoptysis. These symptoms of pulmonary edema, although characteristic of heart failure, may also be due to previously undiagnosed congenital or rheumatic heart disease, preeclampsia, embolic disease, intrinsic pulmonary disease, tocolytic use, or sepsis.

10. Answer: a

(see *Gabbe's Obstetrics* 8e: ch42)

Peripartum cardiomyopathy (PPCM) is a rare syndrome of heart failure presenting in late pregnancy or postpartum. The diagnosis is made after excluding other causes of pulmonary edema and heart failure (Box 42.1). Acute treatment of cardiomyopathy is directed at improving cardiac function and, when present, treating the inciting event. Diuretics are used to decrease preload and relieve pulmonary congestion. Digoxin may improve myocardial contractility and facilitate rate control when atrial fibrillation is present. Afterload reduction is achieved with ACE inhibitors postpartum or hydralazine before delivery. β-Blockade in stable, euvolemic patients has been clearly demonstrated to improve cardiac function and survival outside of pregnancy. The mortality rate for PPCM is reported to be 25% to 50%.

BOX 42.1 Diagnostic Criteria for Peripartum Cardiomyopathy

1. Heart failure within the last month of pregnancy or 5 months postpartum
2. Absence of prior heart disease
3. No determinable cause
4. Echocardiographic indication of left ventricular dysfunction
   - Ejection fraction of <45% or fractional shortening of <30%
   - Left ventricular end-diastolic dimension of >2.7 cm/m^2

---

11. Answer: a

(see *Gabbe's Obstetrics* 8e: ch42)

The diagnosis of MI in pregnancy is often delayed because of the rarity of the event and common symptoms of pregnancy. ST-segment elevation is not a normal finding and, in the context of ongoing chest pain, should markedly increase the suspicion of acute MI. While the MB fraction of creatinine kinase isoenzymes may be elevated at delivery, troponin I levels are not. If confusion regarding the appropriate diagnosis exists in the context of a constellation of findings suggestive of MI, an echocardiogram can be used to confirm abnormal ventricular wall motion in the ischemic region. Acute therapy is based on rapid coronary reperfusion. Coronary angioplasty and stenting have been reported in pregnancy and should not be withheld when appropriate for the mother's condition.

12. Answer: a

(see *Gabbe's Obstetrics* 8e: ch42)

The modified WHO classification uses four categories determined largely by diagnosis: Class I—uncomplicated, mild pulmonary stenosis; Class II—unoperated atrial septal defect (ASD) or VSD and repaired tetralogy of Fallot; Class III—mechanical valves, systemic right ventricle, Fontan circulation, unrepaired cyanotic heart disease, and other complex congenital heart disease, Marfan syndrome with an aorta 40–45 mm in width, bicuspid aortic valve with aorta 45–50 mm; and Class IV—pulmonary hypertension/Eisenmenger syndrome, systemic ejection fraction <30%, systemic dysfunction NYHA class III–IV, severe mitral stenosis, severe symptomatic aortic stenosis, Marfan syndrome with aorta >45 mm, bicuspid valve with aorta >50 mm, native severe coarctation (Table 42.1, Box 42.2).

TABLE 42.1 Modified World Health Organization Classification of Maternal Cardiovascular Risk: Principles.

Risk Class	Risk of Pregnancy by Medical Condition
I	No detectable increased risk of maternal mortality and no/mild increase in morbidity
II	Small increased risk of maternal mortality or moderate increase in morbidity
III	Significantly increased risk of maternal mortality or severe morbidity. Expert counseling required. If pregnancy is decided upon, intensive specialist cardiac and obstetric monitoring needed throughout pregnancy, childbirth, and the puerperium.
IV	Extremely high risk of maternal mortality or severe morbidity; pregnancy contraindicated. If pregnancy occurs, termination should be discussed. If pregnancy continues, care as for class III.

Adapted from Thorne S, MacGregor A, Nelson-Piercy C. Risks of contraception and pregnancy in heart disease. *Heart*. 2006;92: 1520-1525.

BOX 42.2   Modified WHO Classification of Maternal Cardiovascular Risk: Application

Conditions in which pregnancy risk is WHO I
- Uncomplicated, small or mild
  - Pulmonary stenosis
  - Patent ductus arteriosus
  - Mitral valve prolapse
- Successfully repaired simple lesions (atrial or ventricular septal defect, patent ductus arteriosus, anomalous pulmonary venous drainage)
- Atrial or ventricular ectopic beats, isolated

Conditions in which pregnancy risk is WHO II or III

WHO II (if otherwise well and uncomplicated)
- Unoperated atrial or ventricular septal defect
- Repaired tetralogy of Fallot
- Most arrhythmias

WHO II–III (depending on individual)
- Mild left ventricular impairment
- Hypertrophic cardiomyopathy
- Native or tissue valvular heart disease not considered WHO I or IV
- Marfan syndrome without aortic dilation
- Aorta <45 mm in aortic disease associated with bicuspid aortic valve
- Repaired coarctation

WHO III
- Mechanical valve
- Systemic right ventricle
- Fontan circulation
- Cyanotic heart disease (unrepaired)
- Other complex congenital heart disease
- Aortic dilation 40–45 mm in Marfan syndrome
- Aortic dilation 45–50 mm in aortic disease associated with bicuspid aortic valve

Conditions in which pregnancy risk is WHO IV (pregnancy contraindicated)
- Pulmonary arterial hypertension of any cause
- Severe systemic ventricular dysfunction (LVEF <30%, NYHA III–IV)
- Previous peripartum cardiomyopathy with any residual impairment of left ventricular function
- Severe mitral stenosis, severe symptomatic aortic stenosis
- Marfan syndrome with aorta dilated >45 mm
- Aortic dilation >50 mm in aortic disease associated with bicuspid aortic valve
- Native severe coarctation

European Society of Gynecology (ESG); Association for European Paediatric Cardiology (AEPC); German Society for Gender Medicine (DGesGM), Regitz-Zagrosek V, Blomstrom Lundqvist C, Borghi C, Cifkova R, Ferreira R, Foidart JM, Gibbs JS, Gohlke-Baerwolf C, Gorenek B, Iung B, Kirby M, Maas AH, Morais J, Nihoyannopoulos P, Pieper PG, Presbitero P, Roos-Hesselink JW, Schaufelberger M, Seeland U, Torracca L; ESC Committee for Practice Guidelines. ESC Guidelines on the management of cardiovascular diseases during pregnancy: the Task Force on the Management of Cardiovascular Diseases during Pregnancy of the European Society of Cardiology (ESC).Eur Heart J. 2011 Dec;32(24):3147-97.
Adapted from Jastrow N, Meyer P, Khairy P, Mercier LA, Dore A, Marcotte F, Leduc L. Prediction of complications in pregnant women with cardiac diseases referred to a tertiary center, Int J Cardiol, 2010.

43

Respiratory Disease in Pregnancy

Alyssa Stephenson-Famy

(See *Gabbe's Obstetrics: Normal and Problem Pregnancies*, 8e: ch43)

QUESTIONS

1. What percentage of cases of community-acquired pneumonia (CAP) in pregnancy is due to viral infections?

   a. 5%–10%

   b. 10%–20%

   c. 30%–40%

   d. 60%–80%

2. A 30-year-old woman is intubated in the intensive care unit with acute bacterial pneumonia at 28 weeks gestation. She has a history of asthma with recent oral steroid use. She was diagnosed with bacteremia when she was admitted. What acute obstetrical complication is she most likely to develop?

   a. Preterm labor

   b. Preeclampsia

   c. Gestational diabetes

   d. Placental abruption

   e. Fetal macrosomia

3. A 23-year-old female presents at 34 weeks gestation with productive cough, dyspnea, chest pain, and fever. Examination shows decreased breath sounds and crackles in the right lower lung. What is the most appropriate initial test in her evaluation?

   a. Sputum culture

   b. Blood culture

   c. Chest X-ray

   d. Chest CT

   e. ventilation perfusion (VQ) scan

   f. Thoracentesis

4. A 26-year-old female at 20 weeks gestation presents with fever, chills, headache, and cough for the last 12 hours. She spent the last several days with her father, who had a confirmed diagnosis of influenza A after his visit. What is the most appropriate management of this patient?

   a. Influenza A vaccine

   b. Oseltamivir

   c. Azithromycin

   d. Ceftriaxone

   e. Supportive care

5. Which complication occurs more frequently with isoniazid (INH) therapy for tuberculosis during pregnancy?

   a. Renal insufficiency

   b. Bone loss

   c. Rash

   d. Transaminitis

   e. Peripheral neuropathy

6. An 18 year-old-female presents with wheezing and shortness of breath at 24 weeks gestation. She has a history of asthma, for which she is currently taking no medications. She describes feeling short of breath daily but is able to do most of her usual activities and has nighttime exacerbation at least once per week. Her peak flow is 70% of her predicted value. What is the classification of her asthma severity?

   a. Mild intermittent asthma

   b. Mild persistent asthma

   c. Moderate persistent asthma

   d. Severe persistent asthma

7. A 24-year-old with a history of mild intermittent asthma presents for a new obstetric visit at 8 weeks. She stopped taking all medications when she found out she was pregnant. What is the most appropriate prescription to provide her for treatment of her asthma?

   a. Short-acting β-agonist

   b. Long-acting β-agonist

   c. Inhaled corticosteroid

   d. Oral corticosteroid

   e. Leukotriene receptor antagonist

8. A 30-year-woman with asthma presents for labor induction at 41 weeks gestational age. At the time of admission, she is found to have gestational hypertension. Which medication should be strongly avoided during her delivery?

   a. Magnesium sulfate

   b. Labetalol

   c. Prostaglandin (E_2 or E_1)

   d. **Carboprost** (15-methyl PGF2α)

   e. Oxytocin

9. A 26-year-old woman at 30 weeks gestation is admitted with pyelonephritis and sepsis. She goes on to develop acute onset of hypoxic respiratory failure that is not responsive to oxygen therapy. Chest X-ray is most likely to demonstrate which findings:

   a. Perihilar interstitial infiltrates

   b. Bilateral diffuse infiltrates

   c. Upper lobe cavitation

   d. Lobar consolidation

   e. Pleural effusion

   f. Cardiomegaly

10. A 29-year-old woman with cystic fibrosis is considering pregnancy. She has been using mucolytic therapy and she had a forced expiratory volume in 1 second (FEV_1) of 60% of predicted 1 year ago. She has intermittent antibiotic requirement for *Pseudomonas* bronchiectasis. Her nutritional status has improved after starting to take pancreatic enzymes. She was recently hospitalized with respiratory failure and found to have pulmonary hypertension. Which clinical condition puts her at highest risk for mortality in a future pregnancy?

    a. Maternal age

    b. Diminished FEV_1

    c. Bronchiectasis

    d. Pancreatic deficiency

    e. Pulmonary hypertension

ANSWERS

1. **Answer: b**

   (See *Gabbe's Obstetrics* 8e: ch43)

   Pneumonia can be classified as either community acquired or hospital acquired, according to the Infectious Disease Society of America's guidelines.[1] CAP occurs in patients who have not been hospitalized recently and have not had regular exposure to the health-care system.[2] CAP is the most common form of pneumonia in pregnancy. CAP is most commonly caused by bacteria (60%–80% of cases); up to 20% may be associated with atypical bacteria (*Mycoplasma pneumoniae, Chlamydophila pneumoniae, Legionella pneumophila*). The remaining 10%–20% of cases are due to viral infections.

2. **Answer: a**

   (See *Gabbe's Obstetrics* 8e: ch43)

   Preterm labor and preterm delivery are significant complications of pneumonia and more likely in women with bacteremia, who required mechanical ventilation, or who had a serious underlying maternal disease. This may be due to the enhanced prostaglandin production and host inflammatory response due to infection.

3. Answer: c

(See *Gabbe's Obstetrics* 8e: ch43)

All pregnant patients with high suspicion of pneumonia should undergo a chest X-ray. The estimated fetal radiation after a chest radiography is less than 0.01 mGy and has not been associated with any short- or long-term complications. Radiographic findings consistent with bacterial pneumonia include lobar consolidation, cavitation, air bronchograms, and pleural effusion. Other testing, including blood/sputum cultures and thoracentesis, should be performed only if special circumstances are present (Table 43.1).

TABLE 43.1 Recommended Diagnostic Testing for Community-Acquired Pneumonia.

Indication	Blood Culture	Sputum Culture	Legionella UAT	Pneumococcus UAT	Other
Intensive care unit admission	X	X	X	X	a
Failure of outpatient antibiotic therapy		X	X	X	
Cavitary infiltrate	X	X			b
Leukopenia or Chronic severe liver disease	X			X	
Severe obstructive‚Äâ/‚Äâstructural lung disease		X			
Asplenia	X			X	
Pleural effusion	X	X	X	X	c

UAT, Urinary antigen test.
a, Endotracheal aspirate if intubated; b, fungal and tuberculosis cultures; c, thoracentesis and pleural fluid cultures.

4. Answer: b

(See *Gabbe's Obstetrics* 8e: ch43)

The Centers for Disease Control and Prevention estimate that influenza has infected between 9 million and 35 million people, caused 140,000 to 710,000 hospitalizations, and resulted in 12,000 to 56,000 deaths annually since 2010.[3] Once influenza infection is suspected in pregnant patients, within 48 hours of symptom onset, an antiviral medication should be started. Oseltamivir is preferred, but the alternative therapy, zanamivir, is also reasonable.

5. Answer: d

(See *Gabbe's Obstetrics* 8e: ch43)

The recommended prophylaxis is INH 300 mg/day, starting after the first trimester and continuing for 6–9 months.[4] INH should be accompanied by pyridoxine (vitamin B_6) supplementation, 50 mg/day, to prevent peripheral neuropathy associated with INH treatment. INH is associated with an increased risk of hepatitis when taken during pregnancy and postpartum. The absolute risk for liver inflammation in pregnancy from INH use is rare, and therefore, this therapy should be instituted when the risk for conversion to active disease is high.[5] Monthly monitoring of liver function tests may prevent this adverse outcome. Among individuals receiving INH, 10%–20% develop mildly elevated liver function tests. These changes resolve once the drug is discontinued.

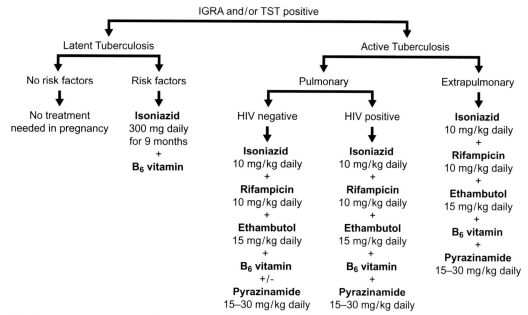

Fig. 43.1 Management of tuberculosis during pregnancy. Risk factor, recent exposure or immunocompromised. *IGRA*, Interferon-gamma release assay; *TST*, tuberculin skin testing.

6. Answer: c

(See *Gabbe's Obstetrics* 8e: ch43)

Asthma may be classified as *mild intermittent, mild persistent, moderate,* and *severe.*[6] The FEV_1 or peak expiratory flow rate (PEFR) values for moderate asthma are usually between 60% and 80% and below 60% in patients with severe asthma.[7] Table 43.2 summarizes the current classification of asthma. Moderate persistent asthma is defined as daily symptoms, nighttime exacerbation at >1 time/week, some interference in normal activities, and a FEV_1/peak flow of 60%–80% of predicted.

TABLE 43.2   Classification of Asthma Severity and Control in Pregnant Patients.

Asthma Control	Well Controlled	Not Well Controlled		Very Poorly Controlled
Asthma severity	*Mild intermittent*	*Mild persistent*	*Moderate persistent*	*Severe persistent*
Symptom frequency, albuterol use	≤2 days/week	>2 days/week but not daily	Daily symptoms	Throughout the day
Nighttime awakening	≤2 times/month	>2 times/month	>1 time/week	≥4 times/week
Interference with normal activity	None	Minor limitation	Some limitation	Extremely limited
FEV_1 or peak flow (% predicted/ personal best)	>80%	>80%	60%–80%	<60%

FEV_1, Forced expiratory volume in 1 second.
Modified from National Heart Lung and Blood Institute, National Asthma Education and Prevention Program Asthma and Pregnancy Working Group. NAEPP expert panel report. Managing asthma during pregnancy: recommendations for pharmacologic treatment—2004 update. *J Allergy Clin Immunol.* 2005;115(1):34–46.

7. Answer: a

(See *Gabbe's Obstetrics* 8e: ch43)

Mild asthma is characterized by a FEV_1 or peak expiratory flow rate (PEFR) above 80% of the personal/predicted best value. Mild asthma may be intermittent (two or fewer daily exacerbations per week or two or fewer nightly exacerbations per month) or persistent (if exacerbations are more frequent than the latter). Patients with mild intermittent asthma will not require maintenance medication and are treated with short-acting β_2-agonists (albuterol) as needed.

8. Answer: d

(See *Gabbe's Obstetrics* 8e: ch43)

Carboprost (15-methyl PGF2α) or hemabate should be avoided in asthmatics due to a risk of bronchospasm. β-Blockers could be a trigger for bronchospasm in theory but are not absolutely contraindicated. Prostaglandins are thought to be safe for cervical ripening or use for uterine atony.

9. Answer: b

(See *Gabbe's Obstetrics* 8e: ch43)

The acute respiratory distress syndrome (ARDS) is a form of noncardiogenic pulmonary edema secondary to an inflammatory response triggered by either pulmonary (e.g., pneumonia, aspiration, pulmonary contusions, smoke inhalation, massive transfusion) or nonpulmonary (sepsis, pancreatitis, burn injuries) insults. In either case, inflammatory mediators lead to diffuse endothelial and alveolar injury with "leakage" of proteins and fluid into the alveolar space. In its pure form, the left ventricular function is normal so that the development of pulmonary edema is not secondary to increased hydrostatic pressure. Bilateral diffuse infiltrates are classically seen with ARDS.

10. Answer: e

(See *Gabbe's Obstetrics* 8e: ch43)

Gravidae with poor nutritional status, pulmonary hypertension (cor pulmonale), and deteriorating pulmonary function early in gestation should consider therapeutic abortion because the risk for maternal mortality may be unacceptably high.

CHAPTER 43

REFERENCES

1. Mandell LA, Wunderink RG, Anzueto A, et al. Infectious Diseases Society of America/American Thoracic Society consensus guidelines on the management of community-acquired pneumonia in adults. *Clin Infect Dis.* 2007;44(Suppl 2):S27-S72.

2. Musher DM, Thorner AR. Community-acquired pneumonia. *N Engl J Med.* 2014;371(17):1619-1628.

3. Centers for Disease Control and Prevention. Disease burden of influenza | seasonal influenza (flu). Accessed February 1, 2020. https://www.cdc.gov/flu/about/disease/burden.htm.

4. Targeted tuberculin testing and treatment of latent tuberculosis infection. American Thoracic Society. *MMWR Recomm Rep.* 2000;49(RR-6):1–51.

5. Nahid P, Dorman SE, Alipanah N, et al. Official American Thoracic Society/Centers for Disease Control and Prevention/ Infectious Diseases Society of America Clinical Practice Guidelines: Treatment of drug-susceptible tuberculosis. *Clin Infect Dis.* 2016;63(7):e147-e195.

6. National Heart Lung and Blood Institute, National Asthma Education and Prevention Program Asthma and Pregnancy Working Group. NAEPP Expert Panel report. Managing asthma during pregnancy: recommendations for pharmacologic treatment—2004 update. *J Allergy Clin Immunol.* 2005;115(1):34-46.

7. National Asthma Education and Prevention Program. Expert Panel report 3: guidelines for the diagnosis and management of asthma—full report 2007. 2007. http://www.nhlbi.nih.gov/files/docs/guidelines/asthgdln.pdf.

44

Renal Disease in Pregnancy

Thaddeus P. Waters

(See *Gabbe's Obstetrics: Normal and Problem Pregnancies*, 8e: ch44)

QUESTIONS

1. All of the following are known maternal physiologic changes to the renal system in pregnancy except:

a. Enlargement of the kidneys

b. Dilatation of the ureters and renal pelvises

c. Increase in renal plasma flow by 50%

d. An increase in serum creatinine in the first trimester

2. A 20-year-old G1P0 presents at 10 weeks for prenatal care. She has no significant past medical history. As part of her initial prenatal laboratory tests, you recommended screening for asymptomatic bacteriuria (ASB). Which of the following is a correct statement regarding ASB in pregnancy?

a. Treatment of ASB may reduce the risk of adverse pregnancy outcomes.

b. The predominant organism identified is *Klebsiella*.

c. Empiric antibiotics are not indicated for women with symptoms of a urinary tract infection before results of a culture.

d. Culture results showing mixed gram-positive bacteria, regardless of bacteria species identified, do not warrant treatment.

3. A 19-year-old G1P0 at 35 weeks gestation presents to the labor and delivery unit with fevers, chills, and dysuria back pain. Her temperature is 101.5°F/38.61 C., her heart rate is 114, and her blood pressure is 87/51. Her evaluation is consistent with pyelonephritis. The fetal heart rate is 170 with minimal variability. All of the following are an appropriate part of her management except:

a. Initiating antibiotic coverage with a third-generation cephalosporin

b. Consultation with intensive care unit services

c. Initiation of intravenous fluid resuscitation

d. Cesarean delivery

4. A 38-year-old G4P2103 at 33 weeks presents with left back pain that radiates to her left groin. She denies symptoms, including fevers, chills, or obstetric complains such as contractions or leakage of fluid. Which of the following is the most appropriate test to order at this time?

a. Transvaginal ultrasound of the cervix

b. Renal ultrasound

c. Urinalysis with culture

d. Complete blood count

5. A 44-year-old G1P0 presents at 33 weeks gestation with headaches, visual changes, and new-onset hypertension (165/104). All of the following are consistent with concern for acute kidney renal injury (AKI) except:

a. Serum creatinine of 1.5 mg/dL

b. A protein/creatinine ratio of 1.2

c. Urine output of 0.3 mL/kg per hour

d. A doubling of the serum creatinine from the patient's baseline

6. A 17-year-old G1P0 has new-onset hypertension and proteinuria (400 mg in a 24-hour urine collection) at 36 weeks gestation. A renal biopsy obtained from this patient at this time would most likely show which of the following?

a. Glomerular endotheliosis

b. Hypertensive changes

c. Normal renal architecture

d. Mesangial immune complex deposits

7. A 41-year-old G5P3013 presents at 12 weeks for prenatal care. Her history is significant for chronic kidney disease (CKD) with hypertension. The patient is currently taking Hydrochlorothiazide (HCTZ), labetalol, and Procardia. Her blood pressure is 120/78 and her serum creatinine is 1.4 mg/dL. A baseline 24-hour urine collection is significant for 5700 mg of protein and her glomerular filtration rate (GFR) is 62 mL/min/1.73 m2. Which of the following is the correct staging of her CKD?

a. Stage 1

b. Stage 2

c. Stage 3

d. Stage 4

8. A 27-year-old G2P1001 presents for preconception counseling. The patient has a history of a renal transplant 2 years ago. Her blood pressure is 110/60, her serum creatinine is 1.4 mg/dL, and a 24-hour urine collection notes 121 mg of protein. She is currently taking mycophenolate mofetil. Which of the following is the most appropriate counseling for this patient?

a. The patient is a good candidate for attempting pregnancy at this time and should continue her immunosuppressive therapy.

b. Her serum creatinine is a relative contraindication to pregnancy.

c. The patient is a good candidate for attempting pregnancy but should discuss altering her immunosuppressive therapy prior to conception.

d. Pregnancy for this patient carries a risk of rejection of her transplant.

ANSWERS

1. **Answer: d**

(see *Gabbe's Obstetrics* 8e: ch44)

Pregnancy is associated with significant anatomic and functional changes in the kidney and its collecting system (Table 44.1). The kidneys enlarge due to increased renal vasculature and interstitial volume. The renal pelvises and ureters dilate by midgestation. Glomerular hyperfiltration in pregnancy results in reduced levels of serum creatinine and blood urea nitrogen.

2. **Answer: a**

(see *Gabbe's Obstetrics* 8e: ch44)

Screening for ASB is warranted because the risk of developing acute urinary tract infection or pyelonephritis is significantly increased in the setting of untreated bacteriuria during pregnancy. Cultures showing mixed gram-positive bacteria, lactobacilli, and *Staphylococcus* species (other than *S. saprophyticus*), may be presumed to be contaminated and therefore are not treated. *Escherichia coli* is the organism responsible for most cases of both ASB and acute urinary tract infection during pregnancy.

TABLE 44.1 **Summary of Renal Changes in Normal Pregnancy.**		
Alteration	**Manifestation**	**Clinical Relevance**
Increased renal size	Renal length is about 1 cm greater on radiographs	Postpartum decreases in size should not be mistaken for parenchymal loss.
Dilation of pelvises, calyces, and ureters	Dilation resembles hydronephrosis on ultrasound or IVP and is usually more prominent on the right side.	Should not be mistaken for obstructive uropathy. Upper urinary tract infections can be more virulent.
Changes in acid-base metabolism	The renal bicarbonate reabsorption threshold decreases.	Serum bicarbonate is 4 to 5 mM/L lower in pregnancy. PCO_2 is 10 mm Hg lower in normal pregnancy. PCO_2 of 40 mm Hg represents retention in pregnancy.
Renal water osmoregulation	The osmotic threshold for AVP release decreases.	Serum osmolarity is decreased by approximately 10 mOsm/L.

AVP, arganine vasopressin; *IVP*, intravenous pyelogram.
Modified from Lindheimer M, Grünfeld JP, Davison JM. Renal disorders. In: Barron WM, Lindheimer M, eds. *Medical Disorders During Pregnancy*, 3rd ed. St. Louis: Mosby; 2000:39-70.

3. Answer: d

(see *Gabbe's Obstetrics* 8e: ch44)

An intravenous antibiotic regimen with broad coverage for gram-negative and gram-positive organisms is recommended. A third-generation cephalosporin is favored over first- or second-generation cephalosporins, such as cefazolin, but the choice of antibiotic should be guided by local microbiology and susceptibility data as well as expected patient tolerance. Complications from w include acute kidney injury, pulmonary edema, acute respiratory distress syndrome, sepsis or septic shock, and spontaneous preterm birth. In this patient, management of her suspected urosepsis is recommended and is not an indication for delivery.

4. Answer: b

(see *Gabbe's Obstetrics* 8e: ch44)

Kidney stones (urolithiasis or nephrolithiasis) complicate 0.03%–0.4% of pregnancies, similar to the rate seen in nonpregnant women. In many cases, there is no prior history of kidney stones. In pregnancy, increased urinary excretion of lithogenic substances such as calcium, uric acid, and oxalate, as well as increased urinary stasis, may contribute to stone formation. Like the general population, calcium stones are most common. Renal ultrasound is recommended as the initial imaging modality when a kidney stone is suspected in pregnancy. Ultrasound detects 60%–88% of stones in the kidney or ureter, avoids radiation exposure, and is excellent for the evaluation of hydronephrosis and hydroureter.

5. Answer: b

(see *Gabbe's Obstetrics* 8e: ch44)

Increased levels of serum creatinine above the normal range (>1.1 mg/dL in most reference labs), or doubling of the serum creatinine concentration from baseline, has been used most often to define AKI in pregnancy. Oliguria is most commonly defined as <400–500 mL in 24 hours, or <0.5 mL/kg per hour, and its presence usually reflects more severe kidney impairment.

6. Answer: a

(see *Gabbe's Obstetrics* 8e: ch44)

Renal biopsies from women with preeclampsia have shown glomerular endotheliosis, a specific lesion characterized by glomerular endothelial swelling, loss of endothelial fenestrae, and occlusion of capillary lumens.

7. Answer: b

(see *Gabbe's Obstetrics* 8e: ch44)

CKD is commonly divided into stages by GFR. Stage 1 represents kidney damage but with normal GFR (≥ 90 mL/min per 1.73 m^2), while stages 2–5 are defined by progressively worsening GFR (mL/min per 1.73 m^2): stage 2, 60–89; stage 3, 30–59; stage 4, 15–29; and stage 5, <15. End-stage renal disease refers to advanced-stage CKD requiring dialysis or renal transplant.

8. Answer: c

(see *Gabbe's Obstetrics* 8e: ch44)

A Consensus Conference organized by the Women's Health Committee of the American Society of Transplantation concluded that pregnancy is usually safe after the first transplant year, provided that renal allograft function is stable (creatinine <1.5 mg/dL and no or minimal proteinuria) and that no rejection episodes have occurred in the year before conception. It is critical that renal transplant recipients continue their immunosuppressive therapy during pregnancy. Any discontinuation of treatment increases the risk for renal allograft rejection and pregnancy complications. Except for medications with major contraindications (e.g., mycophenolate mofetil and sirolimus), the risks of treatment are usually outweighed by the benefits, namely reduced renal allograft rejection.

45

Diabetes Mellitus Complicating Pregnancy

Audrey Merriam

(See *Gabbe's Obstetrics: Normal and Problem Pregnancies*, 8e: ch45)

QUESTIONS

1. Which of the following metabolic changes *does not* occur in early pregnancy?
   a. Decreased leptin
   b. Increased insulin clearance
   c. Decreased free fatty acids
   d. Increased fat stores
   e. Decreased hepatic glucose production

2. Which of the following transporters is the primary glucose transporter in the placenta and how is glucose transported across the placenta?
   a. GLUT4/simple diffusion
   b. GLUT4/facilitated diffusion
   c. GLUT1/simple diffusion
   d. GLUT1/facilitated diffusion
   e. GLUT1/active transport

3. Insulin sensitivity _____ over the course of pregnancy.
   a. Increases
   b. Decreases
   c. Stays the same
   d. Increases only in women without gestational diabetes
   e. Decreases only in women with gestational diabetes

4. Maternal triglycerides _____ throughout gestation and then _____ postpartum.
   a. Decrease/increase in breastfeeding women
   b. Decrease/increase in women who bottle feed
   c. Increase/decrease in breastfeeding women
   d. Do not change/decrease in women who bottle feed
   e. Do not change/increase in breastfeeding women

5. You are covering the labor and delivery unit when a 30-year-old white G1 presents at 34 weeks gestation with decreased fetal movement. Her pregnancy has been complicated by type 1 diabetes and her most recent hemoglobin A1c was 7.5%. She has no other significant medical or surgical history. The nurses cannot find the fetal heart rate (HR) with the monitor and ask you for an ultrasound. On your ultrasound, you confirm a fetal demise. What is the most likely etiology of the fetal demise?
   a. Chronic intrauterine hypoxia
   b. Previously undiagnosed congenital cardiac defect
   c. Previously undiagnosed myelomeningocele
   d. Fetal growth restriction
   e. Viral infection

6. A 23-year-old Hispanic G2P0010 presents at 12 weeks for her first prenatal visit and nuchal translucency scan. She has type 2 diabetes that she has not been taking any medication for. This is an unplanned pregnancy and she is worried about risks to her baby because her diabetes has not been under control. What is the greatest risk to the fetus that could potentially be seen on ultrasound today?
   a. Cardiac defect
   b. Anencephaly
   c. Macrosomia
   d. Clubbed feet
   e. Holoprosencephaly

7. You are seeing a 33-year-old G3P2002 at 37 weeks gestation. She had a growth ultrasound immediately prior to her visit, giving an estimated fetal weight of 4638 g. She has had two prior vaginal deliveries of infants weighing approximately 3800 g and 4000 g. Both pregnancies were prior to her diagnosis of type 2 diabetes. Her only other pregnancy complication is maternal obesity as she had a prepregnancy body mass index (BMI) of 49 kg/m^2, with a weight gain of 18kg in pregnancy. Her glucose control is suboptimal. Her fasting blood sugars are typically in the 100–110 mg/dL range and her postprandial blood sugars are usually 120–160mg/dL. Which of the following is not a risk factor for fetal macrosomia in this patient?

   a. Prepregnancy BMI

   b. Excessive weight gain in pregnancy

   c. Poor glucose control leading to fetal hyperinsulinemia

   d. Maternal weight gain in pregnancy, leading to increased free fatty acids

   e. Birth weights of her previous children

8. You are seeing a 36-year-old G1P1001 for a postpartum visit. She delivered at 38 weeks following induction of labor for poorly controlled A2 gestational diabetes. She tells you that her infant spent time in the neonatal intensive care unit (NICU) for "heart issues." You review her anatomy ultrasounds and growth ultrasounds and note that the heart appeared normal on ultrasound during those visits. He is currently out of the NICU and home with her. What is the most likely cardiac anomaly given this clinical scenario?

   a. Hypoplastic left heart syndrome

   b. Hypertrophic cardiomyopathy

   c. Tetralogy of Fallot

   d. Transposition of the great arteries

   e. Trucus arteriosus

9. A 34-year-old G1P0 comes to see you in consultation as she has recently been diagnosed with gestational diabetes. She is an internal medicine physician and is very concerned about all the potential neonatal complications of diabetes. She is committed to having excellent glucose control but has questions about other potential neonatal issues like calcium and magnesium derangements, hyperbilirubinemia, polycythemia, and respiratory distress syndrome. Which of these complications is most commonly seen despite tight glucose control during pregnancy and delivery?

   a. Hypocalcemia

   b. Hypomagnesemia

   c. Polycythemia

   d. Hyperbilirubinemia

   e. Respiratory distress syndrome

10. A 30-year-old nulliparous woman who has type 1 diabetes treated with an insulin pump comes for preconception counseling; she is trying to optimize her health prior to attempting conception. Her control currently is very good and a recent hemoglobin A1c is 7.2%; however, in college, she was less strict about her control and this resulted in the development of hypertension and renal disease. Her blood pressure (BP) in your office is 135/86 mm Hg and she was recently switched to Nifedipine 60 mg XL daily from her angiotensin-converting enzyme (ACE) inhibitor. You look at the other laboratory tests performed by her endocrinologist and see that her creatinine was 1.5 mg/dL and has been between 1.2 and 1.7 mg/dL over the past year. What is her White classification of diabetes in pregnancy and what is your greatest concern during pregnancy?

   a. Class D/congenital anomalies due to elevated hemoglobin A1c

   b. Class D/need for dialysis during pregnancy

   c. Class F/development of preeclampsia

   d. Class F/congenital anomalies due to elevated hemoglobin A1c

   e. Class F/need for dialysis during pregnancy

11. A 31-year-old G1P0 at 15 weeks with type 1 diabetes is undergoing an ophthalmologic examination. During the examination, the ophthalmologist diagnoses progressive retinopathy and she would normally perform laser photocoagulation for treatment. She is asking your advice about how to proceed. What do you tell her?

   a. She needs to terminate the pregnancy before proceeding.

   b. He should wait until 20–22 weeks gestation because that is the optimal time to perform surgery in pregnancy.

   c. It is safe to perform laser photocoagulation in pregnancy, but he should administer betamethasone for fetal lung maturity first.

   d. He should wait until 28 weeks gestation when fetal monitoring can be performed more easily during the procedure.

   e. It is safe to perform laser photocoagulation in pregnancy at this gestational age.

12. A 40-year-old G5P4004 presents for her first prenatal visit at 13 weeks gestation. Her BMI is 24 kg/m². Her last two pregnancies were complicated by gestational diabetes. She denies a history of hypertension, pregestational diabetes, or cardiovascular disease. She had a Pap smear with human papillomavirus typing 2 years ago and you also see a hemoglobin A1c from 2 years ago, which was 5.4%. She has declined genetic screening because she would not terminate any pregnancy. In addition to routine prenatal labs, which other lab should you order?

a. 1-hour glucose to screen for gestational diabetes

b. Baseline liver function tests (LFTs), creatinine and urine protein:creatinine ratio

c. Electrocardiogram

d. Cell-free fetal DNA screening

e. Thyroid stimulating hormone (TSH)

13. You are seeing a woman with A1 gestational diabetes in the office at 32 weeks. This is her first pregnancy and she has been managing her diabetes with diet and exercise since her diagnosis 4 weeks ago. She has seen the nutritionist and is keeping a food diary in addition to recording her fasting and 1-hour postprandial blood sugars. Her blood sugar logs over the past 2 weeks are as follows:
Fasting: 7/14 elevated (range 93–102)
Breakfast: 9/14 elevated (range 122–152)
Lunch: 4/14 elevated (range 126–148)
Dinner: 14/14 elevated (range 141–176)
You review her food diary and find that she is following a consistent carbohydrate plan and her food choices are appropriate. You discuss that you think she needs medication, but she hates needles and would like to avoid insulin. Her mother, who has type 2 diabetes, is managed on glyburide and she asks you if she can just take that. What is your primary concern about glyburide use in pregnancy?

a. Glyburide crosses the placenta.

b. Glyburide is teratogenic.

c. Glyburide has been associated with increased fetal growth restriction compared with treatment with insulin or metformin.

d. Glyburide has been associated with an increased risk for macrosomia compared with treatment with insulin or metformin.

e. Glyburide should only be used in women with type 2 diabetes.

14. You are seeing a woman with type 2 diabetes in the office at 18 weeks. This is her first pregnancy and she has been managing her diabetes with diet and exercise. She has seen the nutritionist and is keeping a food diary in addition to recording her fasting and 1-hour postprandial blood sugars. Her blood sugar logs over the past 2 weeks are as follows:
Fasting: 0/14 elevated (range 83–94)
Breakfast: 1/14 elevated (range 122–145)
Lunch: 0/14 elevated (range 116–134)
Dinner: 10/14 elevated (range 137–162)
You review her food diary and find that she is following a consistent carbohydrate plan and eating the recommended number of carbohydrates at dinner. How should you manage her moving forward?

a. Initiate weight-based intermediate acting insulin, such as isophane insulin (NPH), at night only.

b. Initiate a rapid-acting insulin, such as lispro, immediately before dinner.

c. Initiation of an oral medication, such as metformin, at night only.

d. Recommend a no-carbohydrate diet.

e. Continue to manage as an A1 gestational diabetic because most of her blood sugars are at goal.

15. A 28-year-old G2P1001 comes to see you for a prenatal visit at 16 weeks gestation. She did not know she was pregnant until last week. Her medical history is significant for obesity (weight 124 kg) and type 2 diabetes. She has been monitoring her finger sticks more frequently since discovering she was pregnant and all of her values are elevated for fasting (range 98–120) and 1 hour postprandial (152–188). She states she needed insulin in her first pregnancy to help control her blood sugars and assumed she will need it in this pregnancy. She is comfortable with injections or taking pills. You wish to begin treatment today. What is the insulin dose and regimen you start her on?

a. 15 units of NPH twice a day

b. Metformin 1000 mg twice a day

c. 124 units of insulin total divided between NPH dosed twice a day and short-acting insulin at meal times

d. 124 units of insulin total divided as 62 units of NPH dosed twice a day

e. 86 units of insulin total divided between NPH dosed twice a day and short-acting insulin at meal times

16. A 20-year-old G1P0 with type 1 diabetes presents at 34 weeks gestation with right flank pain, fevers, nausea, and vomiting. She has been feeling ill for the past 24 hours and has not gotten better despite taking acetaminophen at home. She has had moderate control with her diabetes this pregnancy and uses an insulin pump. Her initial vital signs in triage are as follows: temperature 102.3°F (39.1C), HR 118, respirations 20, BP 112/67. You get an initial finger stick that is 274. You place the fetus on the monitor and the tracing is as follows: baseline 155, minimal variability, no accelerations, one late deceleration. What should not be considered as an early step in management?

a. Placement of large-bore IV cannulas for fluid resuscitation.

b. Obtaining laboratory tests, including complete blood count, complete metabolic panel (CMP) urinalysis/urine culture, beta-hydroxybutyrate, and an arterial blood gas

c. Emergent cesarean delivery for nonreassuring fetal status

d. Discontinuing insulin pump in favor of insulin drip

e. Correction of electrolyte abnormalities

17. You are seeing a 32-year-old G1P0 at 29 weeks gestation with newly diagnosed gestational diabetes. She is upset by the diagnosis because she is thin and takes care of herself. You explain that the initial steps in the management of gestational diabetes include diet and exercise. Which of the following is not recommended in women with gestational diabetes who are managing with diet and exercise?

a. A ketogenic diet (low/no carbohydrates and high fat)

b. Substitution of complex carbohydrates for simple carbohydrates

c. Moderate-intensity exercise for at least 30 minutes five times a week

d. Carbohydrate intake set around 40% of the total daily calorie intake

e. 2000–2500 kcal/d in a woman with a normal BMI

18. A 24-year-old G1P1001 presents for her 6-week postpartum visit. She had a full-term vaginal delivery. The delivery was uncomplicated, but her pregnancy was complicated by A2 gestational diabetes, managed with insulin. She was diagnosed at 22 weeks gestation when she initiated prenatal care. She received a glucose tolerance test (GTT) at that time because her BMI was 38 kg/m². What test could you do today that would diagnose her with diabetes?

a. No test is needed, we can confidently diagnose her with gestational diabetes based on the timing of the test during pregnancy

b. A random plasma glucose of 180

c. Hemoglobin A1c if 5.8%

d. 2-hour (75 g) GTT of 206

e. Fasting plasma glucose of 101

19. You are seeing a 28-year-old G0 for preconception counseling due to gestational diabetes. She also has chronic hypertension that is well controlled on enalapril and her BP in your office today is 124/78. She takes metformin for her type 2 diabetes. Her last hemoglobin A1c was 1 year ago and was 7.5%. She has no significant surgical history. Which of the following is not indicated as part of a preconception workup?

a. Repeat hemoglobin A1c

b. Cardiac stress test

c. Electrocardiogram

d. Baseline assessment of liver function, renal function, and proteinuria

e. Ophthalmologic examination

20. You are seeing a 29-year-old G3P1011 at 36 weeks gestation who has a poorly controlled type 2 diabetes. She has not been compliant with checking her blood glucose and she does not bring her glucose log today. You obtained a hemoglobin A1c level 1 week ago that came back as 9.3%, up from her first trimester A1c of 6.7%. Because of this, you obtain a growth ultrasound that gives an estimated fetal weight (EFW) of 4550 g. Her previous child was delivered 5 years ago, before her diagnosis of type 2 diabetes, and weighed 3478 g. She reports many people coming in the room at deliver and someone "mashing on her belly to deliver the baby." You check a random blood glucose in the office and it is 110 despite having not eaten yet today. Based on all this information, what is your recommendation for delivery?

a. Induction of labor now

b. Induction of labor at 39 weeks with twice weekly nonstress tests

c. Cesarean delivery at 39 weeks with weekly biophysical profiles

d. Induction of labor at 37 weeks following fetal lung maturity testing

e. Cesarean delivery at 37 weeks

ANSWERS

1. Answer: e

(see *Gabbe's Obstetrics* 8e: ch45)

Hepatic glucose production is increased in pregnancy. Early gestation is an anabolic state characterized by increases in maternal fat stores and decreases in free fatty acid concentration. Leptin concentrations and insulin clearance are increased in early pregnancy.

2. Answer: d

(see *Gabbe's Obstetrics* 8e: ch45)

Placental glucose transport occurs by facilitated diffusion and is dependent on a family of glucose transporters referred to as the *GLUT glucose transporter family*. The principal glucose transporter in the placenta is GLUT1.

3. Answer: b

(see *Gabbe's Obstetrics* 8e: ch45)

Relatively uniform decreases are apparent in insulin sensitivity with advancing gestation in all women. The changes in insulin sensitivity from the time before conception through early pregnancy were significantly correlated with changes in maternal weight gain and energy expenditure. The relationship between these alterations in maternal glucose insulin sensitivity and weight gain and energy expenditure may help explain the decrease in maternal weight gain and insulin requirements in women with diabetes in early gestation.[1] In summary, the various degrees of decreased insulin sensitivity observed in late pregnancy in women with normal glucose tolerance or gestational diabetes (GDM) are a reflection of their individual prepregnancy insulin sensitivity.

4. Answer: c

(see *Gabbe's Obstetrics* 8e: ch45)

Cholesterol and triglyceride concentrations increase progressively until term, and then a decrease is seen in serum triglyceride postpartum. The decrease was more rapid in women who breastfeed.

5. Answer: a

(see *Gabbe's Obstetrics* 8e: ch45)

Excessive stillbirth rates in pregnancies complicated by diabetes have been linked to chronic intrauterine hypoxia. Extramedullary hematopoiesis is frequently observed in stillborn infants of diabetic mothers and supports chronic intrauterine hypoxia as a probable cause of these fetal demises.

6. Answer: a

(see *Gabbe's Obstetrics* 8e: ch45)

Most studies have documented a two- to six-fold increase in major malformations in infants of mothers with type 1 and type 2 diabetes. Central nervous system malformations—particularly anencephaly, open spina bifida, and holoprosencephaly—are increased 10-fold in women with pregestational diabetes. Cardiac anomalies are the most common malformations seen in infants born to mothers with pregestational diabetes, with ventricular septal defects and complex lesions such as transposition of the great vessels being the most common.

7. Answer: e

(see *Gabbe's Obstetrics* 8e: ch45)

Macrosomia has been variously defined as birthweight greater than 4000 to 4500 g. Insulin is the most important fetal growth hormone, and fetal hyperinsulinemia results in excessive fetal growth. The increased incidence of macrosomia in pregnancies complicated by diabetes is multifactorial and is related to maternal prepregnancy weight and weight gain, maternal hyperglycemia with frequent excursions in blood glucose levels, as well as increased fetal levels of amino acids, triglycerides, and fatty acids.

8. Answer: b

(see *Gabbe's Obstetrics* 8e: ch45)

A transient form of hypertrophic cardiomyopathy may occur in insulin-dependent diabetics. Among symptomatic infants, septal hypertrophy may cause left ventricular outflow obstruction, although most infants are asymptomatic. The cardiac hypertrophy likely results from fetal hyperinsulinemia, which leads to fat and glycogen deposition in the myocardium.

9. Answer: d

(see *Gabbe's Obstetrics* 8e: ch45)

With good glycemic control, the frequency of neonatal hypocalcemia is less than 5%. Decreased serum magnesium levels have also been documented in pregnant diabetic women, as well as in their infants, but are infrequent. The risk for respiratory distress syndrome is no higher in infants born to diabetic mothers with optimal glucose control than that observed in the general population. Hyperbilirubinemia is seen in 25%–53% of infants born to diabetic mothers and can be seen independent of polycythemia.

10. Answer: c

(see *Gabbe's Obstetrics* 8e: ch45)

Renal disease develops in 25% to 30% of women with diabetes mellitus, with a peak incidence after 16 years of diabetes. Class F describes pregnant women with underlying renal disease. Class D is women with diabetes onset <10 years of age or with the diagnosis for more than 20 years. No deleterious effect on the progression of diabetic nephropathy is apparent with a normal baseline serum creatinine and no significant proteinuria is present. In women with diabetic nephropathy, proteinuria increased in 69% and hypertension developed in 73% during pregnancy. Small studies of patients with serum creatinine >1.5 mg/dL suggest that pregnancy may be associated with a more rapid decline in postpartum renal function but not an increased risk of dialysis during pregnancy. This patient is at a much higher risk for development of preeclampsia than a need for dialysis with her baseline creatinine and hypertension.

11. Answer: e

(see *Gabbe's Obstetrics* 8e: ch45)

Women with proliferative changes due to diabetic retinopathy can safely undergo laser photocoagulation treatment during pregnancy at any gestational age. Treatment should not be delayed until later in gestation or postpartum and betamethasone should not be administered. However, some women may require cesarean delivery or limited Valsalva based on their retinopathy. Termination of pregnancy will not alter any current pathology.

12. Answer: a

(see *Gabbe's Obstetrics* 8e: ch45)

The American College of Obstetricians and Gynecologists (ACOG) and the American Diabetes Association (ADA) recommend early pregnancy screening for undiagnosed type 2 diabetes in women with one or more of the following: history of GDM; infant birth weight ≥4000 g; history of impaired glucose metabolism, polycystic ovary syndrome, or cardiovascular disease; obesity (BMI ≥25 kg/m^2); a first-degree relative with diabetes; and members of high-risk race or ethnicity groups.

13. Answer: d

(see *Gabbe's Obstetrics* 8e: ch45)

During the past 20 years, oral hypoglycemic therapy has become a suitable alternative to insulin treatment in women with GDM. Oral agents may be used instead of insulin when patients are reluctant to take injections, when there is concern about their ability to follow a regimen of multiple insulin injections, or when the cost of insulin is prohibitive for them. Metaanalyses have noted increased risks of macrosomia and hypoglycemia with glyburide compared with insulin. Observational data suggest that glyburide may be less successful in obese women and in those with marked hyperglycemia discovered early in gestation.

14. Answer: b

(see *Gabbe's Obstetrics* 8e: ch45)

As more than 50% of her postprandial dinner values are elevated despite following the recommended diet, she would likely benefit from treatment of her gestational diabetes. Metformin is acceptable but would not correct her postprandial dinner values if given at night. Giving an intermediate-acting insulin at night would also not correct her postprandial values. Totally eliminating carbohydrates is also not recommended, as a persistent ketogenic state is not recommended during pregnancy. Although typical insulin dosing involves a combination of intermediate- and short-acting insulins, it may be acceptable to add just mealtime insulin in certain patients to avoid hypoglycemia at other times of the day.

15. Answer: c

(see *Gabbe's Obstetrics* 8e: ch45)

A weight-based regimen may be utilized with adjustments made for the increasing insulin resistance observed as pregnancy progresses: 0.7 to 0.8 units/kg actual body weight in the first trimester, 1.0 units/kg actual body weight in the second trimester, and 1.2 units/kg actual body weight in the third trimester. Half of the total insulin dose is given as basal insulin, usually NPH, and half as prandial boluses, usually lispro or aspart. Many women with type 2 diabetes who enter pregnancy with their disease controlled with metformin will eventually require the addition of insulin to their regimen.

16. Answer: c

(see *Gabbe's Obstetrics* 8e: ch45)

This patient is presenting with likely diabetic ketoacidosis, precipitated by infection. Stabilization of the patient with IV fluids, electrolyte repletion, and insulin drip usually results in resolution of the nonreassuring fetal HR pattern. However, this process can take several hours; regardless, every effort should be made to correct and stabilize the mother's condition before a potential delivery.

17. Answer: a

(see *Gabbe's Obstetrics* 8e: ch45)

Once the diagnosis of gestational diabetes is established, women are begun on a dietary program of 2000 to 2500 kcal daily. Carbohydrate intake should be around 40% of the daily calories. Carbohydrate restriction results in fat substitute and transfer of excess free fatty acids to the fetus, so a high-fat diet is not recommended. Several studies now suggest that more liberal complex carbohydrate consumption may effectively control maternal hyperglycemia, compared with carbohydrate restriction. Women with GDM are advised to exercise daily for 30 minutes at least 5 days a week or a minimum of 150 minutes per week.

18. Answer: d

(see *Gabbe's Obstetrics* 8e: ch45)

Women with GDM have a seven-fold increased risk for developing type 2 diabetes, compared with women who do not have diabetes during pregnancy. ACOG recommends using either a fasting plasma glucose or a 75-g 2-hour oral GTT at 4 to 12 weeks postpartum. Based on the timing of her GTT, we cannot definitively diagnose the patient with pregestational diabetes without a confirmatory test outside of pregnancy.

19. Answer: b

(see *Gabbe's Obstetrics* 8e: ch45)

Prepregnancy counseling includes an assessment of vascular status and glycemic control. At this time, the nonpregnant patient can learn techniques for self-monitoring of blood glucose, as well as the need for proper dietary management. Hemoglobin A1c levels obtained periconception should be used to counsel diabetic women regarding the risk for an infant with anomalies. Replacement of teratogenic medications, such as ACE inhibitors, should occur prior to conception. Baseline assessment of cardiac, liver, and renal function should occur prior to conception or in the first trimester, due to the increased risk of preeclampsia. Cardiac stress testing should be reserved for women with a history of ischemic cardiac disease or those with symptoms concerning for ischemic cardiac disease.

20. Answer: e

(see *Gabbe's Obstetrics* 8e: ch45)

ACOG recommends consideration of cesarean delivery in women with diabetes when estimated fetal weight exceeds 4500 g. The decision to proceed with delivery should be based on confirmation of deteriorating fetal condition by several tests that show abnormal values or by a concern for stillbirth, as evidenced by poor blood glucose control and fetal overgrowth and/or polyhydramnios. Fetal lung maturity testing is rarely needed. Patients with preexisting diabetes or poorly controlled gestational diabetes should have twice weekly nonstress tests for assessment of fetal well-being, due to the increased risk of fetal demise.

46

Obesity in Pregnancy

Vanita D. Jain

(See *Gabbe's Obstetrics: Normal and Problem Pregnancies*, 8e: ch46)

QUESTIONS

1. Based on the 2009 Institute of Medicine (IOM) Guidelines, women who are considered obese (defined as body mass index [BMI] >30), should gain how much total weight during the pregnancy?

   a. 28–40 lb

   b. 25–35 lb

   c. 15–25 lb

   d. 11–30 lb

2. A 25-year-old G1P0 at 12 weeks gestation presents for her first prenatal visit. As a part of your evaluation you notice her BMI is 42 kg/m². You discuss diet and nutrition, but also mention that there are a number of pregnancy complications associated with obesity. All of the following are noted in a pregnancy affected by obesity, except:

   a. Increased risk for miscarriage

   b. Increased risk of recurrent miscarriage

   c. Increased risk for gestational diabetes

   d. Increased risk for placental abruption

3. A 29-year-old G2P1001 presents at 29 weeks for her routine prenatal appointment. Her pregnancy has been overall unremarkable, with a normal screening 1-hour glucose test and third-trimester labs. Her BMI at the start of the pregnancy was 45 kg/m². In addition to answering her questions regarding routine prenatal care, it would be reasonable to discuss which of the following at this visit?

   a. Planning for a fetal growth ultrasound

   b. Starting probiotics to prevent gestational diabetes

   c. Starting vitamins C and E to prevent preeclampsia

   d. Starting aspirin to prevent preeclampsia

4. A 33-year-old G1P0 presents for her Ob visit at 40 weeks and 5 days. Her induction of labor is scheduled for tomorrow evening at 6:00 p.m. You review the plan. Her pregravid BMI is 47 kg/m². During this visit you should also discuss with the patient:

   a. The need to notify anesthesia upon admission to the labor and delivery unit to finalize an anesthetic plan for delivery and in the event of an emergency

   b. Discuss your intent to deliver with forceps

   c. Recommend a primary cesarean section

   d. Recommend she start aspirin tonight

5. A 22-year-old G1P1001 presents to Obstetric Triage (Ob) triage on postoperative day 4 from a cesarean delivery with a complaint of wound pain. On examination the wound is closed but fluctuant and has surrounding erythema and induration. You suspect a seroma. She is also febrile and mildly tachycardic. In addition to planning for inpatient admission, you order IV fluids and antibiotics and open the wound, which was closed with staples. The fascia is intact and a seroma is evacuated. All of the following are acceptable methods for wound management in obese patients except:

   a. Secondary closure with packing that is changed once or twice daily

   b. Secondary closure with a negative pressure wound vac to be changed once daily

   c. Suture the skin closed now in Ob triage before "admitting the patient to the inpatient unit"

   d. Secondary closure without packing if the area is small (1–2 cm)

6. You are seeing a pleasant 26-year-old G0P0 for a preconception visit. Her BMI is 52 kg/m². In addition to discussing planned prenatal care you emphasize the importance of weight management and discuss various maternal risks in pregnancy affected by obesity. All of the following should also be discussed except:

a. Evaluate for presence of CHTN, diabetes, or dyslipidemia.

b. Advise against bariatric surgery prior to pregnancy.

c. Discuss her contraception plans during her evaluation process and birth spacing.

d. Evaluate for obstructive sleep apnea.

ANSWERS

1. Answer: d

(see *Gabbe's Obstetrics* 8e: ch46)

Gestation weight gain (GWG) recommendations are based on the 2009 IOM guidelines (Table 46.1), in which obese women are recommended to gain 11–20 lb during pregnancy.

TABLE 46.1	**BMI and Obesity**		
Definition	**BMI (kg/m²)**	**Obesity Class**	**IOM Weight Gain (lb)**
Underweight	<18.5		28–40
Normal	18.5–24.9		25–35
Overweight	25.0–29.9	I	15–25
Obese	30.0–39.9	II	11–20
Extremely Obese	≥40.0	III	

BMI, Body mass index; *IOM*, Institute of Medicine.
Adapted from Gunatilake RP, Perlow JH. Obesity and pregnancy: clinical management of the obese gravida. *American Journal of Obstetrics & Gynecology*. 2011;204(2):106-119.

2. Answer: d

(see *Gabbe's Obstetrics* 8e: ch46)

Obesity is associated with an increased risk of early miscarriage (OR 1.2, CI 1.01–1.46) and recurrent miscarriage (OR 3.5, CI 1.03–12.01). Obstetric complications that may be increased include gestational hypertension (published odds ratios ranging from 2.5–3.2), preeclampsia (published odds ratios ranging from 1.6–4.82), gestational diabetes (published odds ratios ranging from 2.6–11.0), and obstructive sleep apnea (OR 13.23, CI: 6.25–28.01).

3. Answer: a

(see *Gabbe's Obstetrics* 8e: ch46)

An important use of fetal ultrasound is the assessment of fetal growth. Obese pregnant women are at risk for both fetal growth restriction and macrosomia. Because fundal height measurements provide more limited information in the setting of obesity, ultrasound should be used in the evaluation of fetal growth. Maternal obesity does not appear to impact the accuracy of the fetal weight estimated by sonogram. The use of probiotics or vitamins C and E have not proven to be effective in prevention of pregnancy-related complications. Low-dose aspirin should be started in the late first/early second trimester to be effective for preeclampsia prevention if the patient meets USPTF criteria for initiation.

4. Answer: a

(see *Gabbe's Obstetrics* 8e: ch46)

There is no need to deliver earlier than usual. While obesity is associated with an increased risk of stillbirth, there are no guidelines that propose delivery prior to full term solely for the indication of obesity. In the absence of randomized clinical trial evidence of specific benefit to this group of women, current recommendations are to use usual obstetric indications for timing of delivery. During the planning for the procedure, providers should take into account the potential difficulties in monitoring, need for an emergent delivery, prolonged incision-to-delivery time, and need for adequate anesthesia prior to proceeding with the emergent delivery. Obesity is a risk factor for VTE, however aspirin is not recommended as thromboprophylaxis for this situation. Mechanical prophylaxis, however, may be indicated.

5. Answer: c

(see *Gabbe's Obstetrics* 8e: ch46)

After discharge from the hospital, approximately 2%–3% of obese women will have a postpartum readmission. Unfortunately, closure with staples increases the risk for postoperative infection. A metaanalysis of 12 randomized clinical trials that evaluated skin closure, which included 3112 women, found absorbable suture when compared to nonabsorbable staples was associated with a reduction in composite wound complications, including infection, hematoma, seroma, wound separation, and readmission. A subgroup analysis of women with BMI >30kg/m^2 confirmed that association in obese women (RR 0.51; 95% CI 0.34–0.75). It is not recommended to close the wound as the seroma will likely recur. Instead, closure by secondary intention is indicated.

6. Answer: b

(see *Gabbe's Obstetrics* 8e: ch46)

All of the following should be discussed. In addition, bariatric surgery may be *beneficial* prior to conception. While behavioral modifications have been advocated and medications used in an effort to lose weight, bariatric surgery remains one of the most effective options. Long-term sustained improvements include durable (>5 years) weight loss, reversal of diabetes, and lipid improvements. Weight reduction after bariatric surgery in between pregnancies is associated with better outcomes in those subsequent pregnancies. Bariatric surgery should be recommended, and contraception planned to time delivery postsurgery appropriately. The most recent practice guidelines (cosponsored by the American Society of Metabolic and Bariatric Surgery, the Obesity Society, and the American Association of Clinical Endocrinology) suggest delaying pregnancy for 12–18 months after bariatric surgery; the American College of Obstetrics & Gynecology (ACOG) recommends a wait of 12–24 months to ensure that pregnancy does not occur during the rapid catabolic weight-loss period, which theoretically may lead to fetal malnutrition and impaired growth.

47

Thyroid and Parathyroid Diseases in Pregnancy

Eva K. Pressman

(See *Gabbe's Obstetrics: Normal and Problem Pregnancies*, 8e: ch47)

QUESTIONS

1. Calcium metabolism is affected by pregnancy in several ways. Which of the following statements is most accurate?

   a. After delivery, urinary calcium excretion is increased.

   b. Blood levels of 1,25(OH)D, the active metabolite of vitamin D, increase in pregnancy.

   c. Calcium loss in lactating mothers leads to the development of osteopenia.

   d. Intestinal absorption of calcium decreases during pregnancy.

   e. Ionized serum calcium increased during pregnancy.

2. A 24-year-old G1P0 woman comes to the office at 8 weeks gestation with nausea, vomiting, fatigue, and daily headaches. She has no known medical problems. No abnormalities are noted on physical examination. Laboratory testing results are shown below. What is the most likely cause of her symptoms?

Glucose	78 mg/dL
Calcium	14 mg/dL
Total protein	6.2 g/dL
Albumin	3.5 g/dL
Chloride	102 mmol/L
Carbon dioxide	18 mmol/L
Potassium	3.9 mmol/L
Sodium	140 mmol/L
alanine aminotransferase (ALT)	18 IU/L
aspartate aminotransferase (AST)	20 IU/L
Bilirubin	0.3 mg/dL
Alkaline Phosphatase	102 IU/L
blood urea nitrogen (BUN)	18 mg/dL
Creatinine	0.7 mg/dL

   a. Autoimmune disease

   b. Normal pregnancy

   c. Parathyroid adenoma

   d. Parathyroid carcinoma

   e. Parathyroid hyperplasia

3. A 28-year-old G2P0010 comes to the office at 8 weeks gestation. She was recently diagnosed with primary hyperparathyroidism after presenting with nephrolithiasis and surgery was recommended. Her serum calcium is 16. Which of the following approaches will minimize potential complications to the patient and the pregnancy?

   a. Delaying surgery until after pregnancy

   b. Intraoperative thyroxine (T4) monitoring

   c. Monitoring serum calcium daily postoperatively

   d. Performing the surgery in the first trimester

   e. Preoperative ultrasonography to localize the adenoma

4. A 26-year-old African woman, G3P2002, comes to the office for a routine prenatal visit at 12 weeks gestation. She recently moved to the northern United States from Ghana. She works as a landscape architect and does not routinely use sunscreen. Which of the following patient characteristics put her at increased risk for vitamin D deficiency?

   a. Current residence

   b. Occupation

   c. Parity

   d. Pregnancy

   e. Sunscreen habits

5. A 29-year-old G2P0010 comes to the office at 10 weeks gestation with concerns about fatigue and a history of hypothyroidism in her mother and sister. She is aware that pregnancy increases the demand for thyroid hormones and that insufficient thyroid hormone levels can be associated with poor pregnancy outcomes. Due to her concerns, a thyroid-stimulating hormone (TSH) and free T4 are measured and are normal for gestational age. From which component of the thyroid gland, shown below, are the additional thyroid hormones secreted?

   a. Both colloid and follicle

   b. Colloid only

   c. Follicle only

   d. Interstitium

   e. None of the above

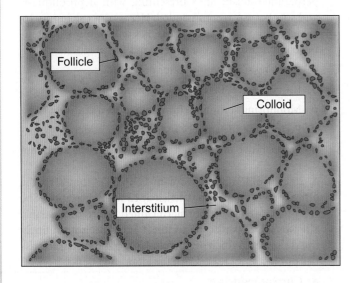

6. Which of the following physiologic changes of pregnancy contribute to an increased demand for thyroid hormone secretion?

   a. Decreased T4-binding globulin (TBG)

   b. Excess iodine availability

   c. Increased concentration of D3 deiodinase

   d. Inhibitory effect of human chorionic gonadotropin (hCG) on the TSH receptor

   e. Transfer of T4 from the fetus

7. A 27-year-old G1P0 woman comes to the office at 7 weeks gestation with recurrent nausea and vomiting. She has been unable to eat anything for 3 days and has only been able to keep down small amounts of water. Laboratory testing shows an hCG of 370,000 IU, a TSH of 1.0 mIU/L, and a free T4 of 2.5 ng/dL. Which of the following findings would not be expected on ultrasound?

   a. Dichorionic twin gestation

   b. Missed abortion

   c. Molar pregnancy

   d. Monochorionic twin gestation

   e. Singleton gestation

8. A 24-year-old G1P0 woman comes to the office for a routine prenatal visit at 20 weeks gestation. Her pregnancy has been uncomplicated and her only medical history is Graves disease that was treated with radioiodine ablation 3 years ago. She has had normal thyroid function tests on stable doses of thyroid hormone replacement both before and during the pregnancy. Thyroid receptor antibody testing is positive. She asks if there is a chance that her history of Graves disease could impact the fetus. Which is the most accurate response?

   a. Because her Graves disease was treated with ablation prior to pregnancy, there is no risk to the fetus.

   b. Because she has had normal thyroid function during pregnancy, there is no risk to the fetus.

   c. Because her thyroid receptor antibodies are positive, there is a risk of thyroid dysfunction in the fetus.

   d. Because she is on thyroid replacement therapy, there is the risk of thyroid dysfunction in the fetus.

   e. It is not possible to determine the risk to the fetus after treatment for Graves disease.

9. A 29-year-old G3P2012 comes to the emergency department at 12 weeks gestation after 4 days of recurrent nausea and vomiting. Prior ultrasound confirmed a viable single intrauterine pregnancy. This is her third visit to the emergency department this pregnancy, and on her last visit 1 week ago, thyroid function tests were obtained. Her TSH was 0.1 IU/mL and her free T4 index was 16. Today, her pulse is 100 bpm and blood pressure is 110/60. Urinalysis shows positive ketones. What is the most appropriate treatment?

   a. IV hydration

   b. Methimazole

   c. Propranolol

   d. Propylthiouracil

   e. Radioactive iodine

10. A 38-year-old G3P2002 at 12 weeks gestation comes to the office for a routine prenatal visit. Thyroid function tests prior to pregnancy showed a TSH of 0.2 IU/mL and a normal free T3 and T4. She was warned that this degree of thyroid abnormality is associated with long-term health risks. What pregnancy outcomes is this condition associated with?

    a. Cognitive delay in her offspring

    b. Increased risk of gestational hypertension

    c. Increased risk of gestational diabetes

    d. Increased risk of preterm delivery

    e. No increased risk of pregnancy complications

11. A 29-year-old G2P0010 comes to the office at 10 weeks gestation for her first prenatal visit. She was diagnosed with Graves disease 2 years ago, 6 months after her last pregnancy. She was prescribed methimazole initially but was switched to propylthiouracil (PTU) when she started to attempt conception. She has struggled with the gastrointestinal side effects of PTU and has not been taking her medication for the last 2 weeks. If her hyperthyroidism remains untreated, risks of which of the following pregnancy complications would increase?

    a. Gestational diabetes

    b. Postterm pregnancy

    c. Maternal hypotension

    d. Fetal macrosomia

    e. Placental abruption

12. What is the most common neonatal morbidity with maternal hyperparathyroidism?

    a. Hypercalcemia

    b. Hyperglycemia

    c. Hypocalcemia

    d. Hypocalcemia

    e. Hyperphosphatemia

13. A 32-year-old nulligravid comes to the office to discuss becoming pregnant. Her medical history includes hyperthyroidism that was diagnosed 6 months ago and is currently well controlled with methimazole, 5 mg TID. She now has regular menses and is hoping to conceive. She plans to breastfeed after delivery. What is the most appropriate treatment during pregnancy and postpartum?

    a. Continue methimazole through pregnancy and lactation.

    b. Continue methimazole for the first trimester and switch to PTU for the remainder of pregnancy and lactation.

    c. Continue methimazole during pregnancy but switch to PTU for lactation.

    d. Switch to PTU through pregnancy and lactation.

    e. Switch to PTU for the first trimester and methimazole for the remainder of pregnancy and lactation.

14. A 29-year-old G1P0010 comes to the office to discuss planning a pregnancy. Her medical history includes a 10-week miscarriage 6 months ago. Since that time, she has only had two menstrual periods and reports continued fatigue, weight gain, and hair loss. A TSH is drawn and returns at 5.2 IU/mL. She has no history of thyroid dysfunction prior to her pregnancy. Which of the following statements is most accurate?

    a. Her recent elevated hCG levels are responsible.

    b. The cause is most likely autoimmune.

    c. There is likely associated pituitary dysfunction.

    d. There is likely hypothalamic involvement.

    e. This is normal physiology after a miscarriage.

ANSWERS

1. **Answer: b**

   (see *Gabbe's Obstetrics* 8e: ch47)

   Blood levels of 1,25(OH)D (calcitriol), the active metabolite of vitamin D, increase early in gestation to twice the nonpregnancy level in the third trimester. This increase comes as a result of stimulation of maternal renal 1α-hydroxylase activity by estrogen, placental lactogen, and parathyroid hormone (PTH), as well as synthesis of calcitriol by the placenta. After delivery, urinary calcium excretion is reduced; ionized serum calcium remains within normal limits; and total calcium, 1,25-hydroxyvitamin D, and serum PTH return to prepregnancy levels. Intestinal absorption of calcium decreases to the nonpregnant rate as a result of the previously mentioned return to normal levels of 1,25(OH)D.[1] Early concern for calcium loss in lactating mothers, with the development of osteopenia, has not been confirmed, and extra calcium supplementation during breastfeeding appears to be unnecessary because calcium supplementation above normal does not significantly reduce the amount of lost bone during gestation.[1] The alteration in calcium and bone metabolism that accompanies human lactation represents a physiologic response that is independent of calcium intake, and the osteopenia appears to be reversible.

2. **Answer: c**

(see *Gabbe's Obstetrics* 8e: ch47)

In pregnancy, because calcium determinations are not routinely performed, clinical manifestations of hyperparathyroidism are present in almost 70% of the diagnosed patients. Common symptoms may include gastrointestinal symptoms such as nausea, vomiting, and anorexia. Also, weakness and fatigue, headaches, lethargy, anxiety, emotional lability, and confusion may occur. There is some overlap with normal pregnancy symptoms. The most common cause of primary hyperparathyroidism (PHPT) in pregnancy is a single parathyroid adenoma, which is present in about 80% of all cases. Primary hyperplasia of the four parathyroid glands accounts for about 15% of the cases reported, 3% are due to multiple adenomas, and only a few cases due to parathyroid carcinoma have been reported in the English literature. Parathyroid cancer is a rare cause of hyperparathyroidism, with very few cases documented in pregnancy. Serum calcium levels are significantly higher than in other cases of PHPT, and perinatal mortality and morbidity are significant. Hypercalcemia with values above 13 mg/dL, in the presence of a palpable neck mass, should raise a strong suspicion of parathyroid carcinoma. Although most young women with hypercalcemia have PHPT, other unusual causes should be ruled out, mainly endocrine disorders, vitamin D or A overdose, the use of thiazide diuretics, or granulomatous diseases.

3. **Answer: e**

(see *Gabbe's Obstetrics* 8e: ch47)

Surgery is the only definitive treatment for PHPT, and the procedure is safe when performed by a surgeon with experience in neck surgery. The cure rate is excellent, and complications due to surgery are low, particularly in the presence of a single lesion. Improvements in the outcome of surgery and avoidance of intraoperative and postoperative complications include (1) preoperative parathyroid adenoma localization by ultrasonography, (2) minimally invasive parathyroidectomy techniques, (3) intraoperative PHPT monitoring to confirm successful surgery, and (4) detection and management of postoperative hypocalcemia. It is preferable to perform the surgery in the second trimester of pregnancy when possible. Medical therapy is reserved for patients with significant hypercalcemia who are not surgical candidates.

4. **Answer: a**

(see *Gabbe's Obstetrics* 8e: ch47)

Vitamin D deficiency is common during pregnancy, especially among high-risk groups that include vegetarians, women with limited sun exposure (e.g., those who live in cold climates, reside in northern latitudes, or wear sun and winter protective clothing), and ethnic minorities, especially those with darker skin. For pregnant women thought to be at increased risk of vitamin D deficiency, maternal serum 25(OH)D level testing can be considered and should be interpreted in the context of the individual clinical circumstance. The American College of Obstetricians and Gynecologists (ACOG) has stated, "At this time there is insufficient evidence to support a recommendation for screening all pregnant women for vitamin D deficiency. For pregnant women thought to be at increased risk of vitamin D deficiency, maternal serum 25(OH)D levels can be considered and should be interpreted in the context of the individual clinical circumstance. When vitamin D deficiency is identified during pregnancy, most experts agree that 1000 to 2000 IU/day of vitamin D is safe."

5. **Answer: b**

(see *Gabbe's Obstetrics* 8e: ch47)

The normal thyroid gland is able to compensate for the increase in thyroid hormone demands by increasing its secretion of thyroid hormones stored as colloid and maintaining them within normal limits throughout gestation. However, in those situations in which there is a subtle pathologic abnormality of the thyroid gland, such as chronic autoimmune thyroiditis, or in women on thyroid hormone replacement therapy, the normal increase in the production of thyroid hormones is not met. As a consequence, the pregnant woman could develop biochemical markers of hypothyroidism such as elevation in serum TSH.

6. **Answer: c**

(see *Gabbe's Obstetrics* 8e: ch47)

In early pregnancy, the maternal thyroid gland is challenged with an increased demand for thyroid hormone secretion, due mainly to (1) the increase in TBG secondary to the effect of estrogens on the liver; (2) the stimulatory effect of hCG on the TSH receptor; (3) high concentrations of type 3 iodothyronine deiodinase (D3), which degrades T4 and triidothyronine to inactive compounds; and (4) the supply of iodine available to the thyroid gland. Active secretion of thyroid hormones by the fetal thyroid gland commences at about 18 weeks gestation, although iodine uptake by the fetal gland occurs between 10 and 14 weeks. Transfer of T4 from mother to embryo occurs from early pregnancy. Maternal T4 has been demonstrated in coelomic fluid at 6 weeks and in the fetal brain at 9 weeks. Maternal transfer continues until delivery but only in significant amounts in the presence of fetal hypothyroidism.

7. Answer: b

(see *Gabbe's Obstetrics* 8e: ch47)

hCG is a weak thyroid stimulator that acts on the maternal thyroid gland TSH receptor; peak hCG values are reached by 9 to 12 weeks gestation. A transient suppression of TSH in the first trimester is common and can be exacerbated by situations in which there is a high production of hCG, such as in cases of multiple pregnancies, or hydatidiform mole. In these conditions, serum free T4 (FT4) concentrations may rise to levels seen in thyrotoxicosis.

8. Answer: c

(see *Gabbe's Obstetrics* 8e: ch47)

Graves disease is caused by direct stimulation of the thyroid epithelial cells by TSH receptor-stimulating antibodies (TSIs, or TRAbs). Highly sensitive and specific assays for detection of TRAbs are now commercially available that are very valuable in assessing fetal and neonatal risk in pregnancy, not only in women with active disease but also in those with a previous history of Graves hyperthyroidism, both in spontaneous remission and after ablation therapy. When hyperthyroidism is properly managed throughout pregnancy, the outcome for mother and fetus is good; however, maternal and neonatal complications for mothers with untreated or poorly controlled hyperthyroidism are significantly increased (Table 47.1).[2]

9. Answer: a

(see *Gabbe's Obstetrics* 8e: ch47)

Gestational hyperthyroidism is defined as transient hyperthyroidism in the first trimester of pregnancy due, with few exceptions, to high titers of hCG secretion that stimulate the TSH receptor. The most common causes of gestational hyperthyroidism are hyperemesis gravidarum, multiple gestation, and hydatidiform mole. Suppressed serum TSH may lag for a few more weeks after normalization of free thyroid hormone levels. Antithyroid medications are not needed. Obstetric outcome is not affected by gestational hyperthyroidism. Birthweight may be slightly lower, but not significantly different, compared with fetuses of control mothers and is related to maternal weight loss.

10. Answer: e

(see *Gabbe's Obstetrics* 8e: ch47)

Subclinical hyperthyroidism is defined as an abnormally low serum TSH with a normal FT4 (and FT3). In a nonpregnant patient population, subclinical hyperthyroidism has been associated with several long-term risks including osteoporosis, cardiovascular morbidity and stroke, cognitive decline, and lower quality of life. Among those identified as having subclinical disease, there was no increase in the rates of maternal, obstetric, or neonatal morbidities when compared to patients who were euthyroid. Interestingly, there was a lower incidence of gestational hypertension among patients with subclinical hyperthyroidism. The findings of this study support the recommendation that antithyroid drugs not be used to treat pregnant patients found to have subclinical hyperthyroidism.

11. Answer: e

(see *Gabbe's Obstetrics* 8e: ch47)

When hyperthyroidism is properly managed throughout pregnancy, the outcome for mother and fetus is good; however, maternal and neonatal complications for mothers with untreated or poorly controlled hyperthyroidism are significantly increased. Fetal and neonatal complications are also related to maternal control of hyperthyroidism. Intrauterine growth restriction, prematurity, stillbirth, and neonatal morbidity are the most common complications (Table 47.1).

TABLE 47.1 Potential Maternal and Fetal Complications of Graves Hyperthyroidism.

Maternal	Fetal
Pregnancy loss	Low birthweight
Pregnancy-induced hypertension	• Prematurity
Preterm delivery	• Small for gestational age
Congestive heart failure	• Intrauterine growth restriction
Thyroid storm	Fetal death
Placental abruption	Thyroid dysfunction
Infection	• Fetal hyperthyroidism
	• Fetal hypothyroidism
	• Neonatal hyperthyroidism
	• Neonatal goiter
	• Neonatal central hypothyroidism

From Patil-Sisodia K, Mestman JH. Graves hyperthyroidism and pregnancy: a clinical update. *Endocr Pract.* 2010;16:118-129.

12. Answer: b

(see *Gabbe's Obstetrics* 8e: ch47)

The two most common causes of neonatal morbidity are prematurity and neonatal hypocalcemia, and the latter is related to levels of maternal hypercalcemia. In early reports, it was often the only clue of maternal hyperparathyroidism. Neonatal hypocalcemia develops between the 2nd and 14th days of life and lasts for a few days.

13. Answer: e

(see *Gabbe's Obstetrics* 8e: ch47)

Although the incidence of both liver toxicity with PTU and embryopathy from methimazole (MMI) are very low, a panel convened by the US Food and Drug Administration and the American Thyroid Association (ATA) recommended the use of PTU only in the first trimester of pregnancy, with a change to MMI in the second trimester. Breastfeeding should be permitted if the daily dose of PTU or MMI is less than 300 mg/day or 20 mg/day, respectively. It is prudent to give the total dose in divided doses after each feeding.

14. Answer: b

(see *Gabbe's Obstetrics* 8e: ch47)

Postpartum thyroiditis (PPT) is defined as transient thyroid dysfunction in the first year after delivery in women who were euthyroid before pregnancy on no thyroid therapy. PPT also occurs following spontaneous or medically induced abortions. The etiology in most cases is autoimmune chronic (Hashimoto) thyroiditis, with a few cases due to hypothalamic or pituitary lesions.

REFERENCES

1. Ficinski M, Mestman JH. Primary hyperparathyroidism during pregnancy. *Endocr Pract*. 1996;2:362.

2. Millar LK, Wing DA, Leung AS, et al. Low birth weight and preeclampsia in pregnancies complicated by hyperthyroidism. *Obstet Gynecol*. 1994;84:946.

48

Pituitary and Adrenal Disorders in Pregnancy

Thaddeus P. Waters

(See *Gabbe's Obstetrics: Normal and Problem Pregnancies*, 8e: ch48)

QUESTIONS

1. All of the following are incorrect regarding the maternal cortisol levels during pregnancy except:

   a. Cortisol levels rise to a level four to five times higher by the end of pregnancy.

   b. Changes in maternal cortisol levels are related to estrogen-induced changes in corticosteroid-binding globulin (CBG) levels and an increase in cortisol production.

   c. While maternal cortisol production increases, there is no change in "free" serum cortisol, urinary free cortisol, and salivary cortisol.

   d. Maternal cortisol levels are unchanged over pregnancy.

2. A 26-year-old G0 presents for prenatal counseling due to a personal history of a pituitary adenoma. The patient is currently taking bromocriptine daily. Which of the following is not correct regarding her management?

   a. Bromocriptine is a teratogen and should be discontinued prior to pregnancy.

   b. Patients with certain types of microadenomas managed with dopamine agonists can have therapy discontinued after conception and be followed clinically during pregnancy.

   c. Patients with large macroadenomas should be assessed monthly for symptoms of tumor enlargement, and visual fields should be formally tested each trimester.

   d. Surgical decompression is a potential option during pregnancy if medical management fails.

3. A 41-year-old G2P0101 presents for prenatal care at 11 weeks gestation. Her history is significant for the development of headaches and loss of both visual fields at 32 weeks in her last pregnancy. The patient was subsequently diagnosed with an enlarged pituitary with hemorrhage and eventual pituitary apoplexy. She subsequently underwent emergent transsphenoidal resection. Which of the following is most accurate regarding hypopituitarism in pregnancy?

   a. Women on thyroxine replacement typically do not require an increase in their dose during pregnancy.

   b. Women on chronic glucocorticoid therapy typically do not require an increase in their dose during pregnancy.

   c. A TSH is always reliable for assessing thyroid replacement therapy in early pregnancy.

   d. Women on chronic glucocorticoids or thyroxine often need an increase in their dose during pregnancy.

4. A 19-year-old G1P1001 has a postpartum hemorrhage with hypovolemic shock immediately following her term delivery. All of the following are true regarding potential complications of this except:

   a. Sheehan syndrome is a common complication of a postpartum episode of hypovolemic shock.

   b. If acute pituitary necrosis is suspected, treatment with saline and stress doses of corticosteroids should be instituted immediately.

   c. An evaluation should include obtaining blood samples for adrenocorticotropic hormone (ACTH), cortisol, prolactin (PRL), and free thyroxine.

   d. Mild variants of pituitary infarction can present months or years later with symptoms of amenorrhea, decreased libido, breast atrophy, or loss of pubic and axillary hair.

5. A 31-year-old G1P0 presents at 13 weeks for prenatal care. Her medical history is significant for central diabetes insipidus (DI). Which of the following is the most accurate statement regarding her medical condition and pregnancy?

   a. DI remains stable over the course of pregnancy for the majority of patients.

   b. DDAVP is a first-line therapy during pregnancy.

   c. Serum sodium concentrations and values for hyponatremia are similar in pregnancy compared to the non-pregnant patient.

   d. Placental vasopressinase is thought to reduce the risk of worsening DI during pregnancy.

6. A 19-year-old G1P0 presents at 16 weeks with severe hypertension (180/110 mm Hg) refractory to parenteral antihypertensive medications. She has symptoms of headaches and palpitations. She denies a history of hypertension outside of pregnancy but reports limited care. An ultrasound of the pregnancy is unremarkable, with normal fetal growth and amniotic fluid volume for the gestational age. All of the following are accurate statements regarding her condition except:

   a. Preeclampsia is the most likely diagnosis for this patient.

   b. A laboratory evaluation including measuring urine metanephrines and catecholamines and plasma metanephrines is indicated.

   c. Labetalol is not recommended for hypertensive control in this situation.

   d. Initial medical management involves α-blockade with phenoxybenzamine or phentolamine.

7. A 22-year-old G2P0010 presents at 17 weeks with severe hypertension (180/110 mm Hg) with headaches, hypokalemia, and proteinuria. Which of the following is most accurate regarding her condition?

   a. Spironolactone is the best therapy for her condition.

   b. A serum aldosterone cannot be used for diagnosis during pregnancy.

   c. The primary cause is often a pituitary adenoma.

   d. Pregnancy complications include growth restriction, preeclampsia, and stillbirth.

8. A 22-year-old G1P0 presents at 23 weeks gestation presents wit new onset severe hypertension. She is noted to have significant hyperglycemia, and physical examination identifies reddish stretch marks on her abdomen with a pronounced fat lump between the shoulders. She also reports worsening muscle weakness. An MRI is notable for an adrenal adenoma. All of the following are accurate statements regarding the patient's condition during pregnancy except:

   a. Medical therapy with metyrapone and ketoconazole are the recommended first-line treatments.

   b. Pregnancy complications are significant, including pregnancy loss, growth restriction, diabetes, and hypertension.

   c. Aggressive medical therapy is indicated to improve pregnancy outcomes.

   d. Transsphenoidal resection of a pituitary ACTH-secreting adenoma and laparoscopic resection of adrenal adenomas have been carried out successfully in several patients during the second trimester.

ANSWERS

1. **Answer: b**

   (see *Gabbe's Obstetrics* 8e: ch48)

   Cortisol levels rise progressively over the course of a normal gestation and result in a two- to three-fold increase by term due to both the estrogen-induced increase in CBG levels and an increase in cortisol production, so that the levels of serum "free" cortisol, urinary free cortisol, and salivary cortisol are also increased.

2. **Answer: a**

   (see *Gabbe's Obstetrics* 8e: ch48)

   Patients with microadenomas and intrasellar or inferiorly extending macroadenomas who were treated only with dopamine agonists and had medication withdrawal after conception need only to be followed clinically throughout gestation. PRL levels may rise without tumor enlargement and may not rise with tumor enlargement; therefore such tests are often misleading[1] and should not be done. Patients with large macroadenomas should be assessed monthly for symptoms of tumor enlargement, and visual fields should be formally tested each trimester. Although data on safety of continuous dopamine agonist therapy during pregnancy are limited, such treatment is probably not harmful. In a separate study of 183 mother-baby outcomes of women receiving a dopamine agonist at some time during their pregnancy, dopamine agonist exposure was associated with an increased frequency of preterm birth, an increased rate of early pregnancy loss, and an insignificant increase in fetal malformations.

3. Answer: b

(see *Gabbe's Obstetrics* 8e: ch48)

Because patients with a hypothalamic/pituitary dysfunction may not routinely demonstrate a rise in their TSH in early pregnancy, it is reasonable to increase the thyroxine supplementation by 0.025 mg after the first 4 to 6 weeks and by an additional 0.025 mg after the second trimester, while continuing to monitor free T4 levels. The dose of chronic glucocorticoid replacement does not usually need to be increased during pregnancy.

4. Answer: a

(see *Gabbe's Obstetrics* 8e: ch48)

Sheehan syndrome consists of pituitary necrosis secondary to ischemia that occurs within hours of delivery, usually secondary to hypotension and shock from an obstetric hemorrhage. The degree of ischemia and necrosis dictates the subsequent patient course (Table 48.1). This syndrome rarely occurs in current obstetric practice.

TABLE 48.1 Symptoms and Signs of Sheehan Syndrome.	
Acute Form	**Chronic Form**
Hypotension	Light-headedness
Tachycardia	Fatigue
Failure to lactate	Failure to lactate
Hypoglycemia	Persistent amenorrhea
Extreme fatigue	Decreased body hair
Nausea and vomiting	Dry skin
	Loss of libido
	Nausea and vomiting
	Cold intolerance

5. Answer: b

(see *Gabbe's Obstetrics* 8e: ch48)

Central DI may develop in pregnancy because of an enlarging pituitary lesion, lymphocytic hypophysitis, or hypothalamic disease. Because of the increased clearance of vasopressin (AVP) by placental vasopressinase, DI usually worsens during gestation, and subclinical DI may become manifest. DDAVP is resistant to vasopressinase and provides satisfactory, safe treatment during gestation. During monitoring of the clinical response, clinicians should remember that the normal sodium concentration is 5 mmol/L lower during pregnancy.

6. Answer: a

(see *Gabbe's Obstetrics* 8e: ch48)

The diagnosis of pheochromocytoma should be considered in pregnant women with severe or paroxysmal hypertension, particularly in the first half of pregnancy or in association with orthostatic hypotension or episodic symptoms of pallor, anxiety, headaches, palpitations, chest pain, or diaphoresis. Laboratory diagnosis of pheochromocytoma relies on measuring urine metanephrines and catecholamines and plasma metanephrines, similar to nonpregnancy state. Initial medical management involves α-blockade with phenoxybenzamine or phentolamine. β-Blockade is reserved for treating maternal tachycardia or arrhythmias that persist after full α-blockade and volume repletion.

7. Answer: d

(see *Gabbe's Obstetrics* 8e: ch48)

Primary aldosteronism has rarely been reported in pregnancy and is most often caused by an adrenal adenoma. The elevated aldosterone levels found in affected patients during pregnancy are similar to those in normal pregnant women, but the plasma renin activity is suppressed. Moderate-to-severe hypertension develops in 85%, proteinuria in 52%, and hypokalemia in 55% of patients; symptoms may include headache, malaise, and muscle cramps. Placental abruption, preterm delivery, intrauterine growth restriction (IUGR), intrauterine fetal death, preeclampsia, small for gestational age, and increase of cesarean section rates are also risks. Spironolactone, the usual nonpregnant therapy for aldosteronism, is contraindicated in pregnancy because it crosses the placenta and is a potent anti-androgen, which can cause ambiguous genitalia in a male fetus.

8. Answer: a

(see *Gabbe's Obstetrics* 8e: ch48)

Diagnosing Cushing syndrome during pregnancy may be difficult, as it mimics other common pregnancy conditions such as preeclampsia. The striae associated with normal pregnancy are usually pale, but they are red or purple in Cushing syndrome. Cushing syndrome is associated with a pregnancy loss rate of 25%, due to spontaneous abortion, stillbirth, and early neonatal death because of extreme prematurity. Medical therapy for Cushing syndrome during pregnancy with metyrapone and ketoconazole is not very effective. IUGR has been reported with ketoconazole and this currently has an FDA-issued black-box warning, due to severe liver toxicity. Transsphenoidal resection of a pituitary ACTH-secreting adenoma and laparoscopic resection of adrenal adenomas have been carried out successfully in several patients during the second trimester.

REFERENCES

1. Divers WA, Yen SS. Prolactin-producing microadenomas in pregnancy. *Obstet Gynecol.* 1983;62:425-429.

49

Hematologic Complications of Pregnancy

Audrey Merriam

(See *Gabbe's Obstetrics: Normal and Problem Pregnancies*, 8e: ch49)

QUESTIONS

1. A 29-year-old G1P0 presents at 30 weeks gestation for a prenatal visit. On reviewing her third-trimester laboratory tests you see her platelets returned as 101,000/mm³ and were 160,000/mm³ at her initial prenatal visit. She denies any history of easy bruising or bleeding in the past or during pregnancy. Her vital signs and physical examination are unremarkable. You counsel the patient that this low platelet count is likely gestational thrombocytopenia. She is very concerned about how it will impact her pregnancy. What do you tell her?

   a. She must have a cesarean delivery to avoid trauma and subsequent bleeding in her infant.

   b. She will need a platelet transfusion at delivery.

   c. methylprednisolone will be initiated at 36 weeks gestation to raise the platelet count.

   d. This is just the result of hemodilution of pregnancy.

   e. You will repeat a complete blood count (CBC) around 34–36 weeks gestation to ensure the platelet count is stable.

2. Which of the following patients would be the best candidate for a platelet transfusion?

   a. A 27-year-old G2P0010 at 40 weeks, in labor with known gestational thrombocytopenia, and an admission platelet count of 100,000/mm³

   b. A 23-year-old G3P2002 at 34 weeks gestation undergoing induction of labor for hemolysis elevated liver enzymes low platelet syndrome (HELLP syndrome) with a platelet count of 60,000/mm³

   c. A 32-year-old G2P1001 at 39 weeks gestation with immune thrombocytopenic purpura (ITP) and a preoperative platelet count of 42,000/mm³

   d. A 38-year-old G1 at 28 weeks gestation with known ITP and a platelet count of 28,000/mm³ on her third-trimester labs

   e. A 24-year-old G2P0010 at 22 weeks gestation with a new diagnosis of thrombotic thrombocytopenic purpura (TTP) and a platelet count of 24,000/mm³

3. A 33-year-old G3P2002 presents at 29 weeks gestation to follow up on her third- trimester laboratory tests. She is accompanied by her youngest child who turned 1 3 days ago. You are reviewing her CBC and notice that her hematocrit is 29% with a mean corpuscular volume (MCV) of 75. Her platelets are normal. You look back at her hemoglobinopathy evaluation as it was normal. You tell her that she is anemic and she asks you what the cause could be. What test do you order to confirm your suspected diagnosis?

   a. Ferritin

   b. B₁₂ level

   c. Folate level

   d. Repeat hemoglobin electrophoresis

   e. Total iron-binding capacity

4. An 18-year-old G1 presents at 24 weeks gestation to the triage area. She has a headache and complains of being extremely fatigued in the past week. She has also noticed her feet swelling. She has been getting routine prenatal care and has had no issues until the past week. Her initial blood pressure is 157/98, pulse 116, respirations 16, and temperature 98.8°F(37.1C). Fetal heart rate is 150 with minimal variability and there are no contractions. You are concerned about preeclampsia and take bloods for laboratory testing and they return as follows: hematocrit 28%, platelets 40,000/mm³, aspartate amniontransferase (AST) 132, alanine aminotransferase (ALT) 117, creatinine 0.8, urine protein 3+, urine red blood cells 2+, lactate dehydrogenase (LDH) 530 IU/L, and uric acid 5 mg/dL. There are schistocytes on the peripheral blood smear and indirect bilirubin is 6 mg/dL. What is the most likely diagnosis and what test can you order to confirm this diagnosis?

   a. Preeclampsia without severe features/no other tests are needed

   b. Preeclampsia with severe features/no other tests are needed

   c. Acute fatty liver of pregnancy/serum glucose

   d. Thrombotic thrombocytopenia purpura (TTP)/ADAMTS13

   e. Placental abruption/fibrinogen

5. Which of the following patients does not require folic acid supplementation of 1 mg?

   a. A 22-year-old at 12 weeks gestation with sickle cell disease

   b. A 30-year-old seeing you for a preconception visit who terminated her first pregnancy at 20 weeks due to spina bifida

   c. A 19-year-old at 8 weeks gestation taking phenytoin for epilepsy

   d. A 28-year-old at 14 weeks with a dichorionic/diamniotic twin gestation

   e. A 34-year-old at 31 weeks gestation with a hematocrit of 29%, an MCV of 102, and a B_{12} level of 650 pg/mL

6. A G1 presents at 34 weeks gestation with increasing pain in her thighs and her back that she attributes to her sickle cell disease. Her pain related to her sickle cell disease has been difficult to manage during this pregnancy and at home she takes scheduled oxycodone extended release and hydromorphone as needed for breakthrough pain. She does not have any other medical problems and does not take any medication besides prenatal vitamins and folic acid. Her initial vital signs are as follows: temperature 101.8°F, pulse 123, respirations 26, oxygen saturation 92% on room air, and blood pressure 116/82. She appears uncomfortable. What is **not** an initial step in your management?

   a. Start supplemental oxygen

   b. Obtain IV access to begin IV hydration

   c. Chest X-ray

   d. Search for a possible infection source—urine culture, blood cultures, possible sputum culture

   e. Withhold pain medication until your examination is complete and you ensure she is not drug seeking

7. A 37-year-old G2P1100 from Southeast Asia presents for preconception counseling. Her first delivery was in Thailand and details are sparse. She thinks she delivered at term and the baby was very big and got stuck on the way out and passed away shortly after delivery. Her second delivery was in the United States and at the time of a growth ultrasound at 24 weeks gestation the fetus was noted to be hydropic, and was a fetal demise at 28 weeks gestation. She has had the same partner for both pregnancies. The only medical history she reports is anemia. She is not on iron because this has never fixed her anemia and she feels well. What is the most likely cause of her pregnancy outcome?

   a. Undiagnosed diabetes

   b. Anti-D antibodies

   c. Mitochondrial disorder

   d. Hemoglobin Bart

   e. Parvovirus B19 infections

8. A 20-year-old G0 originally from the Dominican Republic comes to see you for preconception counseling. Her medical history is significant for sickle cell disease, she has never had acute chest syndrome, and has only needed two transfusions and a handful of hospitalizations for pain management during pain crises. Her hematologist believes her disease is stable right now and it would be an optimal time to attempt pregnancy if she desires. You discuss with her sickle cell disease management in pregnancy and risks of carrying a pregnancy when she has sickle cell disease. Which of the following risks is **not** increased in women with sickle cell disease?

   a. Preterm premature rupture of membranes

   b. Intrauterine fetal demise

   c. Preeclampsia

   d. Deep vein thrombosis

   e. Abruption

9. An 18-year-old G1P1 presents to the emergency department (ED) 5 days postpartum with heavy vaginal bleeding. Approximately 2 hours ago she started having heavy vaginal bleeding while she was sitting down after feeding the baby. She has soaked through three pads since that time and the pants she is wearing now are also soaked. Her vaginal delivery was uncomplicated per her report, but she delivered at another hospital and was brought to your ED by ambulance because it was closest. You have no records on her in your system. The only medical history she reports to you is heavy menses and she says she was given a special medicine after delivery to help control her bleeding for a blood disorder. She is pale and her vitals are as follows: temperature 98.7°F, pulse 132, respirations 18, and blood pressure 97/58. In addition to sending a CBC, fibrinogen, and prothrombin time (PT)/partial thromboplastic time (PTT) what other lab should you send?

   a. ADAMTS13

   b. Factor VIII level

   c. LDH

   d. Factor IX level

   e. Anti-Xa level

10. A 26-year-old white G2P1000 presents at 10 weeks gestation. Her obstetric history is significant for a full-term vaginal delivery where after delivery the neonate was found to have severe grade IV intraventricular hemorrhages and ultimately demised in the first few weeks of life. She is terrified of this happening again. She has no other significant medical history and no one in her family has a problem with bleeding or blood clots. Her blood type is O−, she received Rho(D) immune globulin at the appropriate time intervals, and has never had a blood transfusion. The father of the baby is the same as the first pregnancy. What is the most likely responsible agent?

   a. Traumatic delivery

   b. Primary Parvovirus B19 infection

   c. Anti–HPA-1a antibodies

   d. Anti-D antibodies

   e. Intracranial arteriovenous malformation (AVM)

ANSWERS

1. Answer: e

(see *Gabbe's Obstetrics* 8e: ch49)

In pregnancy, the majority of cases of mild-to-moderate thrombocytopenia are caused by gestational thrombocytopenia. This form of thrombocytopenia has little likelihood of causing maternal or neonatal complications. The obstetrician, however, should rule out other etiologies of thrombocytopenia that are associated with severe maternal or perinatal morbidity. Women with gestational thrombocytopenia generally have a platelet count of $120,000-149,000/mm^3$. No treatment is needed for the mother and vaginal delivery is safe. Platelet transfusions should be reserved for a platelet count below $10,000/mm^3$ or less than $50,000/mm^3$ in the setting of surgery. If platelet counts continue to fall to levels below $50,000/mm^3$, other diagnoses should be entertained.

2. Answer: c

(see *Gabbe's Obstetrics* 8e: ch49)

The obstetrician need not act on the mother's platelet count unless it is below $30,000/mm^3$, if it is below $50,000/mm^3$ with evidence of clinical bleeding, or if surgery is anticipated. In these cases, the treatment depends on the diagnosis. Transfusing platelets in TTP is not recommended as it can worsen the thrombotic potential.

3. Answer: a

(see *Gabbe's Obstetrics* 8e: ch49)

The ferritin level indicates the total status of iron stores. Serum ferritin levels normally decrease minimally during pregnancy; however, a significantly reduced ferritin concentration is indicative of iron-deficiency anemia and is the best parameter to judge the degree of iron deficiency. Serum ferritin has 98% sensitivity and 98% specificity in diagnosing iron deficiency.

4. Answer: d

(see *Gabbe's Obstetrics* 8e: ch49)

To diagnose the hemolytic anemia associated with TTP, the patient must have a negative indirect antiglobulin (Coombs) test. This rules out an immune-mediated cause for the hemolytic anemia. LDH should be elevated, the indirect bilirubin should be increased, and haptoglobin should be decreased, indicating ongoing hemolysis. The neurologic findings in TTP are usually nonspecific. They include headache, confusion, and lethargy. A decrease of ADAMTS13 (the von Willebrand cleaving enzyme) activity is strongly associated with TTP. The platelet decrease with hemolytic uremic syndrome (HUS) is usually milder and commonly presents postpartum.

5. Answer: b

(see *Gabbe's Obstetrics* 8e: ch49)

Prenatal vitamins that require physician prescription contain 1 mg of folic acid, and most nonprescription prenatal vitamins contain 0.8 mg of folic acid. These amounts are more than adequate to prevent and treat folate deficiency. Women with significant hemoglobinopathies, patients taking anticonvulsant medications, women carrying a multiple gestation, and women with frequent conception may require more than 1 mg of supplemental folate daily. Often, 4 mg of folic acid is recommended daily because this is the dose that has been shown to reduce the risk of recurrent neural tube defects (NTDs).

6. Answer: e

(see *Gabbe's Obstetrics* 8e: ch49)

Analgesia, oxygen, and hydration are the clinical foundations for treating these painful crises, and physicians often underestimate the associated pain. Patients have often received many narcotics and may have a tolerance to the usual dosage of these medications. It is crucial to adequately treat this pain.

7. Answer: d

(see *Gabbe's Obstetrics* 8e: ch49)

Homozygous α-thalassemia results in the formation of tetramers of β-chains known as *hemoglobin Bart*. This hemoglobinopathy can result in hydrops fetalis. The American College of Obstetricians and Gynecologists (ACOG) recommends thalassemia screening for pregnant women with a low MCV and no evidence of iron deficiency. This finding is more common in women of Asian descent. α-Thalassemia is also amenable to prenatal diagnosis using quantitative polymerase chain reaction (PCR) or Southern blot analysis.

8. Answer: a

(see *Gabbe's Obstetrics* 8e: ch49)

Cerebral vein thrombosis, pneumonia, pyelonephritis, deep venous thrombosis, transfusion, postpartum infections, sepsis, and systemic inflammatory response syndrome (SIRS) are all more common in women with sickle cell disease. Pregnancy-related complications including hypertensive disorders, antepartum bleeding, abruption, preterm labor, growth restriction, and urinary tract infections are also more common in patients with sickle cell disease.

9. Answer: b

(see *Gabbe's Obstetrics* 8e: ch49)

Bleeding during pregnancy with von Willebrand disease is rare because levels of factor VIII and von Willebrand Factor (vWF) increase during pregnancy. However, shortly after delivery, they drop. If the factor VIII level is less than 50%, treatment during labor and delivery should be initiated. Hemorrhage can also occur several days postpartum. Therefore, factor VIII levels should be checked before the patient goes home after delivery. If a patient experiences a postpartum hemorrhage secondary to vWF, it will probably occur 3–5 days postpartum.

10. Answer: c

(see *Gabbe's Obstetrics* 8e: ch49)

This results in severe neonatal thrombocytopenia and possibly fetal intracranial hemorrhage. The mother, however, will have a normal platelet count. The most common antibodies noted in these patients are anti–HPA-1a antibodies, although several other antibodies have been identified. If this disorder is suspected, the mother's blood should be sent to a reference laboratory with experience in diagnosing neonatal alloimmune thrombocytopenia.

50

Thromboembolic Disorders in Pregnancy

Thaddeus P. Waters

(See *Gabbe's Obstetrics: Normal and Problem Pregnancies*, 8e: ch50)

QUESTIONS

1. Which of the following is most accurate regarding inheritable thrombophilias?

  a. MTHFR mutation is considered a "low-risk" thrombophilia.

  b. The majority are inherited in an autosomal recessive manner.

  c. Factor V Leiden is the least common mutation in the general population.

  d. Homozygosity for a thrombophilia mutation compared with heterozygosity increases the risk for a patient to have a venous thromboembolism (VTE).

2. A 40-year-old G1P1001 is 2 hours post cesarean delivery after a failed induction of labor. You are called to see her for bleeding from her incision site and vaginal bleeding. Upon assessing the patient, you evacuate 1000 mL of clot from the uterus and estimate her total blood loss with surgery to be 2200 mL. Her incision is actively bleeding and you also notice bleeding from her IV sites. In the setting of a substantial vascular insult, which of the following is inaccurate?

  a. Platelet action alone is often sufficient to provide hemostasis.

  b. Fibrin plug formation is a critical process to restore hemostasis.

  c. The key event of hemostasis occurs when thrombin cleaves fibrinogen to fibrin.

  d. Clotting is initiated by the binding of tissue factor to factor VII.

3. All of the following are accurate regarding the physiologic changes to the maternal hemostatic system except:

  a. Increases are seen in concentrations of fibrinogen and factors VII, VIII, IX, X, and XII.

  b. There is a 40%–60% decrease in the levels of free protein S, conferring an overall resistance to activated protein C.

  c. Levels of prothrombin and factors V, XIII, and XI double during pregnancy.

  d. Coagulation parameters begin to normalize as early as 3 weeks postpartum and return to baseline by 6–12 weeks postpartum.

4. A 25-year-old G2P0020 presents for prenatal care at 6 weeks. She reports a history of two prior spontaneous abortions at 6 weeks and 11 weeks. She denies any other significant medical history, including no personal history of a VTE. She reports her mother had a pulmonary embolism at age 40 while on oral contraceptive pills. Which of the following is most accurate regarding screening for antiphospholipid antibody syndrome (APS) in this patient?

  a. The patient's recurrent first-trimester losses warrant APS testing.

  b. The patient's history of a first-degree relative with a VTE warrants APS testing.

  c. The patient does not have an indication for APS testing.

  d. The patient's history of an 11-week pregnancy loss warrants APS testing.

5. A 36-year-old G3P0020 presents to the emergency room at 8 weeks with vaginal bleeding. An ultrasound is performed that identifies a pregnancy loss. She reports a history of two prior spontaneous losses at 6 weeks and 8 weeks gestation managed with a dilation and curettage (D&C) and no further evaluation. Her medical history is significant for a prior VTE outside of pregnancy and she is not taking anticoagulation at this time. Which of the following is the most appropriate next step in her management?

  a. Cytogenetic testing of the products of conception

  b. Anti-β2-glycoprotein (immunoglobulin G [IgG] and immunoglobulin M [IgM]) testing

  c. Anticardiolipin antibody (IgG and IgM) testing

  d. Testing for inheritable thrombophilias

285

6. A 22-year-old G1P0 at 29 weeks gestation presents to the emergency room complaining of a 2-day history of unilateral calf swelling and pain (left greater than right). Her pregnancy has otherwise been uncomplicated to date and she has no significant past medical history. She denies chest pain or shortness of breath. Which of the following is the most appropriate next step in her evaluation?

    a. Assessment of maternal D-dimer levels

    b. A lower extremity venous ultrasound evaluating for noncompressibility of the venous lumen

    c. Measurement of both lower leg circumferences for a difference of 3 cm or more to identify a high risk of VTE

    d. Obtaining screening for antiphospholipid antibodies and heritable thrombophilias

7. A 35-year-old G7P6006 at 12 weeks is referred to you for a history of a deep vein thrombosis (DVT) in her last pregnancy. Her thrombophilia workup was negative. Which of the following treatment options is most appropriate?

    a. Surveillance without anticoagulation antepartum and postpartum

    b. Prophylactic anticoagulation antepartum and surveillance postpartum

    c. Surveillance without anticoagulation antepartum and prophylactic anticoagulation postpartum

    d. Prophylactic anticoagulation antepartum and postpartum

8. An 18-year-old G2P0010 at 24 weeks is seen for transfer of care. She has a history of antithrombin III deficiency, a history of a DVT outside of pregnancy, and obesity (100 kg). Which is the MOST appropriate anticoagulation regimen for this patient?

    a. Enoxaparin 100 mg subcutaneuous (SC) daily

    b. Heparin 7500 units SC twice daily

    c. Heparin 10,000 units SC twice daily

    d. Warfarin 5 mg orally (po) daily

9. A 25-year-old G1P0 at 35 weeks gestation presents for a routine prenatal visit. Her pregnancy was complicated by a DVT in the first trimester, which has required treatment with therapeutic dosing of enoxaparin. She asks you if she can have an epidural in labor. The most appropriate response is:

    a. Yes, if your last dose of anticoagulation was more than 24 hours prior to your request.

    b. Yes, if your last dose of anticoagulation was at least 6 hours prior to your request

    c. No, because the risk of bleeding is too great

    d. Yes, depending on who the anesthesiologist is at the time of your admission

10. A 19-year-old G1P0 at 26 weeks presents to the emergency department complaining of chest pain and shortness of breath. She has not received prenatal care during this pregnancy. She is tachycardic and hypoxic. You recommend imaging for a suspected VTE. Which of the following imaging modalities has the **least** fetal radiation exposure?

    a. Full unilateral venography without an abdominal shield

    b. Chest X-ray without an abdominal shield

    c. Ventilation-perfusion scan

    d. Spiral computed tomography

ANSWERS

1. **Answer: d**

    (see *Gabbe's Obstetrics* 8e: ch50)

    Factor V Leiden is the most common mutation and accounts for over 40% of inherited thrombophilias in most studies. Most of these genetic mutations act in an autosomal-dominant manner, thus one mutation will incur an elevated risk for VTE and individuals with two mutations will have even higher risks for thrombotic events than those with one. Patients with a strong family history of thrombotic events who have screened negative for the panel of known thrombophilia mutations likely have an as yet unrecognized gene defect in a specific component of the coagulation cascade.

2. Answer: a

(see *Gabbe's Obstetrics* 8e: ch50)

Platelet action alone is insufficient to provide adequate hemostasis in the face of a substantial vascular insult; in this setting, the coagulation cascade—with resultant fibrin plug formation—is required to restore hemostasis.

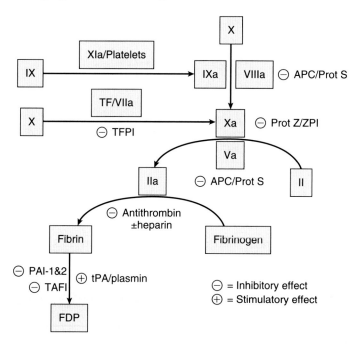

3. Answer: c

(see *Gabbe's Obstetrics* 8e: ch50)

A doubling occurs in circulating concentrations of fibrinogen, and 20%–1000% increases are seen in factors VII, VIII, IX, X, and XII, all of which peak at term in preparation for delivery. Levels of von Willebrand Factor (vWF) also increase up to 400% at term. In contrast, levels of prothrombin and factor V remain unchanged, and levels of factor XIII and XI decline modestly. Concomitantly, there is a 40%–60% decrease in the levels of free protein S, conferring an overall resistance to activated protein C.

4. Answer: d

(see *Gabbe's Obstetrics* 8e: ch50)

Overall, APS is responsible for approximately 14% of thromboembolic events in pregnancy. The diagnosis of APS requires the presence of prior or current vascular thrombosis or characteristic obstetric complications, together with at least one of the following laboratory criteria: anticardiolipin antibodies (IgG or IgM greater than 40 GPL [1 GPL unit is 1 μg of IgG antibody] or 40 MPL [1 MPL unit is 1 μg of IgM antibody] or greater than the 99th percentile), anti–β-2 glycoprotein-I (IgG or IgM greater than the 99th percentile), or lupus anticoagulant.

5. Answer: a

(see *Gabbe's Obstetrics* 8e: ch50)

Recurrent pregnancy loss is a potential clinical obstetric risk factor in the absence of other explanations. In this example, the patient is of advanced maternal age, and an evaluation for cytogenetic causes for her loss should be performed as the first step.

6. Answer: b

(see *Gabbe's Obstetrics* 8e: ch50)

The most accurate ultrasonic criterion for diagnosing venous thrombosis is noncompressibility of the venous lumen in a transverse plane under gentle probe pressure, using duplex and color flow Doppler imaging. The overall sensitivity and specificity of venous Doppler ultrasound (VUS) has been reported at 90%–100% for proximal vein thromboses, but traditionally it has been considered lower for the detection of calf vein thromboses.

7. Answer: d

(see *Gabbe's Obstetrics* 8e: ch50)

Risk stratification based on the likelihoods of recurrence (Table 50.1) is the essential foundation of the recommendations for antepartum and postpartum anticoagulation in patients without recent or active VTE. This issue is also summarized in Table 50.2. After this stratification, appropriate dosing is chosen (Table 50.3).

TABLE 50.1   Inherited Thrombophilias and Association With Venous Thromboembolism in Pregnancy.

Risk	Thrombophilia Type	Prevalence in the European Population	Prevalence in Patients with VTE in Pregnancy	RR/OR of VTE in Pregnancy (95% CI)	Probability of VTE in Pregnant Patients with Personal or Family HX	Probability of VTE in Pregnant Patients Without Personal or Family HX	Study
High risk	FVL homozygous	0.07%[a]	<1%[a]	25.4 (8.8–66)	≥10%	1.5%	1, 2–5
	Prothrombin gene G20210A mutation homozygous	0.02%[a]	<1%[a]	N/A	≥10%	2.8%	6, 7
	Antithrombin III deficiency	0.02%–1.1%	1%–8%	119	11%–40%	3.0%–7.2%	2, 5, 6
	Compound heterozygous (FVL/prothrombin G20210A)	0.17%+	<1%+	84 (19–369)	4.7% (overall probability of VTE in pregnancy)		1, 2, 8
Low risk	FVL heterozygous	5.3%	44%	6.9 (3.3–15.2)	>10%	0.26%	1, 2–4, 9
	Prothrombin G20210A mutation heterozygous	2.9%	17%	9.5 (2.1–66.7)	>10%	0.37%–0.5%	1, 2, 7, 8
	Protein C deficiency	0.2%–0.3%	<14%	13.0 (1.4–123)	N/A	0.8%–1.7%	2, 5, 6, 10
	Protein S deficiency	0.03%–0.13%	12.4%	N/A	N/A	<1%–6.6%	1, 2, 6, 11

[a]Calculated based on a Hardy-Weinberg equilibrium.
CI, Confidence interval; *FVL,* factor V Leiden; *HX,* history; *N/A,* data not available; *OR,* odds ratio; *PREG,* pregnant; *PROB,* probability; *PTS,* patients; *RR,* relative risk; *VTE,* venous thromboembolism.

TABLE 50.2   Anticoagulation in Pregnancy: Indications, Types, and Timing.

Indication	Description	Antepartum	Postpartum
VTE in current pregnancy		Therapeutic LMWH/UFH from diagnosis until delivery	Therapeutic LMWH/UFH regimen until 6 weeks postpartum
High-risk thrombophilia • FVL homozygous • Prothrombin G20210A mutation homozygous • FVL/prothrombin G20210A mutation double heterozygous • Antithrombin III deficiency	History of one prior VTE	Therapeutic or prophylactic LMWH/UFH	Therapeutic or prophylactic LMWH regimen or postpartum warfarin; dosing/level to match antepartum regimen
	No history of VTE	Prophylactic LMWH/UFH	Prophylactic LMWH or postpartum warfarin
Low-risk thrombophilia • FVL heterozygous • Prothrombin G20210A mutation heterozygous • Protein C deficiency • Protein S deficiency	History of one prior VTE	Prophylactic LMWH/UFH or surveillance without anticoagulation	Prophylactic LMWH/UFH or postpartum warfarin
	No history of VTE	Surveillance without anticoagulation or prophylactic LMWH/UFH	Surveillance without anticoagulation or prophylactic LMWH/UFH or postpartum warfarin if patient has additional risk factors
No thrombophilia	History of one prior VTE (pregnancy or estrogen-related)	Prophylactic or therapeutic LMWH/UFH	Prophylactic or therapeutic LMWH/UFH for 6 weeks
	History of one prior VTE (specific event, nonestrogen-related)	Surveillance without anticoagulation	Surveillance without anticoagulation or prophylactic LMWH if the patient has additional risk factors
Two or more prior VTE episodes (thrombophilia or no thrombophilia)	On long-term anticoagulation	Therapeutic LMWH/UFH	Resumption of long-term anticoagulation therapy
	Not on long-term anticoagulation	Therapeutic or prophylactic LMWH/UFH	Therapeutic or prophylactic LMWH/UFH for 6 weeks

FVL, Factor V Leiden; *LMWH,* low-molecular-weight heparin; *UFH,* unfractionated heparin; *VTE,* venous thromboembolism.
Reprinted with permission from Thromboembolism in pregnancy. ACOG Practice Bulletin No. 196. American College of Obstetricians and Gynecologists. *Obstet Gynecol* 2018;132:e1—17.

TABLE 50.3 Example Anticoagulation Regimens.

Type	Drug and Dosing	Surveillance
Prophylactic LMWH	Enoxaparin 40 mg SC once daily	*Consider* target anti-Xa levels of 0.1–0.2 U/mL 4 hours after injection
Therapeutic LMWH	Enoxaparin 1 mg/kg/12 h	Target anti-Xa levels of 0.6–1.0 U/mL tested 4 hours after injection
	Enoxaparin 1.5 mg/kg/24 h	Target anti-Xa levels of 1.2–1.5 U/mL tested 4 hours after injection
Prophylactic UFH	First trimester: UFH 5000–7500 units SC/12 h	aPTT should be in the normal range
	Second trimester: UFH 7500–10,000 units SC/12 h	*Consider* target heparin levels of 0.1–0.2 U/mL
	Third trimester: UFH 10,000 units SC/12 h	
Therapeutic UFH	≥UFH 10,000 U/12 h	Target aPTT in 1.5–2.5× control range tested 6 hours after injection
Warfarin (postpartum, therapeutic)	Begin 5–10 mg oral daily and titrate to INR target	Overlap UFH or LMWH therapy until INR is >2.0 for more than 2 days; target INR, 2.0–3.0
Prophylactic fondaparinux	2.5 mg oral daily	No monitoring guidelines

aPTT, Activated partial thromboplastin time; *INR,* international normalized ratio; *LMWH,* low-molecular-weight heparin; *SC,* subcutaneously; *UFH,* unfractionated heparin; *Xa,* activated factor X.

Modified from American College of Obstetricians and Gynecologists Practice Bulletin no. 196: Thromboembolism in Pregnancy. *Obstet Gynecol.* 2018;132(3):e1-e17; Horlocker TT, Vandermeulen E, Kopp SL, Gogarten W, Leffert LR, Benzon HT. Regional anesthesia in the patient receiving antithrombotic or thrombolytic therapy: American Society of Regional Anesthesia and Pain Medicine Evidence-Based Guidelines (Fourth Edition). *Reg Anesth Pain Med.* 2018;43:263-309.

8. **Answer: c**

(see *Gabbe's Obstetrics* 8e: ch50)

Risk stratification based on the likelihood of recurrence (Table 50.1) is the essential foundation of the recommendations for antepartum and postpartum anticoagulation in patients without recent or active VTE. This issue is also summarized in Table 50.5. After this stratification, appropriate dosing is chosen (Table 50.6).

9. **Answer: a**

(see *Gabbe's Obstetrics* 8e: ch50)

Regional anesthesia is contraindicated within 18–24 hours of therapeutic low-molecular-weight heparin (LMWH) administration. Accordingly, the authors recommend switching to unfractionated heparin (UFH) at 36 weeks or earlier if preterm delivery is expected. Protamine sulfate is not as effective in fully reversing the anti–factor Xa activity of LMWH, although it may reduce bleeding.

10. **Answer: b**

(see *Gabbe's Obstetrics* 8e: ch50)

A chest radiograph exposes the fetus to <0.01 rads. Table 50.3 outlines the fetal radiation exposure of different radiation modalities.

REFERENCES

1. Zotz RB, Gerhardt A, Scharf RE. Inherited thrombophilia and gestational venous thromboembolism. *Best Pract Res Clin Haematol.* 2003;16:243-259.
2. Gerhardt A, Scharf R, Beckmann M, et al. Prothrombin and factor V mutations in women with a history of thrombosis during pregnancy and the puerperium. *N Engl J Med.* 2000;342:374-380.
3. Juul K, Tybjaerg-Hansen A, Steffensen R, Kofoed S, Jensen G, Nordestgaard BG. Factor V Leiden: The Copenhagen City Heart Study and 2 meta-analyses. *Blood.* 2002;100:3-10.
4. Price DT, Ridker PM. Factor V Leiden mutation and the risks for thromboembolic disease: a clinical perspective. *Ann Intern Med.* 1997;127:895-903.
5. Franco R, Reitsma P. Genetic risk factors of venous thrombosis. *Hum Genet.* 2001;109:369-384.
6. Friedrich P, Sanson B, Simioni P, et al. Frequency of pregnancy-related venous thromboembolism in anticoagulant factor-deficient women: implications for prophylaxis. *Ann Intern Med.* 1996;125:955-960.

7. Aznar J, Vayá A, Estellés A, et al. Risk of venous thrombosis in carriers of the prothrombin G20210A variant and factor V Leiden and their interaction with oral contraceptives. *Haematologica.* 2000;85:1271-1276.

8. Emmerich J, Rosendaal FR, Cattaneo M, et al. Combined effect of factor V Leiden and prothrombin 20210A on the risk of venous thromboembolism—pooled analysis of 8 case-control studies, including 2310 cases and 3204 controls. Study Group for Pooled-Analysis in Venous Thromboembolism. *Thromb Haemost.* 2001;86:809-816.

9. Ridker PM, Miletich JP, Hennekins CH, Buring JE. Ethnic distribution of factor V Leiden in 4047 men and women. Implications for venous thromboembolism screening. *JAMA.* 1997;277: 1305-1307.

10. Vossen CY, Conard J, Fontcuberta J, et al. Familial thrombophilia and lifetime risk of venous thrombosis. *J Thromb Haemost.* 2004;2:1526-1532.

11. Goodwin A, Rosendaal FR, Kottke-Marchant K, Bovill EG. A review of the technical, diagnostic, and epidemiologic considerations for protein S assays. *Arch Pathol Lab Med.* 2002;126: 1349-1366.

51

Collagen Vascular Diseases in Pregnancy

Audrey Merriam

(See *Gabbe's Obstetrics: Normal and Problem Pregnancies*, 8e: ch51)

QUESTIONS

1. A 27-year-old G0P0 comes to see you for preconception counseling. She has a diagnosis of systemic lupus erythematosus (SLE) and no significant past surgical history. Her SLE has been difficult to control but she is now on azathioprine and steroid courses as needed for flares. Her last flare was 2 months ago, and she has not needed steroids since then. Her flares typically present with arthritis, thrombocytopenia, oral ulcers, and worsening of her malar rash. Her baseline creatinine is 0.8 mg/dL and she has recently tested positive for SS-A antibodies. She would like to start conceiving immediately and is not currently using anything for contraception with her partner. What is the most predictive factor of how she will do in pregnancy?

   a. Her creatinine level

   b. SS-A antibody positive

   c. Azathioprine use

   d. Flare within the past 6 months

   e. Thrombocytopenia

2. You are seeing a 24-year-old G3P0202 for her first prenatal visit. Her pregnancy history is complicated by two cesarean deliveries at 30 and 32 weeks gestation, respectively, due to preeclampsia with severe features. Her medical history is significant for Systemic Lupus Erythematosus (SLE) complicated by lupus nephritis. This was an unplanned pregnancy but she is pleased about her current pregnancy. Her creatinine is now 2.4 mg/dL, which is close to her baseline of 2.0 mg/dL, and a random urine protein:creatinine ratio is 4.3. What is her greatest risk in this pregnancy?

   a. Fetal growth restriction

   b. Development of preeclampsia

   c. Worsening, irreversible renal disease

   d. Spontaneous preterm delivery

   e. Anuria

3. You are seeing a 34-year-old G1P0 at 35 weeks gestation. Her pregnancy has been complicated by SLE. She had been found to have SS-A and SS-B antibodies in this pregnancy and had been followed by PR intervals on fetal echocardiogram to screen for the development of fetal heart block. She is thrilled that the fetal heart rate has remained normal thus far and is celebrating that she is "in the clear" and that her baby won't be affected by her lupus. How do you counsel her at this time?

   a. The fetus is most likely to develop heart block between 34 weeks gestation and delivery, so you still must monitor the PR interval closely.

   b. There is a 15%–20% chance of the infant developing neonatal lupus, most likely manifesting as a plaque-like rash.

   c. There is a 15%–20% chance of the infant developing neonatal lupus, most likely manifesting as thrombocytopenia, hemolytic anemia, and hepatosplenomegaly.

   d. You celebrate with her and confirm there is no residual risk to the fetus.

   e. The risk for fetal heart block is greatest after delivery when the fibroelastosis develops.

4. You are seeing a 27-year-old woman for her first prenatal visit at 8 weeks gestation. She has had one prior pregnancy that ended in cesarean delivery at 26 weeks due to pre-eclampsia with severe features. The infant subsequently died from complications from necrotizing enterocolitis after a 3-week NICU stay. She has had normal blood pressure since that time. After that delivery she had an-tiphospholipid antibody testing and was found to be sig-nificantly positive for anticardiolipin IgM on two separate occasions 12 weeks apart. She is very nervous about this pregnancy and wants to do everything she can to have a successful pregnancy. What treatment do you offer her?

   a. Aspirin 81 mg beginning at 12 weeks gestation

   b. Aspirin 81 mg with glucocorticoids beginning now

   c. Aspirin 81 mg starting now and prophylactic-dose low-molecular-weight heparin

   d. Aspirin 162 mg and prophylactic-dose low-molecular-weight heparin

   e. Aspirin 162 mg, prophylactic-dose low-molecular-weight heparin and intravenous immunoglobulin (IVIG)

5. You are seeing a 37-year-old G1P0 at 20 weeks gestation for a routine prenatal visit. Her medical history is significant for rheumatoid arthritis (RA). She was taking daily predni-sone and nonsteroidal antiinflammatories (NSAIDs) prior to pregnancy to help control her symptoms. Since becom-ing pregnant she is surprised that she does not have any joint pain despite not taking prednisone or NSAIDs daily. What do you tell her about the likely course of her symp-toms after delivery and long-term, since she is not on medication during pregnancy?

   a. This is a sign her disease will continue to be in remis-sion postpartum and for the rest of her life.

   b. This is a sign her disease symptoms will continue to be under control without medication for 6–12 months after delivery but will return after that.

   c. This is a sign her disease symptoms will continue to be under control without medication for 6–12 months after delivery but her joint disease will worsen after that because pregnancy negatively impacts the long-term course of RA.

   d. Her disease symptoms will likely flare within the first 3 months postpartum and her joint disease will worsen after that because pregnancy negatively impacts the long-term course of RA.

   e. Her disease symptoms will likely flare within the first 3 months postpartum but pregnancy and the potential flare postpartum will not impact her long-term course with RA.

6. A 24-year-old G1 presents for her first prenatal visit at 14 weeks gestation. This is an unplanned but desired preg-nancy. She has not had much medical care since leaving home at 18 years old and does not have any significant medical issues. On your review of systems she admits to drinking a lot of water and using eye drops multiple times a day for dry eyes for the past year. Her BMI is normal, and her examination is unremarkable. In addition to pre-natal laboratory tests, what other tests should you consider ordering, given her symptoms and possible diagnosis?

   a. SS-A and SS-B antibodies

   b. Lupus anticoagulant

   c. Baseline preeclampsia labs (Complete Blood Count [CBC], creatinine, liver function tests [LFTs], and urine protein:creatinine ratio)

   d. C3 and C4 levels

   e. 1-hour glucose challenge test (GCT) to screen for diabetes

7. Which of the following patients would NOT have a diag-nosis of antiphospholipid antibody syndrome (APS)?

   a. A 29-year-old G3P0030 who has had three spontane-ous abortions at 6, 9, and 7 weeks, respectively, and who has positive lupus anticoagulant testing twice on labs drawn 14 weeks apart

   b. A 29-year-old G3P0010 who has a spontaneous demise of a 16-week fetus requiring a dilation and evacuation (D&E), and who has positive β-2–glycoprotein IgG twice on labs drawn 12 weeks apart

   c. A 32-year-old G1P0100 whose previous delivery oc-curred at 28 weeks gestation due to preeclampsia with severe features, complicated by a neonatal birth weight of 550 g and subsequent neonatal demise, who had a positive anticardiolipin IgM at the time of her previ-ous delivery

   d. A 32-year-old G0 with a history of a spontaneous left upper extremity arterial thrombus with positive β-2–glycoprotein IgG twice on labs drawn 1 year apart

   e. A 32-year-old G1P0100 whose previous delivery oc-curred at 28 weeks gestation due to preeclampsia with severe features, complicated by a neonatal birth weight of 550 g and subsequent neonatal demise, who had a positive anticardiolipin IgM at the time of her previ-ous delivery and again 6 months later

8. A 35-year-old G0 comes to see you for preconception counseling. She has a history of rheumatoid arthritis cur-rently controlled on methotrexate. She is getting married next month and wants to start trying to conceive shortly thereafter because she is "old." She is still having regular menstrual cycles every 30 days. She has seen her rheuma-tologist and they plan to switch her from methotrexate to etanercept after her visit with you. How long should she wait between discontinuation of methotrexate and at-tempting to conceive to decrease potential pregnancy risk?

   a. She can attempt conception immediately

   b. 1 month

   c. 3 months

   d. 6 months

   e. 1 year

ANSWERS

1. Answer: d

(see *Gabbe's Obstetrics* 8e: ch51)

Flares in pregnancy most commonly manifest as fatigue, joint pain, rash, and proteinuria. Assessing anti-double-stranded (ds)DNA titers and complement (C3 and C4) levels may provide additional evidence of disease flares in women with clinical symptoms. The routine assessment of anti-dsDNA and complement levels in *asymptomatic* women is of limited utility. Active lupus within 6 months of conception is associated with a four-fold increase in pregnancy loss and 58% risk for flare. Women with SLE should be counseled to delay pregnancy until their disease has been in remission for at least 6 months.

2. Answer: c

(see *Gabbe's Obstetrics* 8e: ch51)

Women with lupus nephritis, particularly active disease, are at especially increased risk for adverse pregnancy outcomes that include hypertensive disorders of pregnancy, disease flares, low birthweight infants, and indicated preterm delivery. How well women tolerate pregnancy is related to disease quiescence at conception. A serum creatinine level of 2.0 mg/dL or greater is considered by some to be an absolute contraindication to pregnancy, because of the risk of pregnancy complications requiring iatrogenic extreme preterm birth (PTB) and the threat to long-term renal function.

3. Answer: b

(see *Gabbe's Obstetrics* 8e: ch51)

Neonatal lupus (NLE) most commonly presents as an erythematous, scaling, plaque-like rash that begins in the early neonatal period and may persist for 1–2 months. Less common manifestations of NLE include hematologic abnormalities (leukopenia, hemolytic anemia, thrombocytopenia) and hepatosplenomegaly. Infants of women with anti-Ro/SS-A and anti-La/SS-B antibodies have a risk of 15%–20% of the newborn developing a manifestation of neonatal lupus.

4. Answer: c

(see *Gabbe's Obstetrics* 8e: ch51)

As defined by the international criteria, at least one clinical criterion and positive antiphospholipid antibodies are required for the diagnosis of definite APS (Box 51.1). The combination of a heparin agent and low dose aspirin (LDA) is the current recommended treatment for APS in pregnancy (Box 51.2) because it serves to provide maternal thromboprophylaxis and may improve pregnancy outcomes. Ideally aspirin is started preconceptionally because of its possible beneficial effects on implantation. Because some patients with APS have immune thrombocytopenia, the platelet count should be assessed prior to starting treatment. Heparin is usually begun in the early first trimester after demonstrating either an appropriately rising serum human chorionic gonadotropin or the presence of a live embryo on ultrasonography.

BOX 51.1   Revised Classification Criteria for the Antiphospholipid Antibody Syndrome[a]

Clinical Criteria

Vascular Thrombosis[b]

1. One or more clinical episodes of arterial, venous, or small-vessel thrombosis in any tissue or organ *and*
2. Thrombosis confirmed by objective, validated criteria (i.e., unequivocal findings of appropriate imaging studies or histopathology) *and*
3. For histopathologic confirmation, thrombosis should be present without significant evidence of inflammation in the vessel wall

Pregnancy Morbidity

1. One or more unexplained deaths of a morphologically normal fetus at or beyond the 10th week of gestation, with normal fetal morphology documented by ultrasound or by direct examination of the fetus *or*
2. One or more premature births of a morphologically normal neonate at or before the 34th week of gestation because of eclampsia or severe preeclampsia or placental insufficiency[c] *or*

3. Three or more unexplained consecutive spontaneous abortions before the 10th week of gestation with maternal anatomic or hormonal abnormalities and paternal and maternal chromosomal causes excluded

Laboratory Criteria

1. Lupus anticoagulant present in plasma on two or more occasions at least 12 weeks apart, detected according to the guidelines of the International Society on Thrombosis and Hemostasis
2. Anticardiolipin antibody of IgG and/or IgM isotype in blood present in medium or high titer (i.e., >40 GPL or MPL or >99th percentile) on at least two occasions at least 12 weeks apart, measured by standardized ELISA
3. Anti-β2–glycoprotein I antibody of IgG and/or IgM isotype in serum or plasma (in titer >99th percentile) present in medium or high titer on at least two occasions at least 12 weeks apart, measured by standardized ELISA

ELISA, Enzyme-linked immunosorbent assay; *GPL, IgG* phospholipid units; *Ig*, immunoglobulin; *MPL*, IgM phospholipid units.
[a]Must meet at least one clinical and one laboratory criterion for diagnosis of "definite" APS.
[b]Superficial venous thrombosis is not included in the clinical criteria.
[c]Features of placental insufficiency may include: (1) abnormal or nonreassuring fetal surveillance, such as a nonreactive nonstress test; (2) abnormal Doppler flow in the umbilical artery (e.g. absent end-diastolic flow); (3) oligohydramnios; or (4) infant birthweight below the 10th percentile for gestational age.
Modified from Miyakis S, Lockshin MD, Atsumi T, et al. International consensus statement on an update of the classification criteria for definite antiphospholipid syndrome (APS). *J Thromb Haemost.* 2006;4:295-306.

BOX 51.2 Recommended Treatment Regimens for Antiphospholipid Syndrome during Pregnancy

Recurrent Preembryonic and Embryonic Loss, No History of Thrombotic Events

Low-dose aspirin alone *or* together with:
- UFH 5000–7500 Units every 12 hours *or*
- LMWH (usual prophylactic doses)

Prior Fetal Death or Preterm Delivery Because of Severe Preeclampsia or Severe Placental Insufficiency, No History of Thrombotic Events

Low-dose aspirin plus:
- UFH 7500–10,000 U every 12 hours in the first trimester and 10,000 U every 12 hours in the second and third trimesters *or*
- UFH administered every 8–12 hours at a dose to maintain the midinterval aPTT[a] at 1.5 times the control mean *or*
- LMWH (usual prophylactic doses)

Anticoagulation Regimens for Women With a History of Thrombotic Events

Low-dose aspirin plus:
- UFH administered every 8–12 hours to maintain the midinterval aPTT[a] or anti-Xa activity in the therapeutic range *or*
- LMWH (preferred)
  - Weight-adjusted therapeutic doses (e.g., enoxaparin 1 mg/kg/12 h or dalteparin 200 U/kg/12 h)

LMWH, Low molecular weight heparin; *UFH*, unfractionated heparin.
[a]Women without a lupus anticoagulant in whom the activated partial thromboplastin time (aPTT) is normal can be monitored with the aPTT. Women with lupus anticoagulant should be monitored with antifactor Xa activity.

5. Answer: e

(see *Gabbe's Obstetrics* 8e: ch51)

The majority of women, perhaps as many as 80%–90%, experience some improvement in their RA symptoms during pregnancy, although only 50% have more than moderate improvement. Improvements in joint pain and stiffness generally begin in the first trimester and persist through several weeks postpartum. Most women who experience an improvement in symptoms during pregnancy will relapse postpartum, typically in the first 3 months. It does not appear that pregnancy has any significant effects on the long-term course of RA.

6. Answer: a

(see *Gabbe's Obstetrics* 8e: ch51)

Sjögren syndrome (SS) is a chronic autoimmune disorder characterized by decreased lacrimal and salivary gland function, which leads to dry eyes and dry mouth. Extraglandular manifestations commonly include fatigue, arthralgias, myalgias, and Raynaud's phenomenon. Women with SS may have a somewhat increased risk of several adverse pregnancy outcomes, including miscarriage, PTB, low birth weight, and neonatal death. Up to 70% of women with SS are positive for anti-Ro/SS-A antibodies, with the accompanying risks for NLE and congenital heart block.

7. Answer: c

(see *Gabbe's Obstetrics* 8e: ch51)

APS diagnosis criteria include at least one of the following clinical criteria: vascular thrombosis, three consecutive spontaneous abortions <10 weeks gestation with normal chromosomes, premature birth of a normal infant complicated by eclampsia, preeclampsia with severe features, or signs of placental insufficiency, and/or one or more unexplained deaths of a normal fetus >10 weeks gestation. In addition, patients must have one of the following laboratory findings: positive lupus anticoagulant, elevated β-2–glycoprotein IgG and/or IgM, or elevated anticardiolipin IgG and/or IgM on two sets of tests drawn 12 weeks apart.

8. Answer: c

(see *Gabbe's Obstetrics* 8e: ch51)

Methotrexate is an abortifacient and is known to be teratogenic. Pregnancy should be delayed three menstrual cycles after drug discontinuation.

52

Hepatic Disorders During Pregnancy

Rini Banerjee Ratan

(See *Gabbe's Obstetrics: Normal and Problem Pregnancies*, 8e: ch52)

QUESTIONS

1. Which of the following laboratory profiles is most consistent with normal physiologic changes in the third trimester of pregnancy?

   a.

Albumin	↓
alanine aminotransferase (ALT)	↔
aspartate aminotransferas (AST)	↔
Alkaline Phosphatase	↑
Total bile acids	↕

   b.

Albumin	↓
ALT	↔
AST	↔
Alkaline Phosphatase	↑
Total bile acids	↕

   c.

Albumin	↓
ALT	↑
AST	↑
Alkaline Phosphatase	↑
Total bile acids	↔

   d.

Albumin	↑
ALT	↓
AST	↓
Alkaline Phosphatase	↓
Total bile acids	↓

2. A 38-year-old G1P0 at 35 weeks gestation presents to her obstetrician's office with generalized pruritis that has been increasing in intensity. She feels itchy all over, but it is worst in her hands and feet and wakes her from sleep at night. She reports good fetal movement. She denies contractions, vaginal bleeding, loss of fluid, or abdominal pain. Physical examination is unremarkable. Blood pressure is 120/70. Her abdomen is soft, nontender, and gravid. Minimal striae are present. Her hands and feet are normal in appearance—no rash is visible. Which of the following laboratory tests is most likely to confirm the diagnosis?

   a. Direct bilirubin

   b. Indirect bilirubin

   c. Bile acids

   d. Alkaline phosphatase

   e. Gamma-glutamyl transpeptidase (GGTP)

3. A 27-year-old G1 P0 woman at 39 weeks gestation presents to the labor and delivery unit with regular, painful contractions every 3–5 minutes. Her past medical history is notable for chronic Hepatitis C. Her liver function tests have been normal during pregnancy, and her viral load is undetectable. Testing for HIV has been negative. Her cervix is 3 cm dilated, 50% effaced, with the vertex at 0/5 station. Spontaneous rupture of membranes for clear fluid occurs upon arrival. Fetal heart rate is category I. What is the risk of vertical transmission of Hepatitis C to the neonate?

   a. <2%

   b. 5%

   c. 20%

   d. 10%–40%

   e. 70%–90%

4. A 34-year-old nulliparous woman presents to her physician's office for preconception counseling. She has a history of portal hypertension and would like to become pregnant. She has had one variceal hemorrhage in the past, requiring endoscopic band ligation of bleeding varices. Her blood pressure in the office is 130/80. Which of the following is the most appropriate recommendation regarding pregnancy for this patient?

   a. Endoscopic evaluation in the first trimester

   b. Caesarean delivery advised to reduce likelihood of bleeding

   c. Risk of splenic artery rupture is high

   d. Risk of recurrent variceal hemorrhage is low

   e. Initiation of beta-blocker therapy to decrease portal pressure

5. A 29-year-old G1P0 with a dichorionic diamniotic twin gestation at 36 weeks gestation presents to the labor and delivery unit with 6 hours of worsening nausea, vomiting, and epigastric abdominal pain. Her pregnancy has been otherwise uncomplicated to date. Both twins are concordant and appropriately grown. She went on vacation to the Caribbean 3 weeks ago. Blood pressure is 140/86. Scleral icterus and jaundice are present and the abdominal examination is notable for epigastric and right upper quadrant tenderness. Deep tendon reflexes are normal. Fetal heart rates are both category I. Serum laboratory studies are shown here:

White Blood Cell Count (WBC) 16.0	ALT 387 u/L	lactate dehydrogenase (LDH) 235 mg%
Hematocrit 36%	AST 428 u/L	Glucose 58 mg/dL
Hemoglobin 11.6 g/dL	Total bilirubin 4.4 μmol/L	Ammonia 105 µmol/L
Platelets 122,000/mm^3	Direct bilirubin 2.6 µmol/L	Creatinine 1.5 mg/dL

   Which of the following is the most likely diagnosis?

   a. characterized by hemolysis, elevated liver enzyme levels and a low platelet count (HELLP) syndrome

   b. Acute fatty liver of pregnancy (AFLP)

   c. Autoimmune hepatitis

   d. Viral hepatitis

   e. Preeclampsia with severe features

6. A 40-year-old G3P2 at 28 weeks gestation presents to the labor and delivery unit with increasing abdominal pain over the past 3 hours. The pain started after she ate fried chicken and French fries for lunch. The pain is in her right upper abdomen and radiates to her back. She says it is beginning to subside now, but she has had several similar episodes over the past 4 weeks, usually after eating. On examination she is afebrile and well appearing. Blood pressure is 120/70. Her abdomen is soft with positive Murphy sign. No rebound or guarding is noted. Fetal heart rate on nonstress test is reactive. complete blood count (CBC) is normal. Serum ALT, AST, and amylase are slightly elevated. Right upper quadrant ultrasound shows a thickened gallbladder wall, pericholestatic fluid, and stones. Which of the following is the most appropriate next step in management?

   a. Amoxicillin-clavulanate therapy

   b. Ursodeoxycholic acid therapy

   c. Magnetic resonance cholangiopancreatography (MRCP)

   d. Expectant management

   e. Laparoscopic cholecystectomy

ANSWERS

1. **Answer: a**

   (see *Gabbe's Obstetrics* 8e: ch52)

   During pregnancy, the serum alkaline phosphatase level normally increases mildly as a result of placental synthesis; the serum albumin level also declines, primarily from hemodilution and secondarily from decreased hepatic synthesis. The serum aminotransferase levels are largely unaffected by pregnancy. Changes of serum levels of common blood tests during pregnancy are summarized in Table 52.1.

TABLE 52.1 Normal Physiologic Changes in Liver Tests in Pregnancy by Trimester.

Test	First Trimester	Second Trimester	Third Trimester
Albumin	↓	↓	↓
ALT	↔	↔	↔
AST	↔	↔	↔
Alkaline Phosphatase	↔	↑	↑
GGT	↔	↓	↓
Total bile acids	↔	↔	↔
Prothrombin time	↔	↔	↔

2. Answer: c

(see *Gabbe's Obstetrics* 8e: ch52)

Intense pruritis that begins in the late second or third trimester of pregnancy, affecting mostly the hands and feet, in the absence of abdominal pain, should lead to an evaluation of intrahepatic cholestasis of pregnancy (ICP). ICP is a diagnosis of exclusion. The most sensitive marker for diagnosis is an elevated serum bile acid level.[1] Patients typically exhibit hyperbilirubinemia that is mild and predominantly conjugated; about 10% of patients develop jaundice. The serum level of alkaline phosphatase is modestly elevated, and the level of GGTP is normal.

3. Answer: a

(see *Gabbe's Obstetrics* 8e: ch52)

Chronic hepatitis C has little impact on pregnancy with overall favorable outcomes. The risk of vertical transmission of hepatitis C from a chronically infected mother with viremia to the neonate is about 5%.[2–5] This rate of vertical transmission is much lower than that for hepatitis B. In women with undetectable viral loads, perinatal transmission is <2%. In contrast, women with HIV coinfection can have hepatitis C transmission rates as high as 20%.[6,7]

4. Answer: e

(see *Gabbe's Obstetrics* 8e: ch52)

In women with portal hypertension considering pregnancy, endoscopy prior to pregnancy can aid in risk assessment of variceal bleeding in pregnancy.[8] In women with preexisting varices, risk of variceal bleeding in pregnancy is higher. Beta-blocker therapy has been shown to decrease portal pressure, thereby decreasing risk of variceal bleeding. Women who do not undergo endoscopic evaluation prior to pregnancy should have an EGD in the early second trimester of pregnancy. Cesarean delivery is typically reserved for routine obstetric indications due to concern for increased surgical bleeding from abdominal and pelvic collateral vessels due to portal hypertension.[8] Pregnant patients with portal hypertension should undergo an ultrasound examination with Doppler studies of the upper abdomen to screen for splenic artery aneurysms at the time of their routine antenatal pelvic ultrasound.

5. Answer: b

(see *Gabbe's Obstetrics* 8e: ch52)

AFLP almost exclusively occurs in the third trimester of pregnancy, with a median gestational age of 36 weeks. Risk factors include primiparity, multiple gestation, and low body mass index[8–10] Presenting symptoms include nausea, vomiting, epigastric abdominal pain, anorexia, and jaundice. On physical examination, women experience right upper quadrant or epigastric pain. Approximately half of these women will have preeclampsia; therefore, there is some overlap with HELLP syndrome.[11–13] Aminotransferase levels can range from slightly above normal to 1000, but usually range between 300–500 units/L.[11] Bilirubin is almost always increased, but usually less than 5 mg/dL. Hypoglycemia and hyperammonemia can occur.

6. Answer: d

(see *Gabbe's Obstetrics* 8e: ch52)

Most cases of biliary colic and some cases of mild acute cholecystitis can be managed conservatively with close observation, expectant management, and deferral of surgery to the immediate postpartum period.[14]

REFERENCES

1. Walker IA, Nelson-Piercy C, Williamson C. Role of bile acid measurement in pregnancy. *Ann Clin Biochem.* 2002;39:105-113.
2. Su GL. Hepatitis C in pregnancy. *Curr Gastroenterol Rep.* 2005;7:45-49.
3. Gibb DM, Goodall RL, Dunn DT, et al. Mother-to-child transmission of hepatitis C virus: evidence for preventable peripartum transmission. *Lancet.* 2000;356:904-907.
4. Polywka S, Pembrey L, Tovo PA, Newell ML. Accuracy of HCV-RNA PCR tests for diagnosis or exclusion of vertically acquired HCV infection. *J Med Virol.* 2006;78:305-310.
5. Mast EE, Hwang LY, Seto DS, et al. Risk factors for perinatal transmission of hepatitis C virus (HCV) and the natural history of HCV infection acquired in infancy. *J Infect Dis.* 2005;192:1880-1889.
6. Polis CB, Shah SN, Johnson KE, Gupta A. Impact of maternal HIV coinfection on the vertical transmission of hepatitis C virus: a meta-analysis. *Clin Infect Dis.* 2007;44:1123-1131.
7. Marine Barjoan E, Berrebi A, Giordanengo V, et al. HCV/HIV coinfection, HCV viral load and mode of delivery: risk factors for mother-to-child transmission of hepatitis C virus? *AIDS.* 2007;21:1811-1815.
8. Tran TT, Ahn J, Reau NS. Corrigendum: ACG Clinical Guideline: Liver disease and pregnancy. *Am J Gastroenterol.* 2016;111:176-194; quiz 196.
9. Reyes H, Sandoval L, Wainstein A, et al. Acute fatty liver of pregnancy: a clinical study of 12 episodes in 11 patients. *Gut.* 1994;35:101-106.
10. Browning MF, Levy HL, Wilkins-Haug LE, Larson C, Shih VE. Fetal fatty acid oxidation defects and maternal liver disease in pregnancy. *Obstet Gynecol.* 2006;107:115-120.
11. Hay JE. Liver disease in pregnancy. *Hepatology.* 2008;47:1067-1076.
12. Moldenhauer JS, O'Brien JM, Barton JR, Sibai B. Acute fatty liver of pregnancy associated with pancreatitis: a life-threatening complication. *Am J Obstet Gynecol.* 2004;190:502-505.
13. Mabie WC. Obstetric management of gastroenterologic complications of pregnancy. *Gastroenterol Clin North Am.* 1992;21:923-935.
14. Date RS, Kaushal M, Ramesh A. A review of the management of gallstone disease and its complications in pregnancy. *Am J Surg.* 2008;196:599-608.

53

Gastrointestinal Disorders During Pregnancy

Thaddeus P. Waters

(See *Gabbe's Obstetrics: Normal and Problem Pregnancies*, 8e: ch53)

QUESTIONS

1. A 40-year-old G2P0 presents at 8 weeks for prenatal care. She has a history of infertility and conceived with in vitro fertilization. In performing a review of systems, the patient reports having a significant change in her diet and she believes her appetite for certain foods has changed. She is very concerned this could reflect an undiagnosed neurologic problem. All of the following are accurate regarding changes in taste perception during pregnancy except:

   a. Changes in taste perception are very common.

   b. The majority of changes in taste perception occur in the first trimester.

   c. Changes in taste reflect an increase in threshold for various taste sensations.

   d. Most women report a greater desire for sour and bitter foods than they might have prior to pregnancy.

2. A 24-year-old G3P1011 presents for a routine obstetric visit at 24 weeks gestation. Her past medical history and prenatal care are uncomplicated to date. The patient reports progressive increase in a burning sensation in her throat, particularly at night, which often leads to a non-productive cough. Which of the following is inaccurate regarding her current condition?

   a. The main alteration to the esophagus during pregnancy is the reduction in lower esophageal sphincter (LES) tone.

   b. Human placental lactogen is believed to mediate changes to the maternal esophagus.

   c. Gastric compression by the enlarged gravid uterus is contributing to the patient's symptoms.

   d. First-line recommendations should be dietary and lifestyle modifications.

3. The patient referenced previously presents at 30 weeks gestation reporting that her initial changes to her diet and limiting food intake close to her bedtime improved her symptoms, however they have now recurred and are persistent throughout the day. As part of her routine obstetric care, the patient also had a recent complete blood count test that noted a hemoglobin of 9.7 g/dL with a mean corpuscular volume of 78. A serum ferritin is 3 ng/mL. All of the following are accurate statements in this situation except:

   a. The patient should initiate treatment with a histamine$_2$ receptor antagonist (H2RA).

   b. Both a H2RA and a proton pump inhibitor (PPI) are recommended with initiation of oral iron with both medications taken at the same time.

   c. Among H2RAs, the most widely studied in pregnancy is ranitidine.

   d. PPIs such as omeprazole are safe to use in all trimesters of pregnancy.

4. A 37-year-old G2P0010 presents for initial obstetric care at 10 weeks gestation. Her past medical history is significant for Crohn disease, for which the patient is taking Humira (adalimumab). All of the following are appropriate counseling for this patient except:

   a. The use of antiintegrin biologics is not recommended as treatment for inflammatory bowel disease (IBD) during pregnancy due to risks of congenital malformations.

   b. Unlike ulcerative colitis, Crohn disease is a transmural process that can involve all of the layers of the bowel wall, with risks of complications such as abscess or fistula formation.

   c. Cesarean delivery is an appropriate recommendation for all women with Crohn disease with active perianal disease.

   d. Adverse pregnancy outcomes for women with IBD may include increased risk of miscarriage, stillbirth, preterm birth, and low birth weight infants.

5. All of the following are accurate regarding nutritional support during pregnancy except:

   a. Enteral nutrition is the preferred method of nutritional support when adequate oral intake is unlikely within 7 days.

   b. Current guidelines recommend consideration of specialized nutritional support for pregnant women when patients are not expected to resume volitional intake within 7 days.

   c. Potential risks of total parenteral nutrition include risks of catheter-related infection.

   d. Parenteral nutrition can be administered from peripheral or central venous access.

6. A 19-year-old G1P0 presents with fever, nausea, vomiting, and abdominal pain. Your clinical examination is significant for abdominal tenderness in the right lower quadrant. Your primary concern is a possible appendicitis. Which of the following is the most accurate in this setting?

   a. Computerized tomography (CT) imaging is the preferred radiologic imaging test to evaluate for an appendicitis.

   b. Ultrasound imaging is an appropriate first-line test, due to a high sensitivity and specificity >80% well described in pregnancy.

   c. Ultrasound findings of an appendicitis include appendiceal mural thickening and periappendiceal fluid.

   d. Appendicitis is reasonably excluded if an abnormal appendix is not identified by ultrasound.

7. All of the following are accurate regarding splenic artery aneurysm rupture during pregnancy except:

   a. Splenic artery aneurysm rupture is rare, with no change in frequency of occurrence during pregnancy and similar distribution of cases by trimester.

   b. Maternal and fetal mortality rates are both >50%.

   c. Treatment consists of volume resuscitation, ligation of splenic artery, and possible splenectomy.

   d. Surgery should be considered even for asymptomatic cases.

8. A 42-year-old obese G1P0 presents for evaluation of nausea and vomiting of pregnancy. Her past medical history is significant for a prior Roux-en-Y procedure 3 years prior. She reports progressive emesis, midline abdominal pain, and decreased appetite. Which of the following is incorrect regarding her situation?

   a. The diagnosis for the patient would be confirmed by radiographic findings of distended bowel loops that contain air-fluid levels, with an abrupt transition between distended and nondistended bowel.

   b. Surgery is recommended in all cases of obstruction due to maternal and fetal risks of expectant care.

   c. Placement of a nasogastric tube is indicated at this time.

   d. Bowel obstruction is a common cause of nonobstetric abdominal emergencies during pregnancy.

ANSWERS

1. Answer: d

(see *Gabbe's Obstetrics* 8e: ch53)

Changes in taste perception and dysgeusia are very common, affecting over 90% of women in some studies. The majority of changes in taste perception occur in the first trimester. For the most part, these changes reflect an increase in threshold for various taste sensations, which may explain why it is common for women to seek out saltier or sweeter foods than they might have prior to pregnancy.

2. Answer: b

(see *Gabbe's Obstetrics* 8e: ch53)

Heartburn occurs in 30%–50% of pregnancies, and is more common later in pregnancy. The development of gastroesophageal reflux disease (GERD) is due to several factors, including: hypotonic LES due to estrogen and progesterone; delayed gastrointestinal transit; gastric compression; and increased intraabdominal pressure by the uterus. Treatment for GERD begins with lifestyle modifications, including avoiding caffeine, alcohol, smoking cigarettes, and nonsteroidal antiinflammatory use.

3. Answer: **b**

(see *Gabbe's Obstetrics* 8e: ch53)

Gastric acid secretions are necessary for absorption of iron, and a large case-control study showed an association between the use of acid-suppressing medications (such as H2RA and PPI medications) and iron-deficiency anemia. This is particularly of concern for women who are already taking oral iron therapy for a diagnosis of iron-deficiency anemia, and they should be instructed to take the two medications at different times from one another.

4. Answer: **a**

(see *Gabbe's Obstetrics* 8e: ch53)

In partnership with the Society for Maternal-Fetal Medicine, the American Gastroenterological Association IBD Parenthood Project Working Group has recently published a care pathway which details recommendations for care throughout pregnancy of the patient with IBD and is available at http://www.ibdparenthoodproject.gastro.org/ (Box 53.1). Newer agents for IBD include antiintegrin biologics (natalizumab and vedolizumab) and ustekinumab (a biologic directed against interleukin (IL) 12/23). For all these newer agents, data are limited, but from both IBD and other registries, there does not appear to be any increased risk for congenital malformations or adverse pregnancy outcomes.

5. Answer: **d**

(see *Gabbe's Obstetrics* 8e: ch53)

Parenteral nutrition describes intravenous delivery of nutrition and calories, bypassing the gastrointestinal tract. It is divided into partial and total parenteral nutrition, depending on whether some or all of the daily nutritional requirements are being given intravenously. Peripheral parenteral nutrition is no longer recommended, so the decision to give parenteral nutrition always requires placement of central

---

BOX 53.1 Preconception Checklist

- Establish care with obstetrician, gastroenterologist, maternal fetal medicine specialist, primary care physician.
- Update health care maintenance including surveillance colonoscopy if needed
- Check labs including complete blood count, iron panel, vitamin D, folate, vitamin b12, baseline fecal calprotectin.
- Adjust regimen to discontinue inappropriate medications (methotrexate, Asacol HD, steroids) and wean off of steroids to achieve steroid free remission
- Ensure IBD is in remission (colonoscopy if appropriate)
- Communicate consistent message among all providers and patient

---

venous access, which brings with it concerns for infection, thrombosis, and other complications.[1]

6. Answer: **c**

(see *Gabbe's Obstetrics* 8e: ch53)

Although CT is the preferred imaging test in nonpregnant patients because of its high diagnostic accuracy, sonography is often the initial imaging test of choice during pregnancy to avoid fetal exposure to radiation from CT. Ultrasound has a reported 86% sensitivity and 81% specificity in the diagnosis of appendicitis in nonpregnant adults or adolescents, but the sensitivity is likely lower in pregnant adults. Diagnostic findings on ultrasound include appendiceal mural thickening, periappendiceal fluid, and a noncompressible tubular structure 6 mm or more in diameter that is closed at one end and open at the other. Appendicitis cannot be excluded if the appendix is not visualized on ultrasound.

7. Answer: **a**

(see *Gabbe's Obstetrics* 8e: ch53)

Splenic artery aneurysm rupture is rare overall but occurs more frequently in pregnancy, especially during the third trimester. Several physiologic changes during pregnancy contribute to this increased risk, including increases in splanchnic and splenic arterial flow related to compression of the aorta and iliac vessels by the gravid uterus, increased blood volume and cardiac output, and the effects of the gestational hormones on the elastic properties of the arterial wall. Patients can range from asymptomatic with incidental findings of splenic artery aneurysms found on imaging studies to sudden diffuse abdominal pain. The diagnosis is made by imaging studies, such as abdominal ultrasound, CT scan, magnetic resonance imaging, or during surgery following a rupture. Treatment consists of volume resuscitation, ligation of splenic artery, and splenectomy for emergency cases. As the maternal mortality rate is as high as 75% and the fetal mortality rate 95%, surgery should be considered even for asymptomatic cases.[2]

8. Answer: **b**

(see *Gabbe's Obstetrics* 8e: ch53)

Along with acute appendicitis and acute cholecystitis, bowel obstruction is among the top three most common causes of nonobstetric abdominal emergencies, with an incidence of 1 per 1500–16,000.[3–6] The approach to intestinal obstruction is the same in pregnancy as in the general population, except that decisions are more urgently required because both the fetus and the mother are at risk. Surgery is recommended for unremitting and complete intestinal obstruction, whereas medical management is recommended for intermittent or partial obstruction.

REFERENCES

1. McClave SA, DiBaise JK, Mullin GE, Martindale RG. ACG clinical guideline: nutrition therapy in the adult hospitalized patient. *Am J Gastroenterol*. 2016;111:315-334.
2. Ha JF, Phillips M, Faulkner K. Splenic artery aneurysm rupture in pregnancy. *Eur J Obstet Gynecol Reprod Biol*. 2009;146:133-137.
3. Bouyou J, Gaujoux S, Marcellin L, et al. Abdominal emergencies during pregnancy. J Visc Surg. 2015;152:S105-115.
4. Connolly MM, Unti JA, Nora PF. Bowel obstruction in pregnancy. *Surg Clin North Am*. 1995;75:101-113.
5. Pandolfino J, Vanagunas A. Gastrointestinal complications of pregnancy. In: and G, ed. *Sciarra JJ*. Philadelphia: Lippincott Williams & Wilkins; 2003:1-14.
6. Perdue PW, John HW Jr, Stafford Pw. Intestinal obstruction complicating pregnancy. *Am J Surg*. 1992;164:384-388.

54

Neurologic Disorders in Pregnancy

Eva K. Pressman

(See *Gabbe's Obstetrics: Normal and Problem Pregnancies*, 8e: ch54)

QUESTIONS

1. The most frequent major neurologic complication encountered in pregnancy is:

   a. Epilepsy

   b. Multiple sclerosis (MS)

   c. Myasthenia gravis

   d. Muscular dystrophy

   e. Stroke

2. A 24-year-old nulligravid woman comes to the office to discuss planning a pregnancy. She has a history of generalized epilepsy since childhood but has not had a seizure in 2 years. She currently takes valproate, which she has been on for many years. She has been using a copper intrauterine device (IUD) for contraception. What is the most appropriate advice regarding her medication therapy?

   a. Continue her current dose of valproate after removing the IUD until she has a positive pregnancy test, then discontinue it rapidly.

   b. Continue her valproate after removing her IUD and throughout pregnancy, increasing her dose if seizures recur.

   c. Work with her neurologist to switch her to lamotrigine prior to discontinuing the IUD and then continue lamotrigine through the pregnancy.

   d. Work with her neurologist to wean her off valproate over the next few months and observe for 9 months prior to removing the IUD.

   e. Advise her that risks to her and her fetus are too high to recommend pregnancy and she should continue using her IUD.

3. The antiepileptic drug (AED) associated with the highest risk of major congenital malformation (MCM) is:

   a. Carbamazepine

   b. Lamotrigine

   c. Levetiracetam

   d. Phenytoin

   e. Valproate

4. A 25-year-old G1P0 presents for prenatal care at 8 weeks gestation. She has a history of seizures and has been stable on lamotrigine, 200 mg twice daily, for 6 months prior to pregnancy and her last lamotrigine level, just prior to pregnancy, was therapeutic at 5 µg/dL. What is the most appropriate plan for therapeutic drug monitoring (TDM)?

   a. Continue her current dose and check levels each trimester.

   b. Continue her current dose and check levels monthly.

   c. Increase her dose by 50% and check levels each trimester.

   d. Decrease her current dose by 50% and check levels monthly.

   e. Discontinue her lamotrigine and do not follow levels.

5. A 28-year-old G2P0010 comes to the office to discuss planning a pregnancy. She has had epilepsy since childhood, which has been well controlled on carbamazepine for the last year, with only one seizure about 3 months ago. She has previously received counseling about the risks of fetal anomalies with epilepsy and carbamazepine but asks if there are other pregnancy complications she should be aware of. Which of the following responses most accurately describes her risks compared with the general population?

   a. She is at increased risk for preeclampsia.

   b. She is at decreased risk for preterm delivery.

   c. She is at increased risk for fetal macrosomia.

   d. She is at decreased risk for postpartum hemorrhage.

   e. Her neonate is at increased risk for intracranial hemorrhage.

6. A 26-year-old nulligravid woman comes to the office for a health maintenance visit. She has a history of epilepsy and reports two seizures in the last 12 months. Her only current medication is levetiracetam. She indicates she would like to get pregnant within the next year. Which of the following statements is most accurate?

   a. Her seizure frequency is likely to be unchanged during pregnancy.

   b. She should switch her medication to valproate prior to pregnancy.

   c. She should be on at least two antiepileptic medications.

   d. The risk her child will have epilepsy is 25%.

   e. Cesarean delivery is recommended to prevent seizure in labor.

7. Folic acid supplementation has been recommended prior to conception and during pregnancy for women who take AEDs for which of the following reasons?

   a. Low folic acid levels decrease the risk of congenital malformations.

   b. AEDs are known to lower folic acid levels.

   c. Folic acid supplementation is associated with lower risk of autism.

   d. Supplementation has been associated with reduction in maternal anemia.

   e. Folic acid supplementation reduces the risk for neural tube defects (NTDs).

8. A 29-year-old G2P0010 is brought to the labor and delivery unit by ambulance after experiencing a generalized seizure at home. She is currently at 38 weeks gestation and has never experienced a seizure before. On arrival she is awake but confused, blood pressure is 140/90, pulse 105, respiratory rate 18, fetal heart rate (FHR) 140 bpm, and reactive. She is no longer seizing. What is the most appropriate treatment at this time?

   a. Initiation of magnesium sulfate

   b. Intubation to protect her airway

   c. Immediate cesarean delivery

   d. Intravenous (IV) antihypertensive therapy

   e. Betamethasone for fetal lung maturation

9. A 24-year-old G1P0 comes to the office at 20 weeks gestation for a routine prenatal visit. Her pregnancy has been uncomplicated. Her medical history includes epilepsy since age 19 that has been well controlled with carbamazepine. She asks about the safety of breastfeeding on her current medications. Which is the best reply?

   a. Breastfeeding on carbamazepine has been associated with better neurodevelopmental outcomes than not breastfeeding.

   b. In general, the risks of neonatal exposure to AEDs through breast milk outweigh the benefits of breastfeeding.

   c. Levels of anticonvulsant medications are expected to fall in the first few weeks after delivery so higher doses will be required.

   d. Pumping breast milk may increase her sleep deprivation which can increase the risk of seizures.

   e. Switching to phenobarbital during breastfeeding is recommended since it has a longer half-life.

10. A 29-year-old G1P0010 comes to the office to discuss planning a pregnancy. Her medical history includes relapsing MS that has been stable for the last 6 months without therapy and she is concerned about how pregnancy might affect the frequency of relapses. Which of the following statements is most appropriate?

    a. MS relapse rates decrease during the first trimester.

    b. MS relapse rates decrease during the third trimester.

    c. MS relapse rates decrease for 3 months postpartum.

    d. MS relapse rates increase in the second trimester.

    e. Pregnancy will increase relapse rates long term.

11. A 27-year-old nulligravid woman comes to the office to discuss planning a pregnancy. She was diagnosed with MS 1 year ago, which is currently well controlled on glatiramer acetate, and she is using a copper IUD for contraception. She asks what she should do about her MS medication in regard to the removal of her IUD. Which is the most appropriate statement?

    a. Continue her current medication after removing the IUD and through her pregnancy.

    b. Discontinue her glatiramer 6 months prior to removing her IUD.

    c. Work with her neurologist to switch her to fingolimod prior to discontinuing the IUD and then continue fingolimod through the pregnancy.

    d. Discontinue her current medication at the same time or shortly before removing her IUD.

    e. Advise her that risks to her and her fetus are too high to recommend pregnancy and she should continue using her IUD.

12. A 24-year-old G1P0 woman comes to the office for a routine prenatal visit at 20 weeks gestation. Her pregnancy has been uncomplicated and her only medical history is migraine headaches, which started 10 years ago, occur once or twice per month, and are preceded by a visual aura. She is not currently on any medication for her migraines, which have decreased in frequency and severity over the last 2 months. Prior to pregnancy she took sumatriptan as needed. She is concerned about adverse pregnancy outcomes related to her migraine headaches. Which of the following statements most accurately reflects her risks relative to patients without migraine headaches?

    a. She is at decreased risk for ischemic stroke in pregnancy.

    b. She is at decreased risk for venous thromboembolism.

    c. She is at increased risk for delivering postdates.

    d. She is at increased risk for preeclampsia.

    e. Her risks for pregnancy complications are not changed.

13. A 29-year-old G3P2012 comes to the Emergency Department 4 days after an uncomplicated vaginal delivery, with a progressive unremitting headache that is worse when she lies down. Her temperature is 37.0°C (98.6 F), blood pressure is 118/68, pulse 88 bpm, and respiration rate 16. She did have an epidural catheter placed for labor analgesia. Laboratory tests are all within normal limits, though her urine specific gravity is 1.032. Which of the following diagnostic tests are most likely to confirm the diagnosis?

    a. CT scan of the lumbar spine

    b. Epidural blood patch

    c. Fundoscopic examination

    d. Lumbar puncture

    e. Magnetic resonance imaging (MRI/MRV) of the brain

14. A 38-year-old G3P2002 at 32 weeks gestation comes to the Emergency Department with headache, acute onset of weakness in her right arm, and difficulty speaking. Her medical history reveals chronic hypertension and hypercholesterolemia. Over the next 30 minutes her symptoms resolve and a noncontrast CT of her head reveals an area of ischemia in the distribution of a distal branch of the left middle cerebral artery. What is the most appropriate treatment for this patient?

    a. Low-dose aspirin

    b. IV recombinant tissue plasminogen activator (tPA)

    c. Embolectomy

    d. Magnesium sulfate

    e. Emergent cesarean delivery

ANSWERS

1. **Answer: a**

   (see *Gabbe's Obstetrics* 8e: ch54)

   Epilepsy affects approximately 1% of the general population and is the most frequent major neurologic complication encountered in pregnancy. Many of the AEDs used to treat epilepsy are also used to treat psychiatric and pain disorders and are commonly prescribed to women of childbearing age; this makes an understanding of their implications for pregnancy imperative for any clinician managing these patients.

2. **Answer: d**

   (see *Gabbe's Obstetrics* 8e: ch54)

   Most women with epilepsy will need to remain on AEDs during their childbearing years and throughout pregnancy. Exceptions include patients with childhood epilepsy, which can remit in adulthood. In select cases of adult-onset epilepsy, patients who have been seizure free for 2–4 years may attempt to wean from seizure medications under a neurologist's supervision. Seizure freedom in the 9 months prior to pregnancy predicts a good chance of seizure control during pregnancy. Thus in an appropriate patient who wanted to stop AED therapy before pregnancy, weaning her off seizure medication should be started at least 1 year before becoming pregnant. Unfortunately, if not carefully counseled, women with epilepsy may abruptly stop all medications as soon as they find out that they are pregnant, which puts both the mother and fetus at risk.

3. Answer: e

(see *Gabbe's Obstetrics* 8e: ch54)

Of these drugs, valproate has been consistently demonstrated to carry a risk of MCMs significantly greater than that of other AEDs and baseline population rates, typically 1%–3% depending on the study population. Compared with control pregnancies, those exposed to valproate monotherapy were at statistically significant increased risk for spina bifida (OR, 12.7), craniosynostosis (OR, 6.8), cleft palate (OR, 5.2), hypospadias (OR, 4.8), atrial septal defects (OR, 2.5), and polydactyly (OR, 2.2). It has also been clearly associated with adverse cognitive and behavioral developmental outcomes.

4. Answer: b

(see *Gabbe's Obstetrics* 8e: ch54)

Many factors—including altered protein binding, changes in plasma volume, changes in the volume of distribution, and even folic acid supplementation—can affect the levels of anticonvulsant medications. Additionally, changes in AED metabolism can be dramatically altered by the pregnant state. In many cases, decreasing AED levels during pregnancy have been associated with loss of seizure control. TDM, or monitoring blood levels and adjusting medication doses correspondingly, is thus useful for many AEDs during pregnancy. Given the interindividual variation in AED metabolism and susceptibility to changes during pregnancy, most experts recommend checking AED drug levels at least monthly for all AEDs and adjusting the patient's dose to keep the patient's level near her prepregnancy therapeutic baseline.

5. Answer: a

(see *Gabbe's Obstetrics* 8e: ch54)

Women with epilepsy may be at increased risk for obstetric complications, though data on obstetric outcomes have been mixed. Population studies from the United States and Norway have associated epilepsy with an increased risk of complications, including a mild to moderate risk of preeclampsia (OR, 1.59–1.7). In a US-based population study there was an increased risk of preterm labor, defined as labor before 37 weeks, in women with epilepsy compared with women without epilepsy (OR, 1.54; 95% CI, 1.50–1.57). Evidence was also sufficient to suggest a near twofold increased risk of small for gestational age infants born to epileptic women taking AEDs compared with infants born to women without epilepsy. A large US-based population study of 5109 women found no difference in rates of postpartum hemorrhage or neonatal bleeding complications when the infant is supplemented with vitamin K.

6. Answer: a

(see *Gabbe's Obstetrics* 8e: ch54)

The patient should be informed that if she has frequent seizures before conception, this pattern will probably continue. Valproate is a poor first choice as an AED for any woman of childbearing age. In addition to the adverse effects on pregnancy, valproate is associated with weight gain, hirsutism, and signs of polycystic ovarian syndrome. On average, the risk of passing on epilepsy is 2.69%–8%. In children of women with generalized epilepsy, the incidence was 8.34% (1.36%–15.36% risk, considering standard error), and if the mother had focal epilepsy, the incidence was 4.43% (1.43%–7.43%). Induction of labor and cesarean delivery should not be recommended to women with epilepsy without specific additional obstetric, medical, or neurologic indications. Most women with epilepsy have successful vaginal deliveries. The risk of seizures during labor in women with epilepsy is 3.5% or less, and seizures are most common in patients who have had seizures during pregnancy.

7. Answer: b

(see *Gabbe's Obstetrics* 8e: ch54)

The 2009 American Academy of Nursing (AAN) practice guidelines recommend folic acid supplementation prior to conception and during pregnancy for all women who take AEDs. These recommendations are largely extrapolated from studies that have demonstrated that folic acid supplementation reduces the risk for NTDs in the general population. Additionally, low first-trimester serum folic acid levels have been correlated with an increased risk for congenital malformations in the offspring of women with epilepsy, and several AEDs are known to lower folic acid levels. A study that surveyed a population-based cohort of Norwegian mothers found that use of folic acid early in pregnancy/preconception was associated with a lower likelihood of language delay at 18 months. A study of women without epilepsy found delayed psychomotor development in children of women exposed to doses greater than 5 mg compared with women who took doses of 0.4–1 mg, which raises concerns about the practice of high-dose supplementation.

8. Answer: a

(see *Gabbe's Obstetrics* 8e: ch54)

Occasionally, seizures are diagnosed for the first time during pregnancy, which may present a diagnostic dilemma. If the seizures occur in the third trimester, they are considered to be eclampsia until proven otherwise and should be treated as such until the physician can perform a proper evaluation. It is often difficult to distinguish eclampsia from an epileptic seizure. The patient may be hypertensive initially after an epileptic seizure and may exhibit some myoglobinuria secondary to muscle breakdown, which will show up as proteinuria on a routine urinalysis. The diagnosis becomes clearer over time, but in either case, rapid, thoughtful action must be undertaken. The first physician to attend a patient after a seizure may not be an obstetrician/gynecologist, and thus magnesium sulfate may not be started acutely; this should be remedied as soon as possible.

9. Answer: a

(see *Gabbe's Obstetrics* 8e: ch54)

The levels of anticonvulsant medications must be monitored frequently during the first few weeks postpartum because they can rise rapidly. The benefits of breastfeeding have been well established and include the promotion of mother-infant bonding. Whereas AEDs taken by the mother are present in breast milk to varying degrees, few data suggest neonatal harm from exposure through breast milk. The Neurodevelopmental Effects of Antiepileptic Drugs (NEAD) study[1] found that infants exposed to carbamazepine, lamotrigine, phenytoin, and valproate in breast milk had higher IQs and language scores at 6 years than those infants whose mothers did not breastfeed. An improvement in parent-reported developmental abilities of children was also noted in breastfed infants in the Norwegian cohort of AED-exposed children at 6 and 18 months, although the effect was not sustained at 36 months.[2] Neither study found adverse effects on developmental outcomes related to breast milk exposure for the studied drugs (carbamazepine, lamotrigine, phenytoin, and valproate). Although further prospective studies of AED exposure via breast milk are necessary, for most AEDs, the theoretic concern of prolonged infant exposure likely does not outweigh the known benefits of breastfeeding. Sleep deprivation associated with trying to feed a newborn may increase the patient's risk for seizures. A key part of managing a pregnancy in women with epilepsy is discussing seizure safety with her and her family. Partners or other members of a patient's support system should assist with night feedings with either pumped milk or formula so that the patient can get a stretch of uninterrupted sleep, typically 6–8 hours depending on the patient.

10. Answer: b

(see *Gabbe's Obstetrics* 8e: ch54)

MS relapse rates decrease during the second and third trimesters of gestation but increase in the first trimester and postpartum. The protective effect of pregnancy may be explained in part by a pregnancy-induced shift from thymus helper 1 (Th 1) cytokines to Th 2 cytokines to facilitate immune tolerance. The Pregnancy in Multiple Sclerosis (PRIMS)[3] study prospectively followed 269 pregnancies in 254 women with MS across 12 European countries. The study found that the annual rate of relapse declined during pregnancy, especially in the third trimester. A rebound of disease activity was noted in the first 3 months postpartum, but subsequently the relapse frequency returned to baseline. Of note, the rate of relapse over the entire pregnancy year—9 months gestation plus 3 months postpartum—did not differ from the baseline rate, and only 28% of patients experienced a postpartum relapse. Despite the transient increase in postpartum relapses seen in women with MS, pregnancy likely has a neutral effect on long-term disease progression.

11. Answer: d

(see *Gabbe's Obstetrics* 8e: ch54)

Patients should be reassured that the vast majority of women with MS can have healthy pregnancies and that MS in the mother does not pose an adverse risk to the fetus. Glatiramer acetate is a large macromolecule that likely does not pass the placenta. While avoiding DMT in pregnancy is preferred, it is increasingly accepted that glatiramer acetate can be continued during pregnancy if needed. Given the long-term effects and half-lives of some oral agents such as fingolimod, it is recommended that they be stopped prior to discontinuation of contraception.

12. Answer: d

(see *Gabbe's Obstetrics* 8e: ch54)

Women with a history of migraine are at increased risk for preeclampsia, gestational hypertension, and thrombotic disorders. A systematic review of 17 studies found that migraine was associated with an increased risk of gestational hypertension (OR, 1.23–1.68), preeclampsia (OR, 1.08–3.5), and ischemic stroke in pregnancy (OR, 7.9–30.7). Only a few studies have examined birth and delivery outcomes in patients with primary headache disorders. One retrospective study from a nationwide population-based database in Taiwan identified 4911 women with migraines who delivered from 2001 to 2003. After adjusting for confounders, a significant increased risk for low birthweight (OR, 1.16; 95% CI, 1.02–1.31) and preterm birth (OR, 1.24; 95% CI, 1.13–1.39) was found.

13. Answer: **e**

(see *Gabbe's Obstetrics* 8e: ch54)

Cerebral venous thrombosis (CVT) is estimated to complicate 9.1%–11.6% of 100,000 pregnancies, and the majority of CVT occur in the postpartum period. In patients with CVT, the chief symptoms are similar to those of idiopathic intracranial hypertension (IIH) because the initial manifestations are due to increased intracranial pressure. Patients typically present with a subacute, progressive, unremitting headache that may be worse when lying down. CVT can be misdiagnosed as a postepidural headache, and this should be considered in the differential diagnosis. When CVT has a positional component, it should be worse lying and better standing, whereas a low-pressure headache often exhibits the reverse. MRI and MRV of the brain are the diagnostic tests of choice, and IV contrast is not needed to make the diagnosis.

14. Answer: **a**

(see *Gabbe's Obstetrics* 8e: ch54)

Ischemic stroke typically presents with acute focal neurologic symptoms. Headache can be present in 17%–34% of cases. The workup should be done swiftly and starts with a noncontrast CT of the head. In most cases of acute ischemic stroke where tPA would reduce morbidity and mortality outside of pregnancy, tPA should be considered after careful counseling of the patient and/or her caregiver(s). For strokes due to small vessel disease/atherosclerosis, low-dose aspirin is usually recommended.

REFERENCES

1. Meador KJ. Breastfeeding and antiepileptic drugs. *JAMA*. 2014;311(17):1797-1798. doi:10.1001/jama.2014.967.
2. Veiby G, Engelsen BA, Gilhus NE. Early child development and exposure to antiepileptic drugs prenatally and through breastfeeding: a prospective cohort study on children of women with epilepsy. *JAMA Neurol*. 2013;70(11):1367-1374. doi:10.1001/jamaneurol.2013.4290.
3. Confavreux C, Hutchinson M, Hours MM, Cortinovis-Tourniaire P, Moreau T. Rate of pregnancy-related relapse in multiple sclerosis. Pregnancy in Multiple Sclerosis Group. *N Engl J Med*. 1998;339(5):285-291.

55

Malignant Diseases and Pregnancy

Thaddeus P. Waters

(See *Gabbe's Obstetrics: Normal and Problem Pregnancies*, 8e: ch55)

QUESTIONS

1. A 39-year-old G2P1001 was scheduled for laparoscopic surgery for an ovarian mass suspicious for malignancy but her surgery was cancelled due to a positive urine pregnancy test. She comes to your office for a consult and you confirm that she is 15 weeks pregnant. Which of the following is an inaccurate statement?

    a. Surgery may be safely performed during all three trimesters.

    b. Surgery in the second trimester is preferred to limit the risk of first-trimester loss but allow for adequate visualization.

    c. Data suggests that pregnant patients may safely undergo laparoscopic surgery during pregnancy.

    d. The minimum pneumoperitoneum pressure required in pregnancy is 10–13 mm Hg.

2. A 32-year-old had thyroidectomy and radiation therapy 3 days prior. You are called for an urgent consult because her urine pregnancy test today was positive. Transvaginal ultrasound demonstrates a small empty gestational sac consistent with 3–4 weeks. Which of the following is most accurate for this patient?

    a. She needs a diagnostic laparoscopy for suspected ectopic pregnancy.

    b. If the pregnancy continues, it is likely to be normal due to an "all or none" phenomenon.

    c. Dilitation and curetage (D&C) is recommended for her miscarriage due to her surgery and radiation exposure.

    d. The recommended limit of radiation exposure in pregnancy is 0.1–0.2 Gy.

3. A 41-year-old G3P0020 at 24 weeks is admitted for chemotherapy. You are attending a multidisciplinary conference with oncology and pharmacy to discuss the pharmacokinetics of her chemotherapy. Which of the following is most accurate regarding her chemotherapy?

    a. Enhanced renal clearance and hepatic metabolism of pregnancy may reduce active drug concentrations.

    b. The amniotic fluid may act as a pharmacologic third space, decreasing maternal and/or fetal toxicity.

    c. Decreased gastrointestinal motility will improve the absorption of orally administered medications.

    d. Plasma albumin increases in pregnancy, thus increasing the amount of drug binding.

4. A 29-year-old G1P0 at 10 weeks gestation presents for her initial prenatal visit. Her family history is significant for three first-degree relatives diagnosed with breast cancer before the age of 30. On her physical examination, you note minimal blood nipple discharge. She does monthly breast examinations and has never noticed it before today. Which of the following is incorrect?

    a. Breast abnormalities should be evaluated in the same manner as if the patient were not pregnant.

    b. Bilateral serosanguinous nipple discharge may be normal in all trimesters of pregnancy.

    c. The risk of congenital malformations is estimated to be 10%–25% when chemotherapy is administered in the first trimester.

    d. The risk of teratogenicity from chemotherapy in the second and third trimester is likely no different from pregnant women who are not exposed to chemotherapy.

5. A 32-year-old G1P0 at 30 weeks gestation is seen in triage for complaints of night sweats, pruritis, and weight loss. Examination demonstrates a palpable lymph node in her neck. Biopsy is consistent with Hodgkin lymphoma (HL). Which of the following is most accurate regarding this patient?

    a. Splenectomy is required during pregnancy to improve maternal outcomes.

    b. Termination of pregnancy is routinely recommended when diagnosed prior to viability.

    c. Routine evaluation includes a single anterior/posterior view chest radiograph with abdominal shielding.

    d. The survival rate for early-stage HL is about 50%, thus treatment should not be withheld during pregnancy.

6. A 39-year-old G2P0010 presented to prenatal care at 8 weeks gestation. She reported spotting within the last week. Her pap smear result was high-grade squamous intraepithelial lesion (HGSIL). She was referred to gynecology oncology who performed a colposcopy and cervical biopsy. Endocervical curettage (ECC) was not performed. Pathology demonstrated microinvasion. She had a cone biopsy performed at 16 weeks with a prophylactic cerclage placed. Pathology demonstrated microinvasion <3 mm in depth with negative margins. She had a chest X-ray with abdominal shielding, renal ultrasound, and noncontrast MRI performed for staging. Her staging was IA1. She is now 20 weeks gestation, with a normal level II ultrasound. Which of the following is most accurate regarding this patient's management?

   a. In patients with stage I disease with negative margins, delays in therapeutic intervention have not been reported to increase recurrence rates.
   b. Definitive therapy with pregnancy termination is recommended given her staging and gestational age.
   c. ECC should have been performed in order to avoid delay of diagnosis.
   d. Cone biopsy during pregnancy should ideally be performed during the first trimester to avoid risks of periviable delivery.

7. You are called to the Emergency Department to evaluate a 49-year-old G2P1001 who presented complaining of severe nausea/emesis and abnormal vaginal discharge. Her examination was significant for a fundal height of 20 cm and a speculum examination with dark grape-like discharge. Transvaginal ultrasound demonstrates a uterine cavity filled with a heterogeneous mass with a "snowstorm" appearance and without an identifiable pregnancy. Which of the following is most accurate regarding this patient?

   a. Her recurrence risk is 25% with her next pregnancy.
   b. Cytogenetics on the products of conception are consistent with a 46,XY paternal homologous chromosomal pattern.
   c. Following evacuation of the uterus, she will need weekly β-human chorionic gonadotropin (β-hCG) until the hCG titer is within normal limits for 3 months, then monthly for 6–12 months.
   d. The risk of requiring chemotherapy is about 20%.

8. A 33-year-old G2P0010 presents at 7 weeks gestation for her initial prenatal visit. She has no significant history. Her physical examination is significant for a raised, irregular mole on her upper shoulder which she believes has increased in size over the last year. You send her to dermatology, and a biopsy confirms malignant melanoma. Which of the following is most accurate?

   a. The incidence of malignant melanoma has been decreasing, with an incidence of about 1%–3% in pregnant or lactating women.
   b. Treatment of localized disease during pregnancy is surgical excision with appropriate margins, with sentinel or complete lymph node dissection if indicated.
   c. Melanoma in pregnancy is associated with an aggressive clinical course even when correcting for tumor thickness.
   d. Therapeutic abortions for advanced disease in the first trimester have demonstrated survival benefit.

9. Delays in diagnosis of malignancy in pregnancy are common for various reasons, except:

   a. Many of the presenting symptoms of cancer are often attributed to pregnancy.
   b. Many of the physiologic changes of pregnancy can compromise the physical examination.
   c. Serum tumor markers, such as α-fetoprotein (AFP), are decreased during pregnancy.
   d. The physician's ability to optimally perform imaging or invasive diagnostic studies may be altered in pregnancy.

10. Which of the following cancers is the most frequently associated with placental and fetal metastasis?

    a. Breast cancer
    b. Lung cancer
    c. Sarcoma
    d. Melanoma

ANSWERS

1. **Answer: d**

(see *Gabbe's Obstetrics* 8e: ch55)

Though surgery may be safely performed during all three trimesters, the second trimester is preferred for patients requiring an abdominal or pelvic procedure, to limit the risk of first-trimester pregnancy loss and preterm labor while allowing for adequate visualization of the abdominal anatomy. Data suggests pregnant patients may safely undergo laparoscopic surgery during pregnancy, though there are no randomized controlled trials comparing approaches. It is recommended that the duration of surgery be minimized, the pneumoperitoneum be kept at a maximum intraabdominal pressure of 10–13 mm Hg, and an open entry technique (Hasson technique) be utilized to gain access to the peritoneal cavity. If oophorectomy or ovarian cystectomy is required in the first trimester, thus compromising the corpus luteum, progesterone supplementation is recommended.

2. Answer: b

(see *Gabbe's Obstetrics* 8e: ch55)

Ionizing radiation is a known teratogen and the developing pregnancy is particularly sensitive to its effects. Critical factors include gestational age, radiation field extent, and the fetal dose. In general, the potential effects of radiation exposure in pregnancy include pregnancy loss, congenital malformations, mental retardation, and cancer induction. Risk is thought to arise if exposed to radiation above the threshold dose of 0.1–0.2 Gy, and thus the recommended limit in pregnancy is 0.05 Gy. Exposure to ionizing radiation above this threshold dose during the first 2 weeks after conception results in an "all or none" phenomenon. If the pregnancy survives, it will likely be normal. During organogenesis and early fetogenesis, doses higher than 0.20 Gy are considered teratogenic and increase the risk of miscarriage.

3. Answer: a

(see *Gabbe's Obstetrics* 8e: ch55)

The pharmacokinetics of chemotherapeutic agents can be influenced by the physiologic changes of pregnancy, which may ultimately impact the efficacy of systemic therapy. In brief, decreased gastrointestinal motility and delayed gastric emptying may alter absorption of orally administered medications. Blood volume expansion occurs early in pregnancy and continues well into the third trimester. This volume expansion, combined with the enhanced renal clearance and faster hepatic metabolism in pregnancy, may reduce active drug concentrations. Plasma albumin decreases in pregnancy, increasing the amount of unbound active drug, whereas estrogen exposure during pregnancy increases other plasma proteins, which might decrease active drug fractions. Lastly, amniotic fluid may act as a pharmacologic third space.

4. Answer: b

(see *Gabbe's Obstetrics* 8e: ch55)

Because the breast changes become more pronounced in later pregnancy, it is important to perform a thorough breast examination at the initial visit. Breast abnormalities should be evaluated in the same manner as if the patient were not pregnant. The most common presentation of breast cancer in pregnancy is a painless lump discovered by the patient. Although bilateral serosanguinous nipple discharge may be normal in late pregnancy, less common presentations include bloody nipple discharge, which should be evaluated with mammography and ultrasound.

5. Answer: c

(see *Gabbe's Obstetrics* 8e: ch55)

The routine evaluation for HL during pregnancy includes a single anterior/posterior view chest radiograph with shielding, liver function tests, serum creatinine clearance, complete blood count, erythrocyte sedimentation rate, lymph node, and bone marrow biopsy. Evaluation of the abdomen is compromised by the gravid uterus, and, if needed, MRI is preferred because it can accurately assess nodes, liver, and spleen. MRI (preferred) or CT scan of the mediastinum may be necessary to evaluate nodal enlargement in the chest. Isotope scans of the liver and skeletal system are best avoided during pregnancy.

6. Answer: a

(see *Gabbe's Obstetrics* 8e: ch55)

Cervical cancer is the most common gynecologic malignancy associated with pregnancy, occurring in approximately 1–2 per 2000–10,000 pregnancies, and approximately 3%, or 1 in 34 cases, of all invasive cervical cancers occur during pregnancy. In patients with small volume, stage I disease, delays in therapeutic intervention have not been reported to increase recurrence rates.

7. Answer: d

(See *Gabbe's Obstetrics* 8e: ch55)

The two clinical risk factors that carry the highest risk of a molar pregnancy are (1) the extremes of the reproductive years (age 50 or older carries a relative risk of over 500) and (2) the history of a prior complete hydatiform mole (CHM) (the risk for development of a second molar pregnancy is 1%–2%, and the risk of a third after two is approximately 25%). For the patient with a CHM, the risk of requiring chemotherapy for persistent gestational trophoblastic disease (GTD) is approximately 20%. Clinical features that increase this risk include delayed hemorrhage, excessive uterine enlargement, theca-lutein cysts, serum hCG greater than 100,000 mIU/mL, and maternal age older than 40.

8. Answer: b

(see *Gabbe's Obstetrics* 8e: ch55)

For localized disease, surgical excision with appropriate margins remains the most effective modality for the treatment of melanoma. Sentinel or complete lymph node dissection can also be safely performed in pregnancy.

9. Answer: **c**

(see *Gabbe's Obstetrics* 8e: ch55)

Delays in diagnosis of cancer during pregnancy are common for various reasons, including the following: (1) many of the presenting symptoms of cancer are often attributed to the pregnancy; (2) many of the physiologic and anatomic alterations of pregnancy can compromise physical examination; (3) serum tumor markers, such as β-hCG, AFP, and cancer antigen 125 (CA 125), are increased during pregnancy; and (4) the ability to optimally perform either imaging studies or invasive diagnostic procedures may be altered during pregnancy.

10. Answer: **d**

(see *Gabbe's Obstetrics* 8e: ch55)

Malignant melanoma is the most frequently reported tumor metastatic to the placenta, which also has a high rate of fetal metastases. Other malignancies that have been reported to metastasize to products of conception include hematologic malignancies, breast cancer, lung cancer, sarcoma, cancer of unknown primary, and gynecologic cancers. When the diagnosis of cancer in pregnancy is present, recommendations include the following: (1) a thorough macroscopic and microscopic evaluation of the placenta; (2) cytologic examination of maternal and umbilical cord blood; and (3) neonates should be examined every 6 months for 2 years with physical examination, chest radiograph, and liver function tests.

56

Skin Disease and Pregnancy

Audrey Merriam

(See *Gabbe's Obstetrics: Normal and Problem Pregnancies*, 8e: ch56)

QUESTIONS

1. You are seeing a 23-year-old G2P0010 at 27 weeks gestation. Her pregnancy has been uncomplicated. Her prenatal laboratory tests were normal. Her only concern is that her gums are bleeding very easily when brushing her teeth in the past 3 weeks. She does not have a history of bleeding excessively with her menses or of easy bruising. She does not think there is anything wrong with her mouth, but she has not been to a dentist since she graduated from high school. In addition to the complete blood count (CBC) you are getting with her third-trimester laboratory tests, what other order do you place?

   a. Referral to a dentist

   b. Referral to hematology

   c. Fibrinogen, PT/PTT tests

   d. Inherited thrombophilia workup

   e. Urine drug screen

2. An 18-year-old G3P0020 at 12 weeks gestation presents for her first prenatal visit. The pregnancy is unplanned but desired, and she is happy about being pregnant. The only medical issue for which she regularly sees a physician is acne. She says her dermatologist told her that all topical medications should be fine in pregnancy. You ask her about which topical medication she uses because you remember that there is one medication that is not recommended due to theoretical risks to the fetus. Which acne medication is contraindicated in pregnancy?

   a. Benzoyl peroxide

   b. Azelaic acid

   c. Erythromycin

   d. Clindamycin

   e. Tretinoin

3. A 40-year-old G1P0 at 34 weeks with an in vitro fertilization gestation presents to triage with 3 days of a fever and malaise. As you are placing her on the monitor you notice a rash in her groin and below her breasts that is erythematous with groups of pustules. Based on the appearance of the rash and the symptoms, you suspect impetigo herpetiformis. Which of the following is a risk factor for this disease?

   a. Hypercalcemia

   b. Psoriasis

   c. Recent viral infection

   d. Recent contact with children with impetigo

   e. History of HSV-1 or 2

4. A 32-year-old G4P2012 woman at 30 weeks gestation presents for an urgent obstetric (OB) visit in your office. Over the past 24 hours she has developed "red blotches" that started on her abdomen, she thinks at her navel, and these have spread over her trunk and arms. The lesions on her abdomen have started to become fluid-filled and are itchy. She denies any new soaps, detergents, or lotions and she has no history of allergies. You perform a small skin biopsy and send it to a dermatopathologist at your hospital which reveals linear C3 deposition along the basement membrane. What is the diagnosis and treatment?

   a. Pemphigoid gestationis, treat with topical corticosteroids

   b. Pemphigoid gestationis, treat with oral corticosteroids

   c. Pemphigoid gestationis, no treatment

   d. Polymorphic eruption of pregnancy (PEP), no treatment

   e. PEP, treat with oral corticosteroids

5. A 30-year old G2P0010 comes for a routine prenatal visit at 37 weeks gestation. Her pregnancy has only been complicated by gestational diabetes, for which diet and exercise have provided adequate glycemic control. She states that over the past week she has developed small, red bumps in her stretch marks and they are quite itchy. It is keeping her up at night. She denies any new soaps or detergents. She has been using cocoa butter to try to prevent stretch marks since 24 weeks gestation and is dismayed that this has developed too. What do you recommend for treatment?

   a. Oral corticosteroids

   b. Delivery

   c. Stopping the applications of cocoa butter

   d. Topical antihistamine cream

   e. Ultraviolet-B (UVB) lights

6. A 39-year-old G4P3003 presents for consultation because of a recent diagnosis of melanoma on her left arm at 23 weeks gestation. She is scheduled for a wide local excision and sentinel lymph node dissection. At this time her oncologist is not recommending further treatment if stage II or less is confirmed, but she is concerned about the effects of pregnancy on the course of her disease because she has three children at home and knows the legal limit of termination in your state is 24 weeks gestation. She would like to know if the pregnancy will make the melanoma worse because if it would she would terminate in efforts to maximize her chance of survival. What do you tell her?

a. Due to the increased estrogen the prognosis of melanoma is worse in pregnancy.

b. There is limited data on pregnancy and melanoma because it is such a rare cancer for this age group.

c. She should undergo pregnancy termination so that the chemotherapy she will need after treatment will not harm the fetus.

d. Pregnancy does not impact the disease course of melanoma and if it is stage II or less treatment is with wide local excision.

e. Melanoma is universally fatal so the fact that she is pregnant does not matter.

ANSWERS

1. **Answer: a**

(see *Gabbe's Obstetrics* 8e: ch56)

Gum hyperemia and gingivitis are common and frequently result in mild bleeding during brushing. This is most prominent during the third trimester and resolves postpartum. Good dental hygiene will minimize symptoms. Regularly scheduled teeth cleaning is safe in all trimesters. Periodontal disease has been associated with adverse pregnancy outcomes, so women without a recent dental examination should be referred for a dental examination.

2. **Answer: e**

(see *Gabbe's Obstetrics* 8e: ch56)

Use of topical tretinoin has not been studied in a large-enough sample to draw conclusions about increased fetal risk during development, although case-control studies have not shown an increased risk. As theoretic concern remains, its use during pregnancy is not recommended.

3. **Answer: c**

(see *Gabbe's Obstetrics* 8e: ch56)

Impetigo herpetiformis is a rare variant of generalized pustular psoriasis that develops primarily during pregnancy, often in association with hypocalcemia, low serum levels of vitamin D, or various infections during pregnancy. The eruption usually develops in the third trimester but can also start in earlier trimesters and postpartum. Diagnosis of impetigo herpetiformis is based on histopathology and treatment is with oral steroids (prednisone 20–40 mg/d).

4. **Answer: b**

(see *Gabbe's Obstetrics* 8e: ch56)

Pemphigoid gestationis is a rare autoimmune disease that usually presents in the second or third trimester with pruritic urticarial lesions that typically begin on the abdomen and trunk and commonly involve the umbilicus. These lesions progress to widespread bullous lesions. Diagnosis is based on immunofluorescence of perilesional skin that demonstrates linear C3 deposition along the basement membrane zone, which is absent in PEP. Most patients respond to treatment with oral corticosteroids.

5. **Answer: d**

(see *Gabbe's Obstetrics* 8e: ch56)

This rash is consistent with PEP, also known as *pruritic urticarial papules and plaques of pregnancy (PUPPP)*. It is the most common dermatologic condition in pregnancy. Lesions are polymorphic and typically begin in abdominal striae and spare the periumbilical area. Mild cases can be treated with antipruritic topical medications, topical steroids, and oral antihistamines. Severely symptomatic cases may require a short course of oral prednisone.

6. **Answer: d**

(see *Gabbe's Obstetrics* 8e: ch56)

Melanoma is the most common malignancy in pregnancy. Many epidemiologic studies evaluating the effect of pregnancy status at diagnosis suggest that the 5-year survival rate is not affected after controlling for confounding factors. The major prognostic determinants of survival for localized melanoma are tumor (Breslow) thickness and ulceration status, and level of invasion is only significant in women with tumors >1 mm thick. If a woman presents with advanced disease prior to viability, termination may be offered; however, there are no guidelines since pregnancy does not affect the outcome of melanoma in the mother and there is a low risk of fetal metastasis.

57

Maternal and Perinatal Infection in Pregnancy—Viral

Alyssa Stephenson-Famy

(See *Gabbe's Obstetrics: Normal and Problem Pregnancies*, 8e: ch57)

QUESTIONS

1. Which mechanism best describes how viral infection leads to signs and symptoms of fever, rash, arthralgias, and myalgias?

   a. Release of virions from host cells

   b. Host cell apoptosis

   c. Oncogenic transformation of host cells

   d. Suppressed function of uninfected host cells

   e. Activation of host immune response (immune cells, release of cytokines, chemokines, and antibodies)

2. A pregnant woman is diagnosed with a new HIV infection that she most likely acquired through heterosexual contact. She and her partner both live in the United States and have not recently traveled. Her partner is a former intravenous (IV) drug user. Which HIV subtype is she most likely infected with?

   a. HIV-1, group M, clade A

   b. HIV-1, group M, clade B

   c. HIV-1, group M, clade C

   d. HIV-1, group N

   e. HIV-1, group O

3. A 22-year-old college student presents for her first prenatal visit. She has had three lifetime male sexual partners and a negative screen for sexually transmitted illnesses 6 months prior to this planned conception. She has no history of intravenous drugs or incarceration. What is the recommendation from American College of Obstetricians and Gynecologists (ACOG) and Centers for Disease Control (CDC) with regards to HIV screening for her in this pregnancy?

   a. No HIV screen is indicated.

   b. Encourage her to "opt out" of prenatal HIV screening.

   c. Perform first-trimester mandatory HIV screen only.

   d. Recommend first-trimester HIV screen and repeat HIV screen in the third trimester if indicated.

   e. Recommend rapid HIV screening in labor.

4. An HIV-positive woman presents for preconception counseling regarding maternal-child vertical transmission of HIV. Which laboratory test is the most important for estimating the rates of vertical transmission?

   a. CD4 count

   b. HIV RNA copy number/mL plasma

   c. HLA-B*5701

   d. HIV resistance testing

   e. Hepatitis B e antigen

5. A 32-year-old G1P0 at 26 weeks gestation calls the clinic with fever, myalgias, cough, and shortness of breath that started 2 to 3 days ago. She received routine influenza vaccination 5 months ago. She works in a school with potentially multiple sick contacts. What is the recommended treatment at this time?

   a. No treatment as she received the influenza vaccine

   b. No treatment as she had onset of symptoms >48 hours ago

   c. No treatment without a positive influenza swab

   d. Empiric treatment with oseltamivir or zanamivir

   e. Empiric chemoprophylaxis with oseltamivir or zanamivir

6. A pregnant woman at 20 weeks has a confirmed exposure and seroconversion to parvovirus B19. She is scheduled for ultrasound surveillance with middle cerebral artery (MCA) Doppler and evaluation for fetal hydrops. This surveillance should continue for which duration of time following maternal infection?

   a. 1 week

   b. 2 weeks

   c. 4 weeks

   d. 8 weeks

   e. 16 weeks

7. A pregnant woman who recently immigrated to New York City from South East Asia with unknown immunization history develops fever, malaise, myalgias, headache, conjunctivitis, and cough. Physical examination demonstrates Koplik spots on the buccal mucosa. What is the most likely cause of her symptoms?

   a. Influenza

   b. Parvovirus

   c. Rubeola

   d. Rubella

   e. Zika virus

8. What is the rate of sensorineural hearing loss in women with subclinical cytomegalovirus (CMV) in pregnancy?

   a. 1%

   b. 5%

   c. 15%

   d. 50%

   e. 90%

9. A 29-year-old G2P1 presents with active labor at term. She has a history of genital herpes simplex virus (HSV), last outbreak was 7 months ago, and she has not been taking antiviral prophylaxis. She has "prodromal" symptoms of an HSV outbreak on her right labia majora, with pain and paresthesia but no lesion. What does ACOG recommend for management?

   a. Normal labor management

   b. Intravenous acyclovir

   c. HSV polymerase chain reaction (PCR) of labia

   d. HSV serologies

   e. Cesarean delivery

10. A 30-year-old female with unknown immunization history presents for routine prenatal care. As part of her prenatal tests, she has a positive hepatitis B surface antigen. Which additional laboratory tests would be most compatible with acute infection?

Answer Choices

Test	A	B	C	D	E
Anti-HBs	−	+	+	−	−
HBeAg	+	−	−	+/−	−
Anti-HBe	−	+/−	−	+/−	+
HBV DNA†	+	−	−	+	+ (low)
ALT	Elevated	Normal	Normal	Normal–elevated	Normal

Alanine aminotransferase (ALT); Antibody to the Hepatitis B surface antigen (anti-HBs); Antibody to the Hepatitis B e antigen (HBe); Hepatitis B e Antigen (HBeAg); *HBV*, hepatitis B virus.
Adapted from Koziel MJ, Thio CL. Hepatitis B virus and hepatitis delta virus. In: Mandell GL, Bennett JE, Dolin R, eds. *Mandell, Douglas, and Bennett's Principles and Practice of Infectious Disease*, 7th ed. Philadelphia: Elsevier; 2010.

11. A 22-year-old G1P0 at 18 weeks returns from a trip to South America in which she had several mosquito bites, a brief febrile illness, and conjunctivitis. Ultrasound of the fetus demonstrates microcephaly. Laboratory testing for which infection should be performed?

    a. Small pox (Variola virus)

    b. Coxsackie virus

    c. Epstein-Barr virus

    d. Zika virus

    e. Ebola virus

12. A 30-year-old G1P0 woman at 8 weeks gestation presents for prenatal care. She is healthy, with no known medical problems. She works as a medical assistant and has a history of work-related needle stick injuries. She has multiple tattoos and piercings. She has traveled extensively in South East Asia. She smokes cigarettes and consumes edible cannabis products but denies illicit substances, IV/intranasal drug use, incarceration, blood transfusion, or high-risk sexual contacts. What is the recommendation for hepatitis screening in pregnancy?

    a. Hepatitis A only

    b. Hepatitis B only

    c. Hepatitis C only

    d. Hepatitis B and C

    e. Hepatitis A, B, and C

13. What precautions are recommended to prevent transmission of Ebola virus disease (EVD) to health-care workers?

    a. Contact precautions only

    b. Droplet precautions only

    c. Environmental precautions only (negative pressure room)

    d. Contact and droplet precautions

    e. Environmental, contact and droplet precautions

14. At 20 weeks' gestation, the results of a fetal anatomy ultrasound show fetal hydrocephalus, echogenic bowel, and microcephaly concerning for congenital CMV infection. What is the most sensitive test for fetal CMV infection?

    a. Maternal serum serologic testing (IgG, IgM)

    b. Maternal serum serologic avidity testing (IgG)

    c. Maternal serum CMV polymerase chain reaction (PCR)

    d. Amniotic fluid CMV PCR before 21 weeks

    e. Amniotic fluid CMV PCR after 21 weeks

ANSWERS

1. Answer: e

(See *Gabbe's Obstetrics* 8e: ch57)

The host immune response to viral infection encompasses both local and systemic effects via activation of immune cells, the induction of an adaptive immune response, and the release of cytokines, chemokines, and antibodies. Thus, the immune response contributes to or causes the signs and symptoms associated with viral infections, including fever, rash, arthralgias, and myalgias.

2. Answer: b

(See *Gabbe's Obstetrics* 8e: ch57)

Most HIV infections in the United States are caused by HIV-1. HIV-1 is divided into three groups: M, N, and O. Over 95% of HIV-1 infections are caused by group M, which is divided into subtypes (or clades) A through K. The predominant type of HIV within the US is clade B, while other clades predominate in other regions of the world.

3. Answer: d

(See *Gabbe's Obstetrics* 8e: ch57)

ACOG and the CDC recommend early prenatal HIV screening using an "opt out" approach, ideally performed at the initial prenatal visit. A second HIV test in the third trimester is recommended for pregnant women with initial negative HIV tests who are at increased risk for HIV acquisition, have history of incarceration, or live in states that require third trimester testing.

4. Answer: b

(See *Gabbe's Obstetrics* 8e: ch57)

Approximately 40,000 Americans are diagnosed with HIV infection annually; women account for 19% of new HIV infections and 23% of existing infections. Women typically acquire HIV infection by heterosexual contact (85%), with 61% of HIV diagnoses occurring in African American women. Achieving HIV RNA <50 copies/mL at the time of delivery is associated with more favorable outcomes for maternal child vertical transmission.

5. Answer: d

(See *Gabbe's Obstetrics* 8e: ch57)

Pregnant women suspected to be infected with influenza should be treated immediately, independent of vaccination status, without waiting for diagnostic confirmation. The recommended treatment for both seasonal and pandemic influenza infection is oseltamivir or zanamivir. Early antiviral treatment (within 48 hours) reduces the duration of the illness, secondary complications, and hospitalizations; treatment should not be withheld if the ideal window is missed.

6. Answer: d

(See *Gabbe's Obstetrics* 8e: ch57)

Serial ultrasounds, including fetal MCA peak systolic velocity assessment, are recommended every 1 to 2 weeks for 8 to 10 weeks following maternal illness to evaluate the fetus for anemia and hydrops. If no signs of hydrops are seen during this period, further evaluation is unnecessary.

7. Answer: c

(See *Gabbe's Obstetrics* 8e: ch57)

Rubeola has an incubation period of 10 to 14 days. Infected individuals first manifest prodromal symptoms, which may include fever, malaise, myalgias, and headache and usually at least one of the three "Cs": cough, coryza, and conjunctivitis. Koplik spots, tiny white spots on a red base on the buccal mucosa lateral to the molar teeth, may appear during the prodrome and are pathognomonic for measles infection.

8. Answer: a

(See *Gabbe's Obstetrics* 8e: ch57)

Congenital CMV is the leading cause of hearing loss in children. While up to 90% of children with congenital CMV infection are asymptomatic at birth, 15% of subclinical, congenital CMV infections in pregnancy can result in hearing loss.

9. Answer: e

(See *Gabbe's Obstetrics* 8e: ch57)

Primary maternal HSV infection, not recurrent infection, accounts for the vast majority of neonatal HSV infections. ACOG recommends elective cesarean delivery for women with demonstrable genital herpes lesions or prodromal symptoms in labor to reduce the incidence of neonatal HSV infection. However, as 60% to 80% of neonatal HSV infections occur following asymptomatic, primary maternal infection, our capacity to prevent neonatal HSV infection by performing cesarean delivery is limited.

10. Answer: a

(See *Gabbe's Obstetrics* 8e: ch57)

Acute infection shows a serologic profile of positive hepatitis B surface antigen, positive Hepatitis B e antigen (HBeAg), present hepatitis B virus DNA, negative anti-Hepatitis B surface antibody, and negative anti-Hepatitis B e antibody. The presence of elevated liver function enzymes also suggests acute infection.

11. Answer: d

(See *Gabbe's Obstetrics* 8e: ch57)

With Zika virus, many patients will be asymptomatic after infection. Symptomatic patients may have low-grade fever, arthralgia, myalgia, maculopapular rash, or conjunctivitis. *Aedes aegypti* and *Aedes albopictus* are the primary mosquito vectors carrying Zika. Microcephaly is the most consistent Zika-virus associated finding on fetal ultrasound.

12. Answer: d

(See *Gabbe's Obstetrics* 8e: ch57)

Hepatitis B screening is recommended for all pregnant women, due to the risk of vertical transmission during pregnancy. While many groups recommend universal screening for hepatitis C, this patient should be screened for hepatitis C due to multiple risk factors. Annual screening for hepatitis C is recommended for IV drug users or persons with ongoing HCV exposure risk factors (Box 57.1).

BOX 57.1   Risk Factors for Hepatitis C

Definite Indications for Screening
Any history of IV drug use (even once)
HIV infection
Unexplained chronic liver disease, including elevated aminotransferase levels
Hemodialysis
Blood transfusion or organ transplant prior to 1992
Receipt of clotting factor concentrates before 1987
Sexual contact with an HIV-, HBV-, or HCV-infected individual
History of incarceration
Intranasal illicit drug use
Individuals born to HCV-infected women
History of unregulated tattooing or body piercing
Health-care worker with history of needle-stick injury
Persons born between 1945 and 1965

Consider Screening (Need Uncertain)
In vitro fertilization from anonymous donors
Known sexually transmitted disease or multiple partners
Steady sex partner of individual with history of injection drug use

---

HBV, Hepatitis B virus; *HCV,* Hepatitis C virus.

13. Answer: e

(See *Gabbe's Obstetrics* 8e: ch57)

While diagnosis of EVD is being considered, the patient should be isolated in a private negative-air flow room with a bathroom. Contact, droplet, and environmental control precautions should be implemented, and appropriate personal protective equipment should be consistently used.

14. Answer: e

(See *Gabbe's Obstetrics* 8e: ch57)

Fetal infection is documented by amniotic fluid culture or PCR as CMV is excreted in urine. Amniotic fluid CMV PCR sensitivity approaches 100% in gestations greater than 21 weeks for fetal CMV infection. Serologic testing is available, but seroconversion can be delayed by 4 weeks and IgM can persist for many months, making interpretation difficult. Avidity testing for IgG can further delineate between primary and recurrent infection; however, these tests are not Food and Drug Administration–approved, due to lack of standardization.

58

Maternal and Perinatal Infection: Bacterial, Chlamydia, Syphilis in Pregnancy

Audrey Merriam

(See *Gabbe's Obstetrics: Normal and Problem Pregnancies*, 8e: ch58)

QUESTIONS

1. A 17-year-old G1P0 presents for a prenatal visit at 36 weeks gestation. She was found to be positive for chlamydia at her previous visit. She received appropriate treatment in the office, but she forgot to tell her partner to get treated and they have had intercourse again since then. In addition to retreating her, you decide to counsel her again on the risks of chlamydia infection in pregnancy. What is the greatest risk of untreated maternal chlamydia infection in pregnancy?

   a. Preterm labor

   b. Preterm premature rupture of membranes (PPROM)

   c. Neonatal pneumonia

   d. Neonatal conjunctivitis

   e. Intrauterine fetal demise (IUFD)

2. Group B streptococcus prophylaxis during labor has been effective at decreasing which of the following?

   a. Late-onset group B streptococcus sepsis

   b. Early-onset group B streptococcus sepsis

   c. Subsequent group B streptococcus colonization in another pregnancy

   d. Urinary tract infections related to group B streptococcus

   e. Chorioamnionitis related to group B streptococcus

3. Which of the following is *not* a risk factor for postoperative wound infection following cesarean delivery?

   a. Removal of pubic hair with clippers

   b. Corticosteroid use

   c. Chorioamnionitis

   d. Scleroderma

   e. Gestational diabetes

4. You are seeing a 31-year-old G2P2002 in the hospital 3 days postpartum from a cesarean delivery. Her surgery and her postpartum course have been uncomplicated except that she had her second fever 102.2F (39.0°C) since delivery. She clinically looks well, and her other vital signs are stable. Her fundus is firm at her umbilicus and nontender. Her incision is intact, with no drainage or surrounding erythema. She does not have any systemic symptoms except feeling slightly sweaty during her two fevers. You order a CT scan and the report states that there is a thrombus in the right ovarian vein. What is your diagnosis and recommended treatment?

   a. Deep vein thrombosis/therapeutic low-molecular weight heparin for 12 weeks

   b. Deep vein thrombosis/warfarin for 6 months

   c. Septic pelvic thrombophlebitis/therapeutic low-molecular-weight heparin for 12 weeks

   d. Septic pelvic thrombophlebitis/therapeutic low-molecular-weight heparin for 10 days

   e. Septic pelvic thrombophlebitis/warfarin for 6 months

5. You are seeing a 25-year-old G1P0 at 16 weeks gestation who is a recent immigrant from the Dominican Republic. During her prenatal testing, toxoplasmosis IgG and IgM were sent and both returned positive, with a low avidity. She is seeing you for consultation regarding these findings. You discuss the risk of congenital toxoplasmosis infection and the next steps to determine the risk to the fetus. What do you tell her about the likelihood of when she was infected and the potential severity of the congenital infection?

   a. This is likely a latent infection and unlikely to cause risk to the fetus.

   b. This is likely a reinfection and unlikely to cause risk to the fetus.

   c. This is likely a new infection and, if fetal infection occurs, which is a lower likelihood because of the earlier gestation, will cause severe fetal effects.

   d. This is likely a new infection and, if fetal infection occurs, which is a higher likelihood because of the earlier gestation, will cause severe fetal effects.

   e. This is likely a new infection and. if fetal infection occurs, which is a lower likelihood because of the earlier gestation, will not cause severe fetal effects.

6. You get called to the emergency department to see a 29-year-old G3P2002 presenting at 15 weeks with right flank pain, fever, and dysuria. She has a history of multiple urinary tract infections and pyelonephritis in a previous pregnancy. At a clinic visit 2 days ago, she was complaining of dysuria, and a urine culture was sent. Her vital signs are as follows: temperature 101°F, pulse 115, respirations 18, and blood pressure 116/72. She does not appear septic but does appear uncomfortable with her back pain. Luckily, the urine culture results are back, and it is positive for *Proteus*. She has a history of hives with ceftriaxone. What is your preferred antibiotic regimen?

   a. Gentamicin IV until 24 hours afebrile, followed by trimethoprim-sulfamethoxazole for 2 weeks

   b. Rifampin IV until 24 hours afebrile, followed by nitrofurantoin for 2 weeks

   c. Gentamicin IV until 24 hours afebrile, followed by Keflex for 2 weeks

   d. Amoxicillin IV until 24 hours afebrile, followed by nitrofurantoin for 2 weeks

   e. Rifampin IV until 24 hours afebrile, followed by trimethoprim-sulfamethoxazole for 2 weeks

7. A 23-year-old G3P0020 presents at 18 weeks gestation for a routine prenatal visit. She states that she has been doing well and just had a cold last week, with a low-grade fever, chills, and a cough, after she attended a Mexican food festival. She feels better this week. You start to listen for fetal heart tones but cannot find them. You bring in an ultrasound and diagnose an IUFD. Which laboratory study would you add to the recommended set of IUFD laboratory tests?

   a. Parvovirus B19

   b. Factor V Leiden genetic testing

   c. Zika virus serology

   d. Gonorrhea

   e. Listeria

8. A 38-year-old G4P2012 presents for her 28-week visit. Her medical history is significant for obesity, Raynaud disease, and syphilis that was treated 8 year ago. She has a penicillin allergy but was desensitized for treatment with penicillin at the time of her diagnosis. Her venereal disease research laboratory (VDRL) titer at the beginning of pregnancy was 1:4. You draw a repeat VDRL titer with her third trimester blood tests, which returns as 1:56. What is your next step?

   a. It is unreliable because she is pregnant, and an autoimmune disease so should just be repeated postpartum.

   b. She should have a lumbar puncture treatment with penicillin and does not need repeat desensitization.

   c. She should have a lumbar puncture and receive repeat treatment with penicillin with desensitization.

   d. The titer is changing as expected after treatment and no further treatment is needed.

   e. She should be delivered now to prevent congenital syphilis.

ANSWERS

1. Answer: c

(see *Gabbe's Obstetrics* 8e: ch58)

Untreated chlamydial infection during pregnancy has been linked with preterm birth, PPROM, low birth weight, and neonatal death in some studies but not in others. Infants born to women with an untreated chlamydial infection of the cervix have a 60% to 70% risk of acquiring the infection during delivery. Untreated *Chlamydia trachomatis* infection may also result in neonatal conjunctivitis (25%–50%) and/or pneumonia (10%–20%).

2. Answer: b

(see *Gabbe's Obstetrics* 8e: ch58)

Streptococcus agalactiae is a gram-positive encapsulated coccus that produces β-hemolysis when grown on blood agar. On average, about 20% to 25% of pregnant women in the United States harbor this organism in their lower genital tract and rectum. Group B streptococcus (GBS) is one of the most important causes of early-onset neonatal infection. The prevalence of neonatal GBS infection now is about 0.5 per 1000 live births. Nationwide group B streptococcus prevention strategies have decreased the number of cases of early-onset GBS sepsis by about 3900 per year and the number of deaths by 200 per year. Treatment has not impacted rates of late-onset group B streptococcus infection in neonates.

3. Answer: e

(see *Gabbe's Obstetrics* 8e: ch58)

About 3% to 5% of patients who have a cesarean delivery develop a wound infection. The major risk factors for this complication are listed in Box 58.1. The principal causative organisms are skin flora (*Staphylococcus aureus*, aerobic streptococci) and the pelvic flora (aerobic and anaerobic bacilli). Pregestational diabetes is a risk factor for wound infection, but gestational diabetes is not. Connective tissue disorders, like scleroderma, increase risk for wound infection.

BOX 58.1   Principal Risk Factors for Post-cesarean Wound Infection

Poor surgical technique such as inadequate preparation of the incision site, removal of hair with a razor rather than electric clippers, failure to close the bottom half of the subcutaneous layer in obese women, use of staples instead of sutures for skin closure

- Low socioeconomic status
- Extended duration of labor and ruptured membranes
- Preexisting infection such as chorioamnionitis
- Obesity
- Pregestational diabetes
- Immunodeficiency disorder
- Corticosteroid therapy
- Immunosuppressive therapy
- Connective tissue disorder
- Smoking

---

4. Answer: d

(see *Gabbe's Obstetrics* 8e: ch58)

Septic pelvic vein thrombophlebitis can initially present similar to endometritis. Patients can also present with temperature instability only and do not appear to be seriously ill. The diagnostic tests of greatest value in evaluating a patient with suspected septic pelvic vein thrombophlebitis are CT scan and MRI. Patients should be treated with therapeutic doses of either IV unfractionated heparin or low-molecular-weight heparin for 7 to 10 days. Long-term anticoagulation with oral agents is probably unnecessary unless the patient has massive clotting throughout the pelvic venous plexus or she has sustained a pulmonary embolism. Patients should be maintained on broad-spectrum antibiotics throughout the period of heparin administration.

5. Answer: c

(see *Gabbe's Obstetrics* 8e: ch58)

Toxoplasmosis testing that suggests an acute infection includes detection of IgM, demonstration of high IgG, and low IgG avidity, OR documentation of IgG seroconversion from negative to positive. Chronic infection is unlikely to cause fetal injury. Congenital infection is most likely to occur when maternal infection develops in the third trimester; however, fetal injury is most likely to be severe when maternal infection occurs in the first half of pregnancy.

6. Answer: a

(see *Gabbe's Obstetrics* 8e: ch58)

Gentamicin has good renal penetration and the patient does not have an allergy to it or a similar class of antibiotic. Rifampin can be used but should be reserved for bacteria with more resistance. Nitrofurantoin is more uniformly effective against the common uropathogens; except for *Proteus* species, then trimethoprim-sulfamethoxazole should be used. Trimethoprim-sulfamethoxazole can be used safely outside of the first trimester and prior to late in the third trimester.

7. Answer: e

(see *Gabbe's Obstetrics* 8e: ch58)

High perinatal morbidity and mortality rates have been reported for listeria infection in pregnancy. The earlier the stage of gestation when maternal infection occurs, the higher the risk of fetal death. Foods that pose a risk of transmitting infection include fresh unpasteurized cheeses, processed meats such as hot dogs, refrigerated pâté and meat spreads, refrigerated smoked seafood, unpasteurized milk, and unwashed raw produce. Patients usually present with a flulike syndrome characterized by fever, chills, malaise, myalgias, back pain, and upper respiratory symptoms.

8. Answer: c

(see *Gabbe's Obstetrics* 8e: ch58)

The VDRL titer should decrease and become negative or very low within 6 to 12 months in early syphilis and within 12 to 24 months in late syphilis (>1 year's duration). A rising titer (defined as a four-fold change in the denominator of the titer) indicates the need for further diagnostic measures, such as a lumbar puncture, and appropriate treatment. The Centers for Disease Control and Prevention recommends that pregnant patients with syphilis in any stage who are allergic to penicillin should be desensitized and then treated with penicillin.

59

Mental Health and Behavioral Disorders in Pregnancy

Anthony Sciscione

(See *Gabbe's Obstetrics: Normal and Problem Pregnancies*, 8e: ch59)

QUESTIONS

1. A 37-year-old G1P0 presents for her first prenatal visit at 12 weeks gestation. She reports that she has a history of major depressive disorder (MDD). She is worried about the effects of MDD on her pregnancy. You counsel her that MDD is one of the most common disorders present in pregnancy. What percent of pregnancies are affected with MDD?

   a. 5%

   b. 8%

   c. 10%

   d. 13%

   e. 16%

2. A 31-year-old primigravida presents for her first prenatal visit at 16 weeks gestation. Her medical history is negative except for a long history of MDD that is controlled by a selective serotonin reuptake inhibitor (SSRI). She is concerned about the risk of adverse outcomes. You counsel her that which of the following is increased in women with MDD during pregnancy?

   a. Preterm birth (PTB)

   b. Placental abruption

   c. Fetal growth restriction

   d. Stillbirth

3. A 20-year-old nulliparous woman presents for her 6-week postpartum visit. She had an uncomplicated vaginal delivery. She states she feels well but is tired, lacks energy, and she is not "her usual self." As per your routine, she is screened for depression using the Edinburgh Postnatal Depression Scale (EPDS). Her score returns consistent with mild MDD. The best next management step is?

   a. Arrange a revisit in 3 months

   b. Refer her for psychotherapy

   c. Begin SSRI therapy

   d. Admit for inpatient therapy

4. A 41-year-old G3P2002 presents for her first prenatal visit at 12 weeks gestation. She has a history of MDD, which is adequately treated with an SSRI. She has read that there is an association with SSRI use and congenital heart defects (CHDs). You counsel her that the risk for CHD in women on a SSRI is?

   a. Not increased

   b. Increased by 3%

   c. Increased by 5%

   d. Increased by 7%

   e. Increased by 11%

5. A 21-year-old nulliparous woman presents for her first prenatal visit at 28 weeks gestation. Her medical history is negative, except for a history of MDD for which she is treated with fluoxetine. She has not seen her psychiatrist in a year and she states that her depressive symptoms have recently increased. You counsel her that SSRI dosing typically has to be increased over which part of pregnancy?

   a. First half of pregnancy

   b. Second half of pregnancy

   c. First and second half of pregnancy

   d. During labor

   e. Postpartum

6. A 26-year-old nulliparous patient presents for preconception counseling. She has a history of bipolar disorder (BD), and she is on treatment that has been effective, and she feels well. Her psychiatrist has counseled her to wean completely off of her pharmacotherapy before anticipated pregnancy. You counsel her that if she is off her medications before pregnancy, the risk for recurrence in pregnancy is:

   a. 40%–50%

   b. 51%–60%

   c. 61%–70%

   d. 71%–80%

   e. 81%–90%

7. A 22-year-old nulliparous woman at 28 weeks gestation presents to the labor and delivery unit complaining of leaking fluid from her vagina. Her prenatal course has otherwise been uncomplicated. Her medical history is negative except for a remote history of panic attacks as a teenager. She is contracting every 3 minutes and her testing confirms rupture of the membranes. Her cervix looks closed on speculum examination. You begin intravenous magnesium sulfate, nifedipine orally, intramuscular betamethasone, intravenous ampicillin, and intravenous erythromycin. Her contractions abate and she is transferred to the antepartum floor after 12 hours of monitoring. You are called from the floor and the nurse states the patient has a panic attack. You treat the panic attack successfully with a benzodiazepine. Which drug likely precipitated her panic attack?

   a. Magnesium sulfate

   b. Nifedipine

   c. Betamethasone

   d. Ampicillin

   e. Erythromycin

8. A 21-year-old nulliparous woman presents for her 6-week postpartum visit. She had a cesarean delivery for breech presentation. Her hospital course was uncomplicated. She states that over the last 3 weeks, she has had a depressed mood and insomnia; otherwise, she feels well. You consider her for the diagnosis MDD. Which of the following statements is true for the diagnosis of MDD according to the *Diagnostic and Statistical Manual of Mental Disorders, Fifth Edition*, criteria?

   a. Diagnostic symptoms must be over 1 week.

   b. Diagnostic symptoms must occur at least three times a week.

   c. You must have at least three of the diagnostic symptoms.

   d. At least one diagnostic symptom must be mood or interest.

   e. There are seven potential diagnostic symptoms.

ANSWERS

1. Answer: d

(see *Gabbe's Obstetrics* 8e: ch59)

Nearly twice as many women (12.0%) as men (6.6%) suffer from an MDD each year. Women are at the greatest risk for MDD between 25 and 44 years, the primary age range for childbearing. The period prevalence of MDD is 12.7% during pregnancy (with 7.5% of women having a new episode) and 21.9% the year after parturition[1]; therefore, MDD is among the most common complications of childbearing. Mothers at increased risk for depression are those who are socioeconomically disadvantaged, have preterm infants, and are adolescents.

2. Answer: a

(see *Gabbe's Obstetrics* 8e: ch59)

In a metaanalysis, Grote and colleagues reported that maternal MDD or depressive symptoms during pregnancy increase the risk of adverse pregnancy outcomes.[2] The associations between antenatal depression and adverse outcomes included PTB (relative risk [RR], 1.13; 95% confidence interval [CI], 1.06–1.21) and low birthweight (LBW) (RR, 1.18; 95% CI, 1.07–1.30). The magnitude of risk for PTB and LBW from MDD was comparable to the risk of smoking 10 or more cigarettes a day but is modest compared to the higher risks associated with black race and substance abuse. Depression and/or anxiety were associated with a three-fold risk for preeclampsia, which may be related to the increased sympathetic activity characteristic of these psychiatric states. Children exposed to maternal MDD in utero have higher cortisol concentrations than do infants of mothers who were not depressed, which constitutes a biochemical change that continues through adolescence and places the offspring at risk for developing mental illness. Children exposed to maternal MDD during fetal life are four times more likely than those not exposed to be depressed at age 16 years. Notably, maternal treatment of MDD during pregnancy normalizes infant cortisol concentrations.

3. Answer: b

(see *Gabbe's Obstetrics* 8e: ch59)

Members of ACOG and the American Psychological Association (APA) developed a consensus document for antidepressant treatment during pregnancy.[3] For mild cases of MDD in pregnant women, psychotherapy is the treatment of choice as the initial intervention. For moderate to severe MDD with marked functional impairment, antidepressant pharmacotherapy or combination therapy (medication and psychotherapy) is appropriate. Established efficacy and tolerability of any antidepressant for the individual woman are strong considerations in drug choice during the risk-benefit decision-making process. Women with chronic or highly recurrent MDD may be on maintenance antidepressant medication when pregnancy occurs. Maintenance antidepressant treatment is recommended after three or more MDDs, due to the near-certain likelihood of recurrence.

4. Answer: a

(see *Gabbe's Obstetrics* 8e: ch59)

Associations between antidepressant use and cardiac defects were attenuated with increasing levels of adjustment, which implies that confounding variables, rather than drug exposure, accounted for much of the impact on congenital malformations. The relative risks (RR) of any cardiac defect with the use of SSRIs were 1.25 (95% CI, 1.13–1.38) in the unadjusted analysis, and markedly attenuated, 1.12 (95% CI, 1.00–1.26), in the analysis restricted to only women who had a diagnosis of MDD. Stratification according to propensity scoring allowed comparisons to be made between population subgroups with nearly identical characteristics (sociodemographics, comorbid disease, drug use, smoking) but who differed on drug exposure. This strategy also addresses the differences in women with psychiatric disorders who choose to continue medication compared with those who do not, on a broad range of potential confounders. After propensity score stratification, the RR was nonsignificant (RR, 1.06; 95% CI, 0.93–1.22). A similar pattern of increased risk for cardiac malformations in unadjusted analyses became insignificant after adjustment was noted for tricyclic antidepressants, serotonin-norepinephrine reuptake inhibitors, bupropion, and other antidepressants.[4] Studies of first trimester SSRI exposure do not demonstrate consistent data to support an increased risk for structural malformations.

5. Answer: b

(see *Gabbe's Obstetrics* 8e: ch59)

All antidepressants are at least partially metabolized by cytochrome P450 (CYP) 2D6, which increases in activity in pregnancy and results in declining plasma drug concentrations. The dose requirements and concentration-to-dose ratios of the SSRIs fluoxetine,[5] citalopram, escitalopram, and sertraline[6] change during pregnancy and postpartum. In the majority of women, the concentrations for the parent compound and metabolites decrease between 20 weeks gestation and delivery. Pharmacogenetic characterization is not currently a standard of care for antidepressant therapy. For most SSRIs, doses must be incrementally increased during the second half of pregnancy to offset greater drug metabolism. Serial administration of a quantitative depression measure (e.g., EPDS or Patient Health Questionnaire-9) is recommended to identify early symptoms of relapse. Early symptoms of relapse require an incremental increase in the dose of the drug (for example, 25 to 50 mg of sertraline).

6. Answer: e

(see *Gabbe's Obstetrics* 8e: ch59)

For women with chronic BD, discontinuation of drug treatment proximal to conception incurred a high risk for recurrence (86%) compared to patients who continued treatment (37%).[7] After birth, all women with BD are at high risk for recurrent mood episodes. Postpartum relapse rates of 66% (95% CI, 57%–75%) without medication treatment compared with 23% (95% CI, 14%–37%) with prophylactic medication compel initiating treatment immediately postpartum to prevent relapse for women who have not been treated in pregnancy.[8]

7. Answer: c

(see *Gabbe's Obstetrics* 8e: ch59)

β-Adrenergic agonists (such as terbutaline) or corticosteroids (such as betamethasone or dexamethasone) may precipitate panic attacks and other anxiety symptoms. Hyperthyroidism is associated with panic attacks and anxiety symptoms and should be considered in the differential diagnosis of postpartum onset anxiety episodes.

8. Answer: d

BOX 59.1   *DSM-5* Criteria for Major Depressive Disorder

Over the last 2 weeks, most of the day nearly every day, five of the following (one symptom must be mood or interest) must cause marked distress or impairment in important areas of functioning:

- Depressed mood
- Markedly diminished interest or pleasure
- Significant weight loss or gain unrelated to dieting
- Insomnia or hypersomnia
- Psychomotor agitation/retardation
- Fatigue or loss of energy
- Feelings of worthlessness/guilt
- Diminished ability to concentrate
- Recurrent thoughts of death

DSM-5, Diagnostic and Statistical Manual of Mental Disorders, Fifth Edition.

REFERENCES

1. Gaynes BN, Gavin N, Meltzer-Brody S, et al. Perinatal depression: prevalence, screening accuracy, and screening outcomes. Evidence report/technology assessment (summary). 2005(119):1-8.

2. Grote NK, Bridge JA, Gavin AR, Melville JL, Iyengar S, Katon WJ. A meta-analysis of depression during pregnancy and the risk of preterm birth, low birth weight, and intrauterine growth restriction. *Arch Gen Psychiatry* 2010;67(10):1012-1024.

3. Yonkers KA, Wisner KL, Stewart DE, et al. The management of depression during pregnancy: a report from the American Psychiatric Association and the American College of Obstetricians and Gynecologists. *Gen Hosp Psychiatry.* 2009;31(5):403-413.

4. Huybrechts KF, Palmsten K, Avorn J, et al. Antidepressant use in pregnancy and the risk of cardiac defects. *N Engl J Med.* 2014; 370(25):2397-2407.

5. Sit D, Perel JM, Luther JF, Wisniewski SR, Helsel JC, Wisner KL. Disposition of chiral and racemic fluoxetine and norfluoxetine across childbearing. *J Clin Psychopharmacol.* 2010;30(4):381-386.

6. Sit DK, Perel JM, Helsel JC, Wisner KL. Changes in antidepressant metabolism and dosing across pregnancy and early postpartum. *J Clin Psychiatry.* 2008;69(4):652-658.

7. Viguera AC, Whitfield T, Baldessarini RJ, et al. Risk of recurrence in women with bipolar disorder during pregnancy: prospective study of mood stabilizer discontinuation. *Am J Psychiatry.* 2007;164(12): 1817-1824; quiz 923.

8. Wesseloo R, Kamperman AM, Munk-Olsen T, Pop VJ, Kushner SA, Bergink V. Risk of postpartum relapse in bipolar disorder and postpartum psychosis: a systematic review and meta-analysis. *Am J Psychiatry.* 2016;173(2):117-127.

INDEX